CT of the Airways

CONTEMPORARY MEDICAL IMAGING

U. Joseph Schoepf, MD, SERIES EDITOR

CT of the Airways, edited by *Phillip M. Boiselle, MD, and David A. Lynch, MB, 2008*

CT of the Airways

Edited by

Phillip M. Boiselle, MD

Beth Israel Deaconess Medical Center and Harvard Medical School, Boston, MA

and

David A. Lynch, MB

National Jewish Medical and Research Center, Denver, CO

꙼ Humana Press

Editors
Phillip M. Boiselle, MD
Department of Radiology
Beth Israel Deaconess Medical Center
  and Harvard Medical School
Boston, MA

David A. Lynch, MB
Division of Radiology
National Jewish Medical and Research Center
Denver, CO

Series Editor
U. Joseph Schoepf, MD
Department of Radiology
Medical University of South Carolina
Charleston, SC

ISBN 978-1-60761-550-7   e-ISBN 978-1-59745-139-0

Library of Congress Control Number: 2007939567

Cover illustration: Courtesy of James A. Cooper, MD. Based on graphic by Amirsys.

Printed on acid-free paper

9 8 7 6 5 4 3 2 1

springer.com

Series Editor's Introduction

Imaging of the airways is a fascinating undertaking and, if done expertly, a true art in medicine. Over the past years, imaging of the airways has become ever more exciting and demanding, as new therapies in pulmonary medicine have become available that require careful imaging assessment of patients to aid management and monitor therapeutic success. The increasing importance of imaging in pulmonary medicine is accompanied by a surge of revolutionary developments in imaging technology that enable ever finer assessment of lung structure and function.

No modality has seen more rapid innovation over the last decade than computed tomography. Current multidetector-row CT technology makes high-resolution imaging of the chest with a spatial resolution of a couple of 100 μm in a matter of mere seconds. Ever more sophisticated post-processing applications enable intuitive, quantitative assessment of lung structure and function in an efficient manner, so that these technologies are increasingly embraced in mainstream medicine to improve patient care.

CT of the Airways, which was so expertly assembled by my dear friends Phil Boiselle and David Lynch, is one of the very first tomes that pays tribute to our new found prowess in airway imaging. The two editors, who are among the most acclaimed thoracic imagers worldwide, did not rest until they had gathered a most distinguished group of contributors from around the globe, who have brought you the cutting edge in pulmonary imaging. As a result, *CT of the Airways* is the most authoritative and up-to-date resource in the field and a splendid, lavish testimony to the editors' and contributors' expertise.

This book fills an immense need in the ever accelerating realm of thoracic imaging. I am certain that *CT of the Airways* will become a trusted resource to many medical imagers around the world, and it is my hope that the editors will continue updating this book with future editions.

U. Joseph Schoepf, MD

To the memory of my father, Phillip R. Boiselle
-PMB
To my wife, Anne, and children Dermot, Eimear, and Eileen
-DAL

Preface

In the past few decades, dramatic technological advancements in CT imaging have revolutionized noninvasive imaging of all thoracic structures, including the airways. With state-of-the-art equipment that is becoming increasingly commonplace, the entire airways can be imaged in only a few seconds, and elegant 3-D reconstructions can be created in only a few minutes. In addition to providing a high-resolution anatomical display of the central and peripheral airways, CT is also establishing itself as the preeminent noninvasive imaging modality for assessing functional airway abnormalities. In parallel, there have also been important advances in diagnostic and therapeutic bronchoscopy and surgery. The information provided by CT has become increasingly essential for establishing accurate diagnoses, guiding and planning procedures, and assessing response to therapy.

Considering the increasingly significant role of CT in airway imaging, there is a need for a comprehensive textbook that addresses CT imaging of the large and small airways. Toward this end, the purpose of this book is three-fold: first, to provide the reader with an up-to-date review of airway anatomy, physiology, pathology, and CT imaging methods; second, to provide the reader with a pragmatic compendium of the state-of-the-art in CT imaging of various common and uncommon airway disorders in adults and children; and third, to introduce the reader to new and emerging techniques that are not yet standard practice, but will likely play an important role in airway imaging in the near future.

This book begins with five introductory chapters devoted to airway physiology, anatomy, pathology, and anatomical and functional CT imaging methods. These chapters are followed by four chapters devoted to large airways disorders in adults, including airway stenoses, neoplasms, malacia, and bronchiectasis. The next section is composed of five chapters devoted to small airways disorders in adults, including asthma, infectious and noninfectious small airways disorders, obliterative bronchiolitis, and smoking-related airway diseases. The final two chapters are devoted to pediatric large and small airway disorders.

This textbook is a collaborative project that has greatly benefited from the contributions of many expert authors from around the globe. We are especially grateful to our contributing authors for sharing their time, expertise, and talents: Ronaldo Baroni, Alan Brody, Pierre-Yves Brillet, Catherine Beigelman-Aubry, Jay Catena, Kathryn Chmura, Edward Chan, Rodrigo Caruso Chate, Thomas Colby, Armin Ernst, Jonathan Goldin, Phillipe Grenier, David Hansell, Stella Hines, Edward Lee, Kyung Soo Lee, Karen Lee, Nestor Müller, John Newell, Daniel Nobrega da Costa, Marilyn Siegel, C. Isabela Silva, Chih-Wei Wang, and Athol Wells. We also thank Dr. James Cooper for the generous contribution of his elegant artwork for the book cover. We are deeply appreciative of the administrative support of Kyle Rutherford and Maxima Baudissin. We also acknowledge the support and guidance of U. Joseph Schoepf, MD, Series Editor, and Mr. Paul Dolgert, Editorial Director, at Humana Press. Finally, we thank our wives, families, and colleagues for their ongoing encouragement and support.

The intended audience for this book is primarily radiologists and pulmonologists, but the content will likely also be of interest to thoracic surgeons, pulmonary pathologists, and other physicians who are involved in the care of patients with airway diseases. It is our hope and intent that the contents of this book will ultimately enhance the care of adults and children who suffer from airway disorders.

Phillip M. Boiselle, MD
David A. Lynch, MB

Contents

xi

Part IV: Pediatric Airways Disorders

Contributors

RONALDO HUEB BARONI, MD, PhD • Department of Radiology, Hospital das Clinicas da Faculdade de Medicina da Universidade de Sao Paulo and Hospital Israelita Albert Einstein, Sao Paulo, Brazil

CATHERINE BEIGELMAN-AUBRY, MD • Department of Radiology, Hôpital Pitie Salpetriere, Paris, France

PHILLIP M. BOISELLE, MD • Department of Radiology, Beth Israel Deaconess Medical Center and Harvard Medical School, Boston, MA

PIERRE-YVES BRILLET, MD • Department of Radiology, Hôpital Avicenne – APHP, Université Léonard de Vinci (Paris XIII), France

ALAN S. BRODY, MD • Department of Radiology, Children's Hospital Medical Center, Cincinnati, OH

JAY CATENA, MD • Department of Radiology, Beth Israel Deaconess Medical Center, Boston, MA

EDWARD D. CHAN, MD • Department of Medicine, National Jewish Medical and Research Center, Denver, CO

RODRIGO CARUSO CHATE, MD • Department of Radiology, Hospital Israelita Albert Einstein, Sao Paulo, Brazil

KATHRYN CHMURA, MD • Department of Medicine, National Jewish Medical and Research Center, Denver, CO

THOMAS V. COLBY, MD • Department of Pathology, Mayo Clinic, Scottsdale, AZ

ARMIN ERNST, MD • Division of Thoracic Surgery and Interventional Pulmonology, Beth Israel Deaconess Medical Center, Harvard Medical School, Boston, MA

JONATHAN G. GOLDIN, MB ChB, PhD • Department of Radiological Sciences, UCLA Medical Center, Los Angeles, CA

PHILIPPE A. GRENIER, MD • Department of Radiology, Hôpital Pitie Salpetriere, Paris, France

DAVID M. HANSELL, MD • Department of Radiology, Royal Brompton Hospital, London, United Kingdom

STELLA HINES, MD • Department of Medicine, National Jewish Medical and Research Center, Denver, CO

EDWARD Y. LEE, MD, MPH • Department of Radiology, Children's Hospital, Boston, MA

KAREN S. LEE, MD • Department of Radiology, Beth Israel Deaconess Medical Center, Boston, MA

KYUNG SOO LEE, MD • Department of Radiology, Samsung Medical Center, Seoul, Republic of Korea

DAVID A. LYNCH, MB • Division of Radiology, National Jewish Medical and Research Center, Denver, CO

NESTOR L. MÜLLER, MD, PhD • Department of Radiology, The University of British Columbia, Vancouver General Hospital, Vancouver, BC

JOHN D. NEWELL, JR, MD • Division of Radiology, National Jewish Medical and Research Center, Denver, CO

DANIEL NOBREGA DA COSTA, MD • Department of Radiology, Hospital Israelita Albert Einstein, Sao Paulo, Brazil

U. JOSEPH SCHOEPF, MD • Department of Radiology, Medical University of South Carolina, Charleston, SC

MARILYN J. SIEGEL, MD • Department of Radiology, Mallinckrodt Institute of Radiology, St. Louis, MO

C. ISABELA S. SILVA, MD, PhD • Department of Radiology, The University of British Columbia, Vancouver General Hospital, Vancouver, BC

CHIH-WEI WANG, MD • Department of Pathology, Chang Gung Memorial Hospital, Taipei, Taiwan

ATHOL U. WELLS, MD • Department of Respiratory Medicine, Royal Brompton Hospital, London, UK

I Introductory

Airway Anatomy and Physiology

Kathryn Chmura, Stella Hines, and Edward D. Chan

1. INTRODUCTION

With inspiration, air travels from the nares through the nasal cavity, nasopharynx, oropharynx, glottis, and the tracheobronchial tree down to the alveoli, where gas exchange occurs. This chapter focuses on the gross and microscopic anatomy of the conducting and respiratory portions of the airways and the physiology of the airways and highlights the development of the tracheobronchial tree and lung parenchyma. The nasal cavity, naso-oropharynx, and larynx will be discussed in less detail. Critical components of the respiratory system that will be discussed only superficially include the respiratory center in the pons, medulla, and the muscles of respiration. Radiologic, pathologic, and/or physiologic correlations will be provided for some key airway diseases although more detailed patho-radiologic discussions of them are provided in subsequent chapters.

2. DEVELOPMENT OF THE LUNGS

The lower airway is derived from the laryngotracheal diverticulum, an endodermal-derived tissue that sprouts from the ventral wall of the foregut at approximately the fourth week of gestation (Fig. 1) *(1)*. The diverticulum progressively branches from the fourth to the seventh weeks of gestation to form the left and right lung buds, left and right main bronchi, secondary lobar bronchi, and the segmental bronchi. The lung stroma, eventually forming the pulmonary interstitium, is derived from the splanchnic mesodermal tissue of the ventral foregut. From the seventh to the tenth weeks of gestation, cartilage rings form in the walls of the trachea and larger bronchi while there is progressive branching of the bronchopulmonary segmental airways. The pulmonary arteries, formed from mesodermal embryonic tissue, branch with the bronchi. During the terminal sac period of lung development (from seventh month gestation to birth), the epithelia at the tips of the segmented bronchi have differentiated from cuboidal to squamous epithelial cells. Subsequent close associations of the distal squamous epithelium with the endothelium of blood vessels and lymphatics form the primitive alveoli.

3. GROSS ANATOMY

3.1. Supraglottic Airway

By definition, the supraglottic airway begins at the nares and oral cavity and ends at the vocal cords (Fig. 2). Upon inspiration through the nose, air travels through the nares, is moisturized by the nasal turbinates, and subsequently traverses the nasopharynx, oropharynx, hypopharynx, and vestibule of the larynx before passing through the vocal cords. From the mouth, air travels from the oral cavity directly into the oropharynx.

From: *Contemporary Medical Imaging: CT of the Airways*
Edited by: P. M. Boiselle and D. A. Lynch © Humana Press, Totowa, NJ

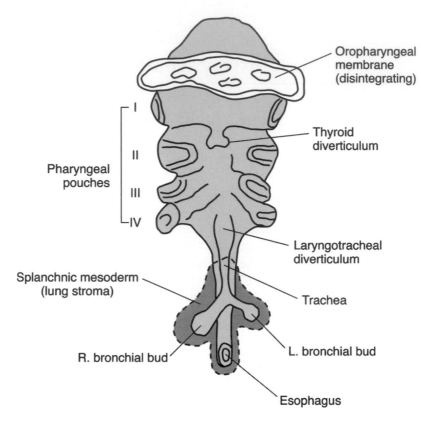

Fig. 1. Ventral view of upper foregut (4–5 weeks' gestation). Adapted from ref. *1*.

3.1.1. Nasal Cavity

The nasal cavity is the space between the roof of the mouth and the cranial base, divided vertically in the middle by the nasal septum. The roof of the nasal cavity is formed by the nasal spine of the frontal bones, nasal bones, cribriform plate of the ethmoid bone, and anterior body of the sphenoid bone. The floor of the nasal cavity is formed by the palatine processes of the maxillae and the horizontal processes of the palatine bones. The nasal septum comprises both bone and cartilage. The bony component of the nasal septum is formed by the vomer and the perpendicular plate of the ethmoid bone. The lateral walls of the nasal cavities are formed by the maxilla, palatine, and ethmoid bones. The lateral walls of the nasal cavity also contain three projections called the inferior, middle, and superior nasal turbinates, which separate the nasal cavity into four air chambers, namely the inferior nasal meatus, middle nasal meatus, superior nasal meatus, and the spheno-ethmoidal recess. The nasal turbinates serve to increase the surface area within the nasal mucosa to facilitate moistening of inspired air. Sensory innervation to the nasal cavity is supplied by the maxillary nerve with a small contribution from the nasociliary branch of the ophthalmic nerve. Autonomic innervation is supplied by the postganglionic sympathetic fibers that innervate the nasal blood vessels and postganglionic parasympathetic fibers from the pterygopalatine ganglion that innervate the nasal glands to release secretions.

3.1.2. Nasopharynx and Oropharynx

The nasopharynx functions to transmit humidified air from the nasal cavity down to the oropharynx. The nasopharynx lies above the soft palate and behind the posterior nares or conchae of the nasal

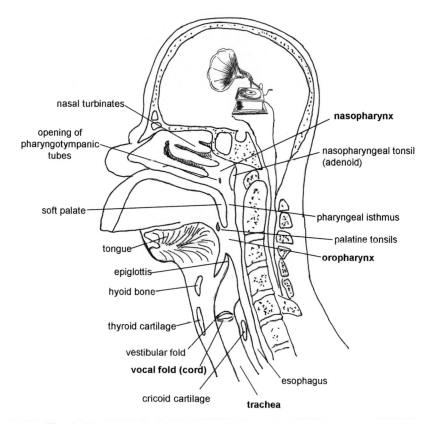

Fig. 2. Key anatomical landmarks of the extrathoracic upper airways.

cavities. Except for the soft palate, the walls of the nasopharynx are rigid and therefore the nasopharyngeal cavity does not obliterate. The pharyngeal isthmus connects the nasopharynx with the more caudal oropharynx. During swallowing, the pharyngeal isthmus may be sealed off from the oropharynx when the soft palate elevates and the superior pharyngeal constrictor muscle contracts (Fig. 2). The lateral walls of the nasopharynx contain the openings of the bilateral pharyngotympanic (Eustachian) tubes. The nasopharynx also contains lymphoid tissues and mucous glands that serve both immune and non-immune host-defense functions. The adenoid or nasopharyngeal tonsil is a mucosa-associated lymphoid tissue (MALT) located in the roof and posterior wall of the nasopharynx. The mucosa of the nasopharynx is supplied by afferent sensory nerves that join the maxillary branch of the trigeminal cranial nerve. The mucous glands in the nasopharynx are supplied by efferent postganglionic parasympathetic fibers whose cell bodies are located in the pterygopalatine ganglion.

The oropharynx extends from the soft palate to the upper border of the epiglottis. Its lateral walls consist of the palatopharyngeal arches and the lymphoid tissue-containing palatine tonsils. Its anterior border is the pharyngeal part of the tongue and its posterior border is the epithelial mucosa that abuts the body of the second and upper part of the third cervical vertebrae. The oropharynx may be viewed as an "intersection" in the aerodigestive tract because it can transmit inspired air into the trachea and liquid or masticated food into the esophagus. The soft palate serves to block swallowed food and liquid from regurgitating up into the nasopharynx, but it also contains mucous glands and taste buds. The soft palate mucous glands are innervated by (i) the lesser palatine nerve (a branch of the maxillary nerve), which contains the secretomotor efferent branches of the postganglionic parasympathetic fibers whose cell bodies are located in the pterygopalatine ganglion, and (ii) postganglionic sympathetic fibers from the carotid plexus. The taste buds are innervated by afferent taste fibers that run in the lesser palatine nerve and through the pterygopalatine ganglion without synapsing to join the greater petrosal nerve, a branch of the facial cranial nerve. Somatic afferent sensory fibers of the soft palate are supplied by the lesser palatine nerve, a branch of the maxillary nerve, whose cell bodies are in the trigeminal ganglion. The palatine tonsils receive their somatic sensory nerve supply from a plexus formed by tonsillar branches of the lesser palatine nerve and tonsillar branches of the glossopharyngeal nerve.

3.2. Larynx

The larynx is a hollow, cartilaginous structure that runs from the inferior border of the epiglottis to the first tracheal ring. Through the actions of the vocal cords, the larynx functions as a sphincter in transmitting air from the oropharynx to the trachea and in vocalization. In addition, the valve-like epiglottis helps to prevent swallowed food and liquid from entering the respiratory passages.

There are two pairs of vocal cords, which project medially from the walls of the larynx, the vestibular folds ("false vocal cords") and the vocal folds ("true vocal cords"). The vestibular and vocal folds divide the larynx into (i) the vestibule (upper chamber), located above the vestibular folds; (ii) the ventricle, the small middle chamber located between the vestibular and vocal folds; and (iii) the infraglottic cavity, which extends from the vocal folds to the lower border of the cricoid cartilage (Fig. 3). The vestibular folds create a triangular-shaped opening, called the rima vestibuli, in the larynx when viewed from above. The vocal folds form a similar but smaller triangular-shaped opening called the rima glottidis. Although "glottis" is often used synonymously with larynx, glottis technically refers to the vocal folds and the rima glottidis aperture between the vocal folds (Fig. 3).

The laryngeal skeleton is formed by nine cartilages (thyroid, cricoid, epiglottis, and paired arytenoid, corniculate, and cuneiform) that are joined by various ligaments and membranes; for example, the thyrohyoid membrane connects the thyroid cartilage to the superiorly located hyoid bone, thereby suspending the larynx. Nine extrinsic laryngeal muscles depress the larynx (omohyoid, sternohyoid, and sternothyroid), elevate the larynx (stylohyoid, digastric, mylohyoid, geniohyoid, and stylopharyngeus), or bring the hyoid bone toward the thyroid cartilage (thyrohyoid). There are seven paired and one single intrinsic muscles of the larynx that are involved in finer movements of the laryngeal parts: two cricothyroid, two posterior cricoarytenoid, two lateral cricoarytenoid, two thyroarytenoid, two thyroepiglotticus, two aryepiglotticus, two oblique arytenoid, and one transverse arytenoid. Thus, there are 8 named and a total of 15 intrinsic laryngeal muscles. Four paired muscles adduct (lateral cricoarytenoids), abduct (posterior cricoarytenoids), tense (cricothyroids), or relax (thyroarytenoids) the vocal cords. All eight named intrinsic muscles of the larynx are innervated by

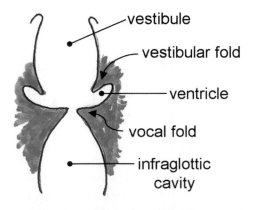

Fig. 3. Coronal section of the larynx.

two motor branches of the vagus nerve: the cricothyroid muscle is supplied by the external laryngeal nerve and the rest are supplied by the recurrent laryngeal nerve.

During normal respiration, the arytenoid cartilages abduct, opening the rima vestibuli and rima glottidis and allowing for passage of air from the laryngeal inlet to the trachea. During forced inspiration, the arytenoid cartilages are rotated laterally by the intrinsic laryngeal muscles (mainly by the posterior cricoarytenoid muscles), which abduct the vocal folds. As a result, the rima glottidis widens from a triangular-shaped opening to a rhomboid-shaped opening, thus increasing further the diameter of the laryngeal airway and allowing more air to enter the trachea.

3.3. Infraglottic Airway

3.3.1. Tracheobronchial Tree

The tracheobronchial tree constitutes the airway below the vocal cords (Fig. 4). The trachea enters the thorax 1–3 cm above the level of the suprasternal notch; its intrathoracic portion is 6–9 cm in length. In normal human adult males, the tracheal diameter is 1.3–2.5 cm in the coronal plane and 1.3–2.7 cm in the sagittal plane; in normal human adult females, the tracheal coronal and sagittal diameters are 1.0–2.1 cm and 1.0–2.3 cm, respectively *(2)*. The trachea is comprised of 16–20 C-shaped cartilaginous rings anteriorly with a soft membrane posteriorly. It bifurcates approximately at the sternal angle (angle of Louis) into the left and right mainstem bronchi. The right mainstem bronchus is wider and shorter and runs more vertically than the left mainstem bronchus *(3)*. As a result, the left mainstem bronchus passes inferolaterally at a more acute angle than the right mainstem bronchus. The left mainstem bronchus is located inferior to the aortic arch and anterior to the esophagus and thoracic aorta. Both mainstem bronchi enter their respective lungs at the hila.

Analogous to the roots of a tree, the mainstem bronchi branch to form lobar bronchi, also known as secondary bronchi. On the right lung, there are three lobar bronchi: right upper lobe bronchus, right middle lobe bronchus, and right lower lobe bronchus. On the left lung, there are two lobar bronchi: left upper lobe bronchus and left lower lobe bronchus. Each of these lobar bronchi divides into several segmental bronchi (tertiary bronchi), which supply the bronchopulmonary segments of

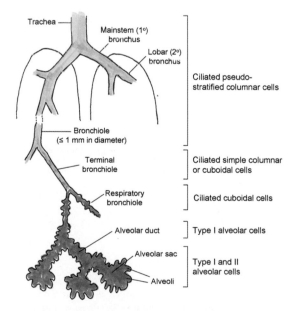

Fig. 4. Schematic demonstration of the tracheobronchial tree. Adapted from ref. *11*.

Table 1
Lobes and Bronchopulmonary Segments of the Lung with Boyden's Schema for Numbering of Bronchi

	Right lung		Left lung	
	Segment	Boyden's number	Segment	Boyden's number
Upper lobe	Apical segment	B1	Apical segment	B1
	Anterior segment	B2	Anterior segment	B2
			Posterior segment	B3
	Posterior segment	B3		
			Superior segment of lingula	B4
			Inferior segment of lingula	B5
Middle lobe	Lateral segment	B4	None	
	Medial segment	B5		
Lower lobe	Superior segment	B6	Superior segment	B6
	Medial basal segment	B7	Anteromedial basal segment	B7, B8
	Anterior basal segment	B8	Lateral basal segment	B9
	Lateral basal segment	B9	Posterior basal segment	B10
	Posterior basal segment	B10		

each lobe (Table 1). Bronchopulmonary segments are the smallest surgically resectable units of the lungs. Beyond these segmental tertiary bronchi, there are 20–25 generations of progressively smaller subsegmental branches that eventually lead to conducting bronchioles → terminal bronchioles → respiratory bronchioles → alveolar ducts → and alveolar sacs. The conducting bronchioles are also anatomically important because they help define the pulmonary lobule, a basic unit of the lung (Fig. 5).

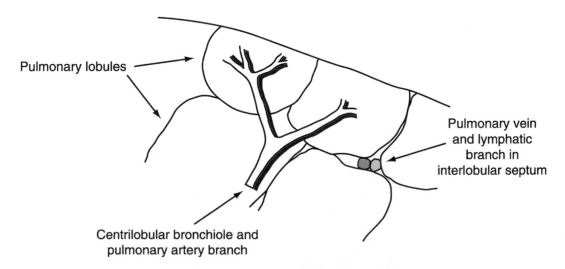

Fig. 5. The pulmonary lobule. The conducting centrilobular bronchioles supply the basic units of the lung, known as pulmonary lobules. As the name implies, note that the centrilobular bronchioles and their accompanying pulmonary artery branches enter at the center of the lobule. By contrast, branches of the pulmonary veins and lymphatics are located at the margins of the lobule, within the interlobular septa.

3.3.2. Blood Supply of the Upper Respiratory Tract and the Tracheobronchial Tree

Blood to the respiratory system is supplied by two different circulations, the pulmonary artery circulation and the bronchial artery circulation. The pulmonary artery circulation is primarily involved with gas exchange whereas the bronchial artery circulation is involved with nutrient delivery. Hence, whereas the pulmonary artery circulation is a high-flow, low-pressure system and serves as the means of gas exchange, the bronchial circulation supplies oxygenated blood and nourishment to the connective tissue of the bronchial tree, lower trachea, airway nerves, and lymph nodes as well as the visceral pleura *(4)*. Blood supply to the trachea is segmental. The upper trachea is perfused by multiple branches of the inferior thyroid artery. By contrast, the lower trachea is supplied by the bronchial arteries. The internal mammary artery can also contribute to the blood supply of the lower trachea *(5)*. Within each bronchopulmonary segment, a branch of the pulmonary artery descends in proximity to the bronchus, following it posterolaterally, and ultimately sends arterial branches to lobar and segmental bronchi on their posterior surfaces. The bronchial arteries also descend along the posterior aspects of the bronchi as far distally as the respiratory bronchioles. The pulmonary veins, while at the bases of bronchopulmonary segments, are found in the interlobular septae, along with lymphatic vessels (Fig. 5). As also shown, these veins are typically as far away from the centrilobular bronchioles as possible, a principle known as "Miller's dictum." A main vein drains each bronchopulmonary segment, and this vein is typically located on the anterior surface of the corresponding bronchus. These veins ultimately converge to drain into the left atrium *(4,6)*.

Knowledge of the blood supply of the airways is important in the management of life-threatening hemoptysis. The two left bronchial arteries arise from the thoracic aorta, one superior to and another inferior to the left mainstem bronchus. The single right bronchial artery often arises as a common trunk with the third or fifth posterior intercostal artery or even from the left bronchial artery *(3)*. As these arteries are part of the high-pressure systemic circulation, it is not surprising that massive hemoptysis most likely originates from the bronchial circulation. Another important pearl is that bronchial arteries can give rise to the anterior spinal arteries in about 5% of patients, and thus embolization of bronchial arteries when controlling massive hemoptysis may result in spinal paralysis. The bronchial arteries enter the lung at the hila and immediately dive into the connective tissue surrounding the bronchi and begin branching. Typically, two or three branches anastomose with each other to form a peribronchial plexus with an elongated and irregular mesh accompanying each division of the conducting airway.

After oxygenated blood is delivered to the airway tissue, this blood is returned to the heart by various pathways. Bronchial veins drain only part, approximately 25–33%, of the blood delivered by the bronchial arteries to the bronchial tree. The right bronchial vein drains into the azygous vein. The left bronchial veins drain into the accessory hemiazygous vein or into the left superior intercostal vein. The remaining 67–75% of the blood delivered by the bronchial arteries returns to the heart via the pulmonary veins draining into the left atrium. Interconnections between the bronchial vessels and precapillary and postcapillary pulmonary vessels called bronchopulmonary veins drain into the pulmonary veins. Blood leaving the capillary bed around the terminal bronchioles flows through anastomoses with the alveolar capillaries and drain into pulmonary veins. Whereas the pulmonary artery circulation receives the entire cardiac output with each cardiac cycle, the amount of blood flow through the bronchial arterial circulation is low. In studies of dogs, the left lung received 1% of cardiac output via the bronchial artery, with 50% of this circulation going to the parenchyma and the remainder supplying the trachea and bronchi. Extrapolating these findings to humans gives an estimate of bronchial blood flow to both lungs of <3% of the total cardiac output. Furthermore, a normal adult lung remains viable without a bronchial circulation as demonstrated in transplanted lungs. Venous blood from the pulmonary arteries supply all the metabolic substrates needed by the lung parenchyma, and oxygen is provided by diffusion from the airspaces *(7)*. However, bronchial circulation remains critical to fetal pulmonary development and may contribute significantly to gas exchange in many congenital cardiac abnormalities and in certain disease states, such as pulmonary fibrosis, where an increase in the size and number of bronchial arteries has been seen *(5)*.

3.3.3. Innervation of the Airways

Nerves to the airways regulate airway caliber size, blood flow, and mucous secretion. Thus, abnormalities in neural control may contribute to airflow limitation and mucous hypersecretion. Simplistically, three main types of airway nerves exist (Table 2): (i) efferent parasympathetic nerves, which release acetylcholine, (ii) efferent sympathetic nerves, which release norepinephrine, and (iii) afferent (sensory) nerves, which release glutamate. The efferent sympathetic and parasympathetic fibers principally affect the bronchial smooth muscles, resulting in either bronchodilatation or bronchoconstriction, respectively *(8)*.

In general, the axons of the preganglionic parasympathetic fibers release acetylcholine that binds to nicotinic receptors located on the postganglionic neuron. In turn, the postganglionic neurons release acetylcholine that binds to muscarinic receptors on the target organ. Thus, increased parasympathetic output to the lungs via the vagus nerve causes the release of acetylcholine, which then triggers bronchoconstriction. Whereas there are four subtypes of muscarinic (M) receptors identified in the lungs, three are presently known to differentially play important roles in airway physiology. First, activation of the M_3-receptors by acetylcholine present on airway smooth muscle cells causes their contraction, resulting in bronchoconstriction. Second, activation of either M_1- or M_3-receptors enhances mucous secretion in the airways. Third, the M_2-receptor is unique in that it is known as an inhibitory muscarinic receptor (also called an autoreceptor). The M_2-receptors are located at the

Table 2
Innervation of the Airways

Nerve type	Location of cell bodies	Neurotransmitter released	Receptor of the released neurotransmitter binds	Effects on the airways
Efferent parasympathetic	Preganglionic nerve: dorsal vagal nucleus of the vagus nerve	Acetylcholine	Nicotinic	Bronchoconstriction except for M_2-receptor, which theoretically may cause bronchodilatation
	Postganglionic nerve: peripheral ganglia in the lungs	Acetylcholine	Muscarinic	
Efferent sympathetic	Preganglionic nerve: intermediolateral cell column in the lateral horn gray matter of T2 to T4 spinal cord	Acetylcholine	Nicotinic	Bronchodilatation
	Postganglionic nerve: paravertebral sympathetic ganglion of T2 to T4	Epinephrine, norepinephrine	Adrenergic	
Sensory afferent	Inferior nodose vagal ganglion			

terminal (the axonic end) of the postganglionic nerve and thus are prejunctional receptors to the airway smooth muscle cells. By an autocrine negative feedback mechanism, activation of M_2-receptors on the presynaptic postganglionic nerve by acetylcholine released by the same nerve serves to inhibit further acetylcholine release.

In contrast to the effects of the parasympathetic output to the airways, the efferent sympathetic nerve causes the release of norepinephrine that results in bronchodilatation. Interestingly, in humans there are few direct sympathetic nerve connections to the airways. Nevertheless, sympathetic nerves relax airway smooth muscles indirectly through modulation of the parasympathetic ganglia; that is, activation of prejunctional β_2-adrenergic receptors on the cholinergic nerves of the airways results in inhibition of acetylcholine release. Furthermore, norepinephrine and epinephrine released systemically can bind to adrenergic receptors that are abundantly present in the airways. The family of adrenergic receptors is comprised of β_1-, β_2-, α_1-, and α_2-receptors. In the airways, β_2-adrenergic receptor stimulation results in an increase in adenylyl cyclase activity, resulting in airway smooth muscle relaxation and bronchial dilatation. Because β_2-adrenergic receptors predominate on bronchial smooth muscles, activation of β_2-receptors by β_2-agonists such as albuterol bronchodilates the airways. Conversely, it is also the reason that non-selective $\beta_1\beta_2$-blockers like propranolol can cause bronchoconstriction in susceptible individuals *(9)*. Because β-adrenergic receptors present on airway smooth muscles are essentially comprised of β_2-adrenergic receptor subtype *(10)*, selective β_1-blockers (e.g., atenolol, metoprolol), which have a 20-fold greater affinity for β_1-adrenergic receptors than β_2-adrenergic receptors, are less likely to induce bronchoconstriction than non-selective $\beta_1\beta_2$-blockers.

Traveling via the vagus nerve, the afferent (sensory) nerves transmit signals from mechano-stretch receptors in the lungs to limit inspiration when an "overstretch signal" is received from the lungs. This reflex to prevent overdistension of the lungs is known as the Hering–Breuer reflex.

4. HISTOLOGY

4.1. Conducting Portion of the Airways

The conducting portion of the airways, comprised of the trachea, bronchi, and the conducting and terminal bronchioles, is lined by ciliated pseudostratified columnar or ciliated cuboidal epithelium. In general, five cell types make up this epithelial layer *(11)*: (i) ciliated columnar or cuboidal cells—the major cell type present; (ii) goblet cells, which secrete mucous; (iii) brush cells with numerous microvilli on their apical surfaces—these cells have afferent nerve endings on their basal surfaces and are considered to be sensory receptors; (iv) basal (short) cells that lie on the basal lamina but do not extend to the luminal surface and are considered to be stem cells that differentiate into other cell types; and (v) small granule cells that resemble the basal cells except that they possess numerous granules.

4.1.1. Trachea and Bronchi

The trachea is lined by the typical respiratory epithelium of the conducting airways, i.e., ciliated pseudostratified columnar epithelium (Fig. 6A). The trachea also contains many goblet cells that secrete viscous mucous and serous glands that produce a more fluid mucous. Sixteen to 20 C-shaped cartilage rings located in the lamina propria serve to keep the tracheal lumen open during respiration. Fibroelastic ligaments and bundles of smooth muscles are bound to the perichondrium to bridge the open ends of the C-shaped cartilage rings. Contraction of smooth muscle in the posterior tracheal membrane during the cough reflex produces marked tracheal luminal narrowing, resulting in rapid acceleration of expelled air and solid bronchial contents.

The epithelia of the mainstem bronchi, lobar bronchi, segmental bronchi, and the subsegmental bronchi are similar to that of the trachea and are comprised mainly of ciliated pseudostratified columnar cells and goblet cells (Fig. 6B). The lamina propria of these larger airways contains

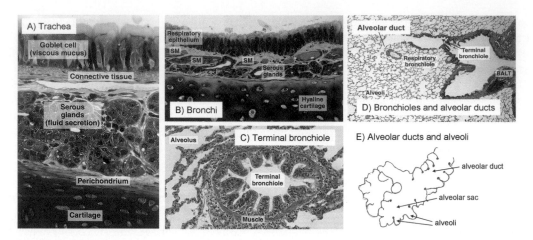

Fig. 6. Histology of the airways. (**A**) Histology of the normal trachea showing the typical pseudostratified columnar ciliated cells, goblet cells, underlying connective tissue, and the serous glands. (**B**) Histology of a bronchus showing the pseudostratified columnar ciliated cells, serous glands, cartilage, and smooth muscles. (**C**) Histology of the terminal bronchiole in which the epithelium is comprised of ciliated simple columnar or cuboidal cells, goblet cells, and Clara cells. Note the well-developed smooth muscle layer in the lamina propria of the terminal bronchiole. (**D**) Histology of the terminal bronchiole, respiratory bronchiole, alveolar ducts, and alveolar sacs. (**E**) Drawing of alveolar ducts, alveolar sacs, and alveoli. From ref. *11*.

crisscrossing bundles of smooth muscles, elastic fibers, serous glands, lymphocytes, and bronchus-associated lymphoid tissue (BALT). In the larger bronchi, the cartilage encircles the bronchi; as the bronchi become smaller, the cartilage rings are replaced by irregular islands of cartilage, mainly at branch points.

4.1.2. Conducting and Terminal Bronchioles

Somewhat arbitrarily, bronchi become bronchioles when cartilage is no longer present in their airway walls. Bronchioles have also been defined as airways with diameters ≤5 mm. Each conducting bronchiole, also known simply as a bronchiole, enters a pulmonary lobule, the basic lung unit (Fig. 5). Pulmonary lobules are pyramid-shaped units, with the apex directed toward the hilum. In the fetus, the lobules are well demarcated from each other by thin connective tissue septa; in adults, the septa are incomplete and thus the lobules are less well delineated. Each bronchiole branches to form five to seven terminal bronchioles, the most distal components of the conducting portion of the airways (Fig. 6C).

The epithelium of the conducting bronchioles is lined with ciliated pseudostratified columnar cells whereas ciliated simple columnar or cuboidal cells line the terminal bronchioles. Mucous-secreting goblet cells are scattered amongst the ciliated epithelial cells. The terminal bronchiole epithelia also contain Clara cells, which secrete proteins that protect the bronchiolar lining against oxidative pollutants and inflammation. The lamina propria of both the conducting and terminal bronchioles contains smooth muscles and elastic fibers. The smooth muscles are innervated by the vagus nerve (which causes bronchoconstriction) and by the sympathetic nerves (which cause bronchodilatation). Unlike the bronchi, there are no serous glands in the bronchioles.

4.2. Respiratory Portion of the Airways

4.2.1. Respiratory Bronchioles

Respiratory bronchioles are the distal continuation of the terminal bronchioles (Fig. 6D). Respiratory bronchioles are the transition between the conducting and respiratory portions of the airways.

The epithelium of respiratory bronchioles is lined by ciliated cuboidal epithelial cells and Clara cells. At the rim of the alveolar openings, the bronchiolar epithelium becomes continuous with the very thin squamous alveolar lining cells, better known as the Type I alveolar cells (*see* Section 4.2.2.). The lamina propria of respiratory bronchioles contains smooth muscles and elastic fibers.

4.2.2. Alveolar Ducts and Alveoli

The walls of alveolar ducts are almost completely occupied by openings to the alveoli (Fig. 6E). Their epithelium is lined by Type I alveolar cells and their lamina propria contains smooth muscle bundles which appear as knobs between adjacent alveoli. In contrast to the more proximal airways, the alveolar ductal and alveolar epithelial cells do not possess cilia. Elastic and reticular fibers form a complex network encircling the openings of the alveoli, which are evaginations of the respiratory bronchioles, alveolar ducts, and alveolar sacs. Alveolar epithelium is lined by Type I alveolar cells, which make up 97% of the alveolar surface with the rest comprised of Type II cuboidal cells. Elastic fibers in the lamina propria of alveoli enable them to expand with inspiration and to contract passively with expiration. Reticular fibers serve to help prevent alveolar overdistension and damage to the delicate capillaries and thin alveolar septa.

5. PHYSIOLOGY

5.1. General Considerations

The neuro–respiratory axis can be metaphorically described as a series of links of a chain, each dependent on the other for full strength and function. At the head of the respiratory chain is the organization of breathing in the central nervous system, i.e., the medulla, pons, and even higher cortical centers of the cerebrum. The control of breathing is divided into the automatic and voluntary controls. In a practical sense, the main function of automatic control is to maintain minute ventilation to a target $PaCO_2$ of ~40 mmHg and blood pH of ~7.40 at sea level. Hypoxia, sensed by chemoreceptors located in the carotid bodies, is another potent stimulus for increased respiration. Hypoxemia-induced afferent impulses travel up the carotid sinus nerve, whose fibers run alongside the glossopharyngeal nerve and the vagus nerve to synapse with the inspiratory neurons to increase minute ventilation. Thus, afferent fibers from peripheral chemoreceptors and also from lung mechano-stretch receptors travel up two cranial nerves to synapse with neurons whose cell bodies are located in two regions of the medulla: the nucleus tractus solitarius and the nucleus ambiguus. Surrounding these two nuclei are inter-neurons known as the reticular activating system that serve to connect the neurons of the automatic control with higher brain centers to control the state of alertness. Efferent fibers from both these nuclei synapse with motor neurons that serve the muscles of respiration.

The diaphragm is the major muscle of inspiration. Its main function upon contraction is to move inferiorly, creating a negative intrathoracic pressure and allowing ambient air to entrail down its pressure gradient along the airways and into the alveolar spaces. Less widely appreciated is that upon contraction, the diaphragm also has expiratory action on the upper rib cage in addition to the well-known inspiratory function on the lower rib cage *(12)*. The sole motor innervation to the diaphragm is supplied by the phrenic nerves, whose efferent motor fibers arise from C3, C4, and C5 (mainly C4) ventral rami of the spinal cord.

5.2. Pulmonary Function Tests

5.2.1. Introduction

Pulmonary physiology is clinically and quantitatively measured by a pulmonary function test (PFT). A complete PFT is comprised of three main components: (i) spirometry to assess airflow limitation, (ii) lung volume measurement, and (iii) a single breath diffusion capacity for carbon monoxide measurement (DLco). Pulmonary function testing helps to (i) classify a lung disorder as obstructive, restrictive, or mixed; (ii) evaluate the degree of respiratory impairment; (iii) assess response to treatment; (iv) determine pulmonary risk with non-pulmonary surgery; and (v) predict degree of respiratory impairment after lung resectional surgery. Normal PFT values are derived from predictive formulae based on an individual's height, weight, age, gender, and race. These normal physiologic values are commonly expressed by their appropriate units (e.g., liters/second) but also as percent of predicted values. In general, the normal predicted range is wide because of normal variation between subjects even after accounting for the aforementioned patient demographics. One important caveat is that although a pulmonary function value may be considered "within normal limits," it may be a significant decrement for that particular individual when compared with a previous value. For example, if at baseline an individual has a lung capacity of 150% of the predicted value but is now 100% of the predicted value, it is a significant decrease in lung capacity despite still being within normal limits. Furthermore, spirometric values and some of lung volume measurements such as total lung capacity (TLC) are effort-dependent. Therefore, for optimal PFT determination, it is essential to have maximum effort by the patient, correctly calibrated equipment, and conduction of the test by knowledgeable and motivated respiratory technicians.

Determining which components of the PFT (i.e., spirometry, lung volumes, and/or diffusion capacity) are necessary for a particular patient should be based on whether a particular type of pulmonary disorder is already known or not and what question is posed. For example, in patients with unexplained dyspnea or interstitial lung disease, a complete testing that includes spirometry, lung volumes, and DLco, both initially and on subsequent exams, is necessary. However, in an asthmatic in whom one is assessing response to therapy, measuring DLco is neither necessary nor cost-effective. By contrast, a DLco measurement in a patient with chronic obstructive pulmonary disease (COPD) will assist in classifying the COPD as either mainly chronic bronchitis (preserved DLco) or emphysema (reduced DLco).

5.2.2. Measurement of Airflow

Spirometry, which plots flow rate as a function of lung volume, is traditionally measured by a volume displacement instrument called a spirometer, with volume as the measured variable and airflow rates derived by dividing volume into timed segments, i.e., airflow = Δvolume/Δtime. Spirometries are more currently obtained by a pneumotach, in which airflow is measured and volume is obtained by integration of the airflow, i.e., volume = $\int$airflow = $\int \Delta$volume/Δtime. Spirometric measurements are reproducible, inexpensive, and widely available. Basic spirometry readings include the amount of air that can be blown out with maximal effort, known as the forced vital capacity (FVC), the volume exhaled in the first second of the FVC maneuver (FEV1), and the FEV1/FVC ratio. Whereas spirometry can be diagnostic of obstructive lung diseases, it is insufficient to diagnose restrictive lung disease but may be suggestive (Table 3). Shown in Fig. 7A is the contour of an idealized normal flow–volume loop with its inspiratory and expiratory limbs. By contrast, Fig. 7B shows only the expiratory limb of a flow–volume loop of one individual with no lung disease but who performed the test with various efforts. As can be seen, spirometric measurements can be very effort-dependent and inaccurate values may be obtained with suboptimal efforts or poor techniques. Note that by convention, the values of the lung volume on the *x*-axis is reverse of the algebraic standard *x*-axis in that the lung volumes increase as one moves leftward toward the origin.

FEV1 is considered to be within normal limits when it is between 80 and 120% of the predicted value. FEV1 <80% of the predicted value and an FEV1/FVC ratio <0.70–0.75 indicate airway obstruction as seen with asthma, COPD, bronchiolitis, and bronchiectasis. Shown in Fig. 8A is the expiratory limb of the flow–volume loop of a normal subject (solid black line) superimposed on one from a patient with obstructive lung disease (dashed red line). Note that in the patient with airway obstruction, there is concavity of the expiratory limb, decreased height of the peak flow, and increased lung volumes such as the residual volume (RV) and TLC. As the names would suggest, RV is the

Table 3
Diagnosis of Ventilatory Impairment

Parameter	Obstructive*	Restrictive
Basic spirometry		
FEV1	Decreased	Normal or decreased
FVC	Normal or decreased but to a lesser degree than the FEV1	Decreased
FEV1/FVC = % FEV1	Decreased	Normal or increased
Lung volumes		
RV	Normal or increased	Decreased
FRC (TGV)	Increased	Decreased
TLC	Normal or increased	Decreased

*FVC, forced vital capacity; FEV1, volume exhaled in the first second of the FVC maneuver; FRC, functional residual capacity; RV, residual volume; TLC, total lung capacity.

volume of air that is remaining in the lung after a maximal expiratory effort whereas TLC is the total volume of air in the lung after a maximal inspiratory effort. Figure 8B shows an obstructive spirogram before bronchodilator treatment (pre-BD) and after treatment (post-BD). Not only have there been improvement in the flow in the expiratory limb and peak flow, but the lung volumes have improved after bronchodilatation, i.e., the TLC has decreased (shifted rightward) because greater amounts of intrapulmonary air can to be expelled after bronchodilator treatment. By definition, an increase in FEV1 by ≥12% plus an absolute increase of at least 200 mL after administration of an inhaled bronchodilator such as albuterol signifies a positive bronchodilator response and is indicative

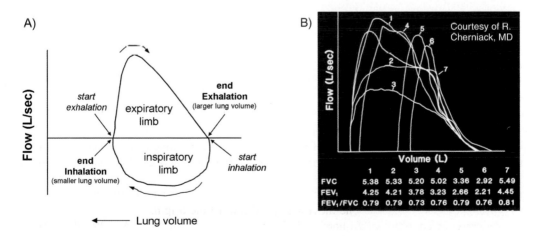

Fig. 7. Optimal and suboptimal flow–volume loops. **(A)** An idealized normal flow–volume loop with the normal contour of the inspiratory and expiratory limbs. **(B)** These actual expiratory flow–volume loops are of a normal individual who performed spirometry with varying degrees of effort and technique to illustrate that this test is effort-dependent. Note that marked differences in FEV1, FVC, and the FEV1/FVC ratio may be obtained with suboptimal efforts. Figure 7B is courtesy of Dr. Reuben Cherniack, National Jewish Medical and Research Center.

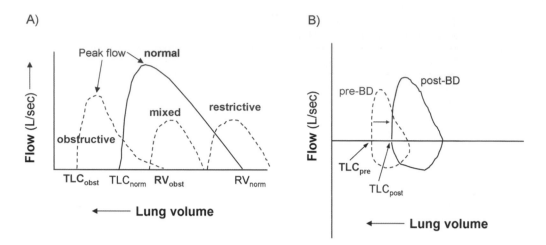

Fig. 8. Abnormal flow–volume loops. **(A)** Comparison of normal (solid black line) and obstructive (dashed red line) expiratory flow–volume loops. Note the hallmarks of airway obstruction on the spirogram: concavity of the expiratory flow loop, the decreased peak flow, and increased lung volumes [residual volume (RV) and total lung capacity (TLC)]. The flow–volume loops of individuals with restrictive lung disease (dashed blue line) and with mixed obstructive-restrictive lung disease (dashed purple line) are shown for comparison. **(B)** Inspiratory and expiratory low–volume loops of a patient with airflow obstruction before bronchodilator (pre-BD) and after inhalation of and response to a bronchodilator (post-BD).

of at least partial reversible airway obstruction. In cases with mild airflow limitation, this provocative bronchodilator test may be the only indication of airflow obstruction.

For comparison, the expiratory limb of a flow–volume loop is shown from a patient with restrictive lung disease (Fig. 8A, dashed blue line) showing decreased lung volumes. In a patient with mixed obstructive-restrictive lung disease (Fig. 8A, dashed purple line), one typically finds decreased TLC and increased RV compared with normal.

5.2.3. Measurement of Lung Volumes

Lung volume determination is necessary to assess restrictive lung disease and evidence of hyperinflation in obstructive lung disease and for measuring diffusion capacity (DLco). The three lung volumes most clinically relevant are the TLC, the functional residual capacity (FRC), and the RV. The tidal volume (TV) is the volume of air inhaled or exhaled during rest breathing. As shown in Fig. 9, FRC is the volume of air remaining in the lungs at the end of a normal expiration (i.e., lung volume at the end of a TV expiration), whereas RV is the volume of air remaining in the lungs at the end of a maximal forced expiration (i.e., lung volume at the end of a FVC maneuver); thus, the RV is the volume of air that remains in the lung even after maximal effort to empty the lungs. Other lung volume measurements include expiratory reserve volume (ERV) and inspiratory reserve volume (IRV) although they are less clinically useful (Fig. 9). Note that lung *capacities* such as inspiratory reserve capacity (IRC), FRC, vital capacity (VC = FVC), and TLC are comprised of the sum of two or more lung *volumes*, e.g., TLC = IRV + TV + ERV + RV.

The normal range for lung volumes are a TLC of 80–120% of the predicted value, FRC of 75–120% of the predicted value, and RV of 75–120% of the predicted value. Increased lung volumes are typically seen with obstructive lung disease and are defined as TLC or FRC =120% of the predicted value. Air trapping is defined by an increase in RV >120% of the predicted value. Hyperinflation is defined as TLC and FRC >120% of the predicted value and an RV >140% of the predicted

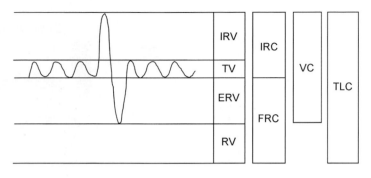

Fig. 9. Lung volumes and capacities. Schematic diagram of lung volumes and capacities. Shown on the respiratory tracing are three tidal breaths flanking a full inspiratory and expiratory effort. IRV, inspiratory reserve volume; TV, tidal volume; ERV, expiratory reserve volume; RV, residual volume; IRC, inspiratory reserve capacity; FRC, functional residual capacity; VC, vital capacity; TLC, total lung capacity.

value. As shown in Fig. 8A, an increase in lung volumes is characterized by a leftward shift of the flow–volume loop.

In contrast to obstructive lung diseases, restrictive lung disease such as pulmonary fibrosis is functionally defined as a reduction in lung volumes and capacities. Hence, the findings in restrictive lung disease are reduced TLC, FRC, RV, and FVC (i.e., <75 or 80% of the predicted value); because the FVC is at least or more severely affected than the FEV1 in restrictive lung disease, the FEV1/FVC ratio is normal or high.

5.2.4. Measurement of Diffusion Capacity

Each alveolus is intimately wrapped by a network of alveolar capillaries (Fig. 10). This anatomy allows the exchange of O_2 and CO_2 between the alveolar and blood compartments by the diffusion of these gas molecules across alveolar–capillary septum, comprised of type 1 epithelial cells, endothelial cells, and their fused basal laminae (Fig. 10). The DLco measures the ability of the lung to transfer gas and saturate the hemoglobin in red blood cells. Because carbon monoxide (CO) is so avidly bound to hemoglobin, it is an ideal gas for assessing the ability of the lung to transfer gas. Thus, CO is used as a surrogate for O_2. The technique involves inhaling a single breath of gas enriched for helium and CO, followed by measurement of CO, often by chromatography, of the expired gas. When there is good gas exchange in the lungs, very little CO is breathed out because much of the CO has diffused across the normal alveolar–capillary membrane, but when there is loss of surface area for gas exchange as seen in emphysema, less CO diffuses into the lungs and hence higher levels are measured in the expired breath.

DLco that is 80–120% of the predicted value is considered to be within normal limits. Causes of an increased DLco (DLco >120% of the predicted value) are generally associated with increased recruitment of the pulmonary vascular bed as seen with exercise, left to right intracardiac shunts, asthma (due to increased pulmonary blood volumes as a result of more negative intrathoracic pressure), extremely high altitudes, and early congestive heart failure, or increased hemoglobin in the lungs (pulmonary hemorrhage) that binds and sequesters the inhaled CO. By contrast, diffusion capacity is decreased (DLco <80% of the predicted value) in conditions that disrupt the alveolar–capillary surface for gas transfer such as pulmonary resection, pulmonary fibrosis, pulmonary thromboembolism, and emphysema. DLco is generally corrected for hemoglobin levels—as polycythemia will increase DLco and anemia will decrease DLco. If both the DLco and lung volumes are decreased, the DLco should be corrected for alveolar volume (V_A). Normally, the TLC (measured by body plethysmography) and V_A (measured by distribution of helium gas) are roughly equal. However, if the decreased DLco

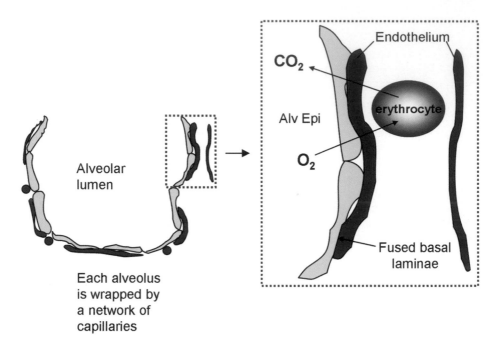

Fig. 10. Alveolar–capillary septa and diffusion capacity. The thin alveolar–capillary septum allows the diffusion of O_2 and CO_2 between erythrocytes in the alveolar capillaries and the alveolar space. This diffusion capacity is measured by the ability of trace amounts of inhaled CO to transfer across the entire alveolar capillary membrane. The blood–air barrier includes the alveolar epithelium, fused basal laminae, and the endothelium.

normalizes after correcting for V_A (DLco/V_A), then there is poor gas distribution accounting for the low DLco. Furthermore, small but otherwise normal lungs because of neuromuscular weakness may also have low DLco that normalizes after correction for V_A.

5.2.5. Pressure–Volume Curves and Lung Compliance

The more compliant the lung, the more easily distensible it is. Conversely, a lung with decreased compliance (= increased elastance) is relatively less distensible. Generation of a pressure–volume curve is a technique to measure the lung compliance. It is performed by measuring lung volumes as a function of the intrathoracic pressure. Thus, compliance is determined by measuring the change in expiratory lung volumes with change in transpulmonary pressure where the transpulmonary pressure = $P_{alveolar\ space}$ (measured at the mouth) − $P_{pleural\ space}$ (measured by esophageal balloon manometer). Thus, when the transpulmonary pressure is graphed on the *x*-axis and the lung volume is graphed on the *y*-axis, the slope of the curve, i.e., the change in volume per unit pressure change ($\Delta V/\Delta P$), is known as the compliance. Shown in Fig. 11A are pressure–volume curves of a normal individual (solid black line) and in a patient with emphysema (red line). Emphysema is an example of a highly compliant lung as evinced by the increased slope ($\Delta V/\Delta P$) of the red compliance curve. Note that compliance is inversely related to elastance; for example, a highly compliant lung due to emphysema has low elastance due to loss of elastic recoil. As a result of the decreased elastic recoil and airway obstruction, the volume of emphysemic lungs is generally larger than normal. By contrast, a non-compliant fibrotic lung, as shown by the blue compliance curve, would have low compliance (as shown by the relative decreased slope of $\Delta V/\Delta P$) but high elastance. Because of this relatively high elastic recoil, the lung volumes in pulmonary fibrosis are decreased. An analogy can be made to rubber bands. As shown in Fig. 11B, the thin, stretchable rubber band (analogous to the hyperinflated

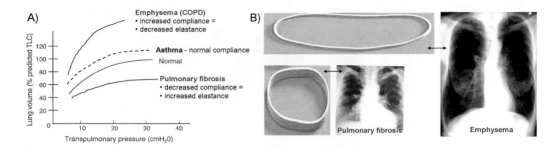

Fig. 11. Compliance and pressure–volume curves. (**A**) Respiratory pressure–volume (compliance) curves of a normal individual and individuals with asthma, emphysema, and pulmonary fibrosis. Whereas asthma and emphysema may be associated with increased lung volumes, the respiratory compliance ($\Delta V/\Delta P$) of the asthmatic patient is normal, while the compliance of the emphysematous patient is increased because of loss of lung elastic tissues. By contrast, pulmonary fibrosis is associated with decreased compliance (decreased $\Delta V/\Delta P$). Note that the PV curve of the emphysematous lung is also truncated because it cannot generate high enough intrathoracic pressure because it has lost elastic recoil. (**B**) Analogy between rubber bands and highly compliant and non-compliant lungs. An old thin rubber band and an emphysematous lung both have high compliance, low elastance, and high volumes. By contrast, a brand new thick rubber band and a fibrotic lung have low compliance, high elastance, and low volumes.

emphysematous lung) is highly compliant but has lost much of its elastic property, whereas the thick, difficult-to-stretch rubber band (analogous to the small fibrotic lung) has low compliance but retains great elastic property. Even in normal lungs, the compliance is lower, as shown by the more horizontal slope of the curve, at high expanding pressures. Another important pearl is that the compliance of the asthmatic patient (dashed line) is normal, i.e., slope of the pressure–volume curve in the asthmatic is normal even though the lung volumes at any given pressure are higher than normal (Fig. 11A). This is because in asthma, the lung parenchyma is intrinsically normal whereas in emphysema, there is parenchymal destruction. We will next discuss some specific disorders that further highlight, in a more clinical way, the significance of the anatomic and physiologic correlations discussed previously.

5.3. Physiologic, Imaging, and Histopathologic Correlations

5.3.1. Larger Airway Obstruction

Larger airway obstruction has characteristic flow–volume loops depending on whether the obstruction is variable or fixed, extrathoracic or intrathoracic.

5.3.1.1. VARIABLE INTRATHORACIC AIRWAY OBSTRUCTION (ASTHMA AND COPD)

Variable intrathoracic obstruction of the larger airways is best exemplified by asthma and COPD. COPD is traditionally divided into chronic bronchitis—defined clinically as chronic sputum production for ≥ 3 months in each of 2 consecutive years in the absence of other causes such as bronchiectasis, tuberculosis, lung cancer, and congestive heart failure—and emphysema—defined anatomically by destruction of alveolar spaces although in reality most patients have varying features of both. As shown previously in Fig. 8A, both asthma and COPD have expiratory airflow limitation and hyperinflated lung volumes. In asthma, however, the lung function may be completely normal during quiescent times, whereas in emphysema, the abnormalities may wax and wane but generally are persistent. Another functional distinction between asthma and emphysema is that the DLco is preserved and may even be increased in asthma, whereas it is decreased in patients with moderate to severe emphysema due to diminished capillary–alveolar surface area necessary for gas exchange.

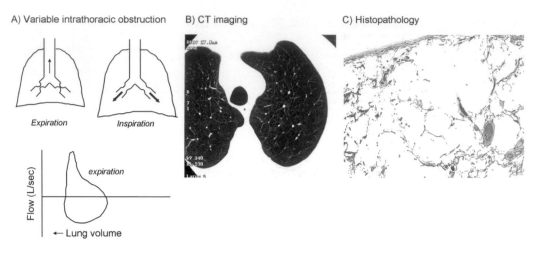

A) Variable intrathoracic obstruction   B) CT imaging   C) Histopathology

Expiration   Inspiration

Flow (L/sec)

expiration

← Lung volume

Fig. 12. Emphysema—variable intrathoracic obstruction. (**A**) With variable intrathoracic airway obstruction, maximal decrease in airflow occurs during forced expiration due to the increased intrathoracic pressure generated. The corresponding flow–volume loop shows decreased airflow in the expiratory limb. (**B**) CT scan of a patient with emphysema demonstrates decreased vascularity with multiple emphysematous spaces. (**C**) Histopathology of emphysema shows alveolar destruction and increase in size of air spaces.

Figure 12A shows that variable intrathoracic obstruction occurs mainly during expiration due to increased pressure generated in the thorax during expiration along with loss of elastic recoil (in emphysema) or bronchoconstriction (asthma); as shown, this airflow obstruction is detected by the abnormal expiratory limb of the flow–volume loop. Figure 12B is the CT scan of a patient with emphysema demonstrating the paucity of vascularity due to destruction of alveolar walls and coalescence of alveolar spaces. Figure 12C is a histopathologic image of an emphysematous lung showing the thin-walled cystic structures as a result of such destruction. This loss of alveolar tissues in emphysema results in the decreased ability of the lung to tether the airways open during expiration, resulting in airflow obstruction and in increased compliance.

5.3.1.2. Variable Extrathoracic Airway Obstruction (Vocal Cord Dysfunction)

Airflow limitation associated with variable extrathoracic obstruction, exemplified by vocal cord dysfunction (VCD), occurs mostly during the inspiratory phase (Fig. 13A), resulting in the truncation of the inspiratory limb of the flow–volume loop (Fig. 13B). Vocal cord dysfunction is a functional condition often mistaken for asthma and characterized by adduction of the vocal cords during inspiration *(13)*. Shown in Fig. 13C are typical laryngoscopic findings seen with VCD. All three glottises are drawn at mid-inspiration. Note that compared with the normal glottic function, patients with VCD have suboptimal and even paradoxical movement of their vocal cords. One important caveat is that not uncommonly, VCD may co-exist with asthma.

5.3.1.3. Fixed and Other Forms of Large Airway Obstruction

Fixed airway obstruction, whether it occurs in the extrathoracic trachea or in the large intrathoracic airways, causes truncation of both the inspiratory and expiratory limbs of the flow–volume loop (Fig. 14A). Examples of fixed obstruction throughout the respiratory cycle include subglottic stenosis, tracheal tumors, and severe epiglottitis (Fig. 14B). Unique types of intrathoracic airway obstruction that may be detected by spirometry are carinal obstruction (Fig. 14C) and collapsible trachea due to relapsing polychondritis or other causes of tracheomalacia (Fig. 14D).

A) Variable extrathoracic obstruction (VCD)   B) Flow-volume loops of VCD

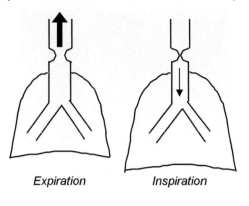

Expiration   *Inspiration*

C) Normal vocal cord movement and VCD

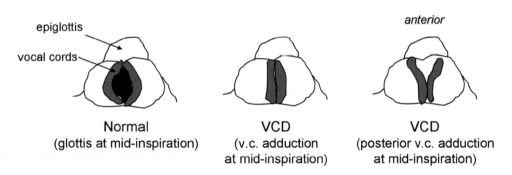

Normal	VCD	VCD
(glottis at mid-inspiration)	(v.c. adduction at mid-inspiration)	(posterior v.c. adduction at mid-inspiration)

Fig. 13. Vocal cord dysfunction—variable extrathoracic obstruction. (**A**) With variable intrathoracic obstruction, maximal decrease in airflow occurs during forced inspiration. (**B**) Two examples of abnormal flow–volume loops in vocal cord dysfunction (VCD) showing the decreased airflow during inspiration. (**C**) Drawings of a normal glottis and of two examples of VCD upon inspiration viewed by laryngoscopy. Note that during inspiration in the presence of VCD, there is increased obstruction due to the paradoxical adduction of the vocal cords inward.

5.3.2. Small Airways Obstruction

There are many different pathologic types of bronchiolitis. As will be discussed in more detail in subsequent chapters, constrictive bronchiolitis and panbronchiolitis are associated with an obstructive pattern and hyperinflation. By contrast, bronchiolitis obliterans organizing pneumonia (cryptogenic organizing pneumonia) and cellular bronchiolitis are typically associated with restrictive physiology *(14)*.

5.3.3. Mixed Restrictive-Obstructive Disease

Mixed restrictive-obstructive disease may be due to a patient having two separate disease processes that cause obstruction and restriction (e.g., having both COPD and lung fibrosis). It may also be due to certain distinct respiratory disorders that have features of a mixed restrictive-obstructive physiology. Such disorders include hypersensitivity pneumonitis, sarcoidosis, lymphangioleiomyomatosis, tuberous sclerosis, neurofibromatosis, and eosinophilic granuloma.

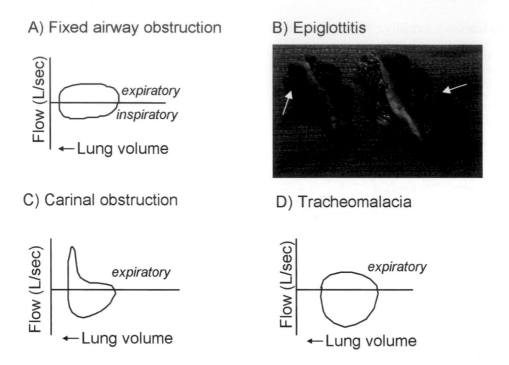

Fig. 14. Fixed and other forms of large airway obstruction. (**A**) Flow–volume loop of fixed large airway obstruction. (**B**) Gross pathologic findings of epiglottitis in an adult. Mid-sagittal view of the epiglottis revealed the lingual (ventral) location of the exophytic mass (arrows). If a flow–volume loop were to be performed in such a patient with severe epiglottitis, the flow–volume loop seen in (A) would be expected. Flow–volume loops of (**C**) a patient with fixed obstruction at the level of the carina and (**D**) a patient with tracheal collapse due to tracheomalacia.

Mixed restrictive-obstructive lung disease is often associated with normal FRC, decreased TLC, and increased RV (Fig. 8A). Moreover, although diffuse interstitial lung diseases typically cause restrictive patterns with normal or high FEV1/ FVC, and reduced lung volumes (TLC, FRC, and RV), airflow limitation may develop in end-stage lung fibrosis. Bronchiectasis usually causes airflow obstruction due to airway inflammation and increased intraluminal mucous accumulation, but reduced volumes may also be seen due primarily to lung fibrosis and/or chronic parenchymal inflammation distal to the bronchiectatic lung segments.

ACKNOWLEDGMENTS

We thank Dr. Carlyne Cool of University of Colorado School of Medicine for the emphysema micrograph.

REFERENCES

1. Cochard LR. 2002. The respiratory system. *Netter's Atlas of Human Embryology*. MediMedia USA, Inc., Teterboro. 113–129.
2. Breatnach E, Abbott GC, Fraser RG. Dimensions of the normal human trachea. *AJR Am J Roentgenol* 1984;142:903–906.
3. Moore KL, Dalley AF. 2006. *Clinically Oriented Anatomy*, 5th ed. Lippincott Williams and Wilkins, Baltimore.
4. Garcia JGN, Malik AB. 2005. Pulmonary circulation and regulation of fluid balance. *In* Mason RJ, Broaddus VC, Murray JF and Nadel JA, editors. *Textbook of Respiratory Medicine*, 4th ed. Elsevier Saunders, Philadelphia. 138–139.
5. Grillo HC. 2000. Surgical anatomy of the trachea and techniques of resection. *In* Shields TW, Locicero J and Ponin RB, editors. *General Thoracic Surgery*, 5th ed. Lippincott Williams and Wilkins, Philadelphia. 873–883.

6. Albertine KJ, Williams MC, Hyde DM. 2005. Anatomy and development of the respiratory tract. *In* Mason RJ, Broaddus VC, Murray JF and Nadel JA, editors. *Textbook of Respiratory Medicine*, 4th ed. Elsevier Saunders, Philadelphia. 3–25.
7. Kuhn C. 1988. Normal anatomy and histology. *In* Thurlbeck WM, editor. *Pathology of the Lung*. Thieme, New York. 11–45.
8. Barnes PJ. 2005. General pharmacologic principles. *In* Mason RJ, Broaddus VC, Murray JF and Nadel JA, editors. *Murray and Nadel's Textbook of Respiratory Medicine*. Elsevier Saunders, Philadelphia. 197–234.
9. McGavin CR, Williams IP. The effects of oral propranolol and metoprolol on lung function and exercise performance in chronic airways obstruction. *Br J Dis Chest* 1978;72:327–332.
10. Carstairs JR, Nimmo AJ, Barnes PJ. Autoradiographic visualization of beta-adrenocepter subtypes in human lung. *Am Rev Respir Dis* 1985;132:541–547.
11. Junqueira LC, Carneiro J. 2005. *Basic Histology – Text and Atlas*, 11th ed. McGraw-Hill, New York.
12. Zakynthinos SG, Koulouris NG, Roussos C. 2005. Respiratory system mechanics and energetics. *In* Mason RJ, Broaddus VC, Murray JF and Nadel JA, editors. *Murray and Nadel's Textbook of Respiratory Medicine*. Elsevier Saunders, Philadelphia. 87–135.
13. Balkissoon R. Vocal cord dysfunction, gastroesophageal reflux disease, and nonallergic rhinitis. *Clin Allergy Immunol* 2007;19:411–426.
14. Chan ED, Kalayanamit T, Lynch DA, Tuder R, Arndt P, Winn R, et al. Mycoplasma pneumoniae-associated bronchiolitis causing severe restrictive lung disease in adults: report of three cases and literature review. *Chest* 1999;115:1188–1194.

2

Radiologic Anatomy of the Airways

Phillip M. Boiselle and David A. Lynch

Summary

Knowledge of normal airway anatomy on CT is a requisite for accurately detecting and characterizing airway disorders. In this chapter, normal anatomy of the upper airways, trachea, and bronchi are illustrated and reviewed on axial, multiplanar, and 3-D reconstruction images. The normal CT anatomy of the small airways is also reviewed.

Key Words: Anatomy; CT; trachea; bronchi; bronchioles.

1. UPPER AIRWAY

Recognition of the standard axial landmarks of the airway is important for evaluating the upper airway (Fig. 1) (1). The first important anatomic landmark is the epiglottis, which forms the superior border of the larynx. On axial slices, it first appears as a horizontally oriented, elliptical soft tissue density (Fig. 1A). Inferiorly, it forms the border between the laryngeal airway and the valleculae, paired ovoid structures seen anterior to the epiglottis. The valleculae are separated by a thin band of tissue, the glossoepiglottic fold (Fig. 1B). The next most important landmarks are the aryepiglottic folds, which appear as triangular-shaped structures located along the anterolateral aspect of the airway. They continue posteriorly and form the border between the laryngeal airway anteriorly and pyriform sinuses posteriorly. Inferiorly, the glottic airway is comprised of the true and false cords. The upper airway at the level of the false cords is visualized as an elliptical structure bounded posteriorly by the base of the aryepiglottic folds (Fig. 1C). The latter can be differentiated by the presence of fat in the surrounding soft tissues. The airway at the level of the true cords is elliptical in shape, bounded anteriorly by the thyroid cartilage and laterally by the homogeneous soft tissue density of the thyroarytenoid muscle (Fig. 1D). The subglottic airway has a more circular shape and is bordered posteriorly by cricoid cartilage (Fig. 1E).

Although axial images are routinely used to evaluate the upper airway, multiplanar reformations (MPRs) in the coronal and sagittal planes are also helpful for evaluating upper airway pathology (Fig. 2) (1). Coronal MPR images are particularly helpful for defining the anatomy of the larynx, with delineation of the aryepiglottic folds, true and false cords, laryngeal ventricles, and subglottic space (Fig. 2A). Sagittal MPR images also enable excellent delineation of upper airway structures, particularly the epiglottis, vallecula, and pyriform sinuses (Fig. 2B) (1). Sagittal shaded-surface displays (Fig. 2C) and volume rendered images (Fig. 2D) are effective 3-D reconstruction techniques for depicting upper airway anatomy and pathology.

From: *Contemporary Medical Imaging: CT of the Airways*
Edited by: P. M. Boiselle and D. A. Lynch © Humana Press, Totowa, NJ

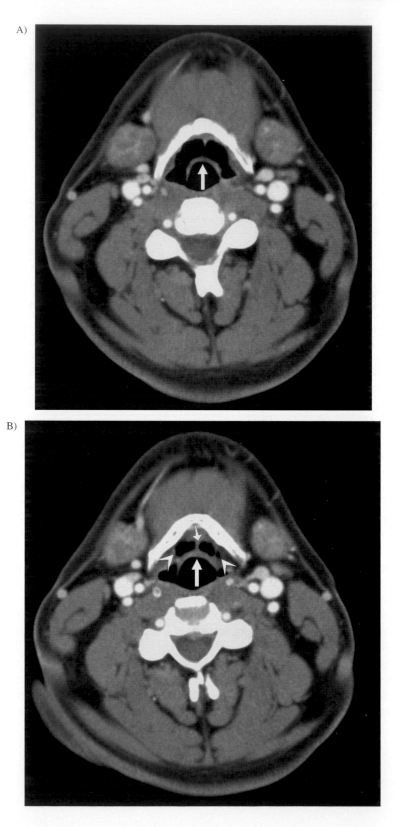

C)

D)

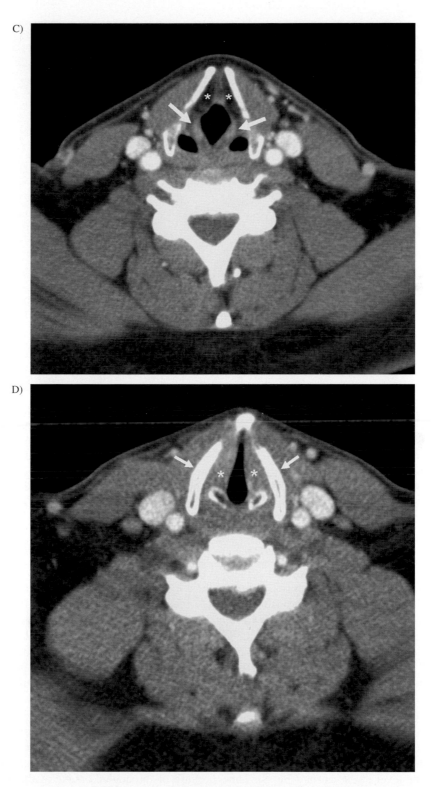

Fig. 1. *(Continued)*

E)

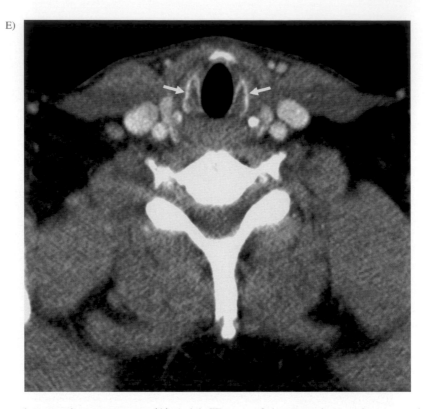

Fig. 1. Normal upper airway anatomy. (**A**) Axial CT scan of the upper larynx shows superior aspect of the epiglottis (arrow). (**B**) Axial CT scan shows the base of the epiglottis (arrow), the valleculae anteriorly (arrowheads) separated by the glossoepiglottic fold (thin arrow). (**C**) Axial CT scan shows the base of the aryepiglottic folds (arrows) and delineates the beginning of the false cords. Note the fat density (asterisks) in the soft tissues lateral to the false cords. (**D**) Axial CT inferior to D shows the level of the true vocal cords (asterisks). The glottic airway is elliptical in shape, bordered anteriorly by thyroid cartilage (arrow) and laterally by thyroarytenoid muscle. (**E**) Axial CT shows the subglottic airway as more ovoid in appearance. Note surrounding cricoid cartilage (arrow). (Reprinted with permission from ref. *1*)

2. TRACHEA

The trachea extends from the inferior margin of the cricoid cartilage to the carina, a keel-like ridge that marks the origin of the main bronchi (Fig. 3) *(2)*. The trachea is comprised of 16–22 C-shaped cartilages, which are linked longitudinally by annular ligaments of fibrous and connective tissue *(2)*. The cartilages are connected posteriorly by the membranous wall of the trachea, which lacks cartilage and is supported by the trachealis muscle, comprised of transverse smooth muscle fibers that narrow the tracheal lumen upon contraction *(2)*. During forced expiration, this results in normal anterior bulging of the posterior membrane, resulting in a mean decrease in anteroposterior dimension of 32% during forced expiration *(3)*.

The trachea is generally midline in position, but it is often displaced slightly to the right at the level of the aortic arch. This displacement may be accentuated in older patients with markedly tortuous, atherosclerotic aortas (Fig. 4). Proximally, the trachea lies close to the skin surface. However, the trachea angles posteriorly as it courses inferiorly in the thorax, eventually achieving a mid-coronal location at the level of the carina (Fig. 5). Thus, because of the angled course of the trachea, axial CT images do not provide a true perpendicular cross section of the tracheal lumen.

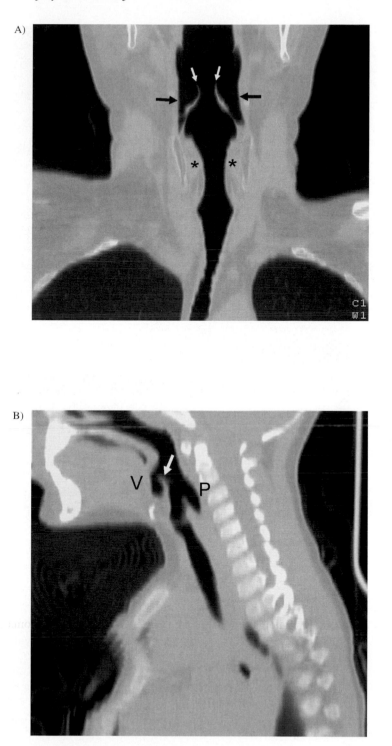

Fig. 2. Three-dimensional reconstruction techniques in the upper airway. (**A**) Coronal multiplanar reformation image shows the upper airway in an adult. Note the delineation of the pyriform sinuses (black arrows), aryepiglottic folds (white arrows), and the glottic airway (asterisks). (**B**) Sagittal multiplanar reformation image of the upper airway in a child. Note the appearance of the epiglottis (arrow), valleculae (V), and pyriform

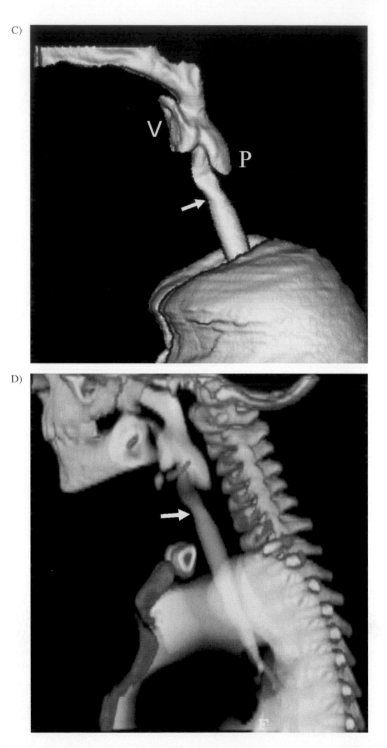

Fig. 2. *(Continued)* sinus (P). (**C**) Sagittal shaded-surface display of the upper airway. Note delineation of the valleculae (V), the pyriform sinuses (P), and the glottic airway (arrow). (**D**) Volume rendered image of the upper airway. This reconstruction technique allows display of both bony landmarks and the airway (arrow). (Reprinted with permission from ref. *1*)

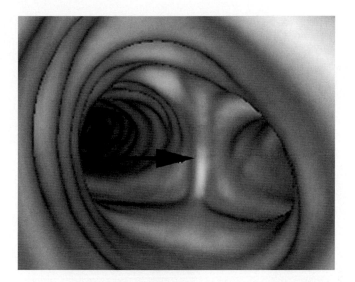

Fig. 3. Virtual bronchoscopic depiction of tracheal lumen. Virtual bronchoscopic (internal rendering) of tracheal lumen depicts carina (arrow), a keel-like ridge that demarcates the origin of the right and left bronchi. Repetitive arcs along anterior and lateral walls represent the C-shaped cartilaginous rings

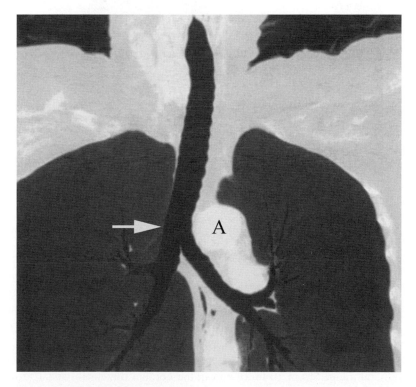

Fig. 4. Accentuated tracheal displacement by tortuous aorta. Coronal oblique multiplanar reformation minimum intensity projection (minIP) image demonstrates accentuated rightward displacement of the trachea (arrow) due to a tortuous, atherosclerotic aorta (A)

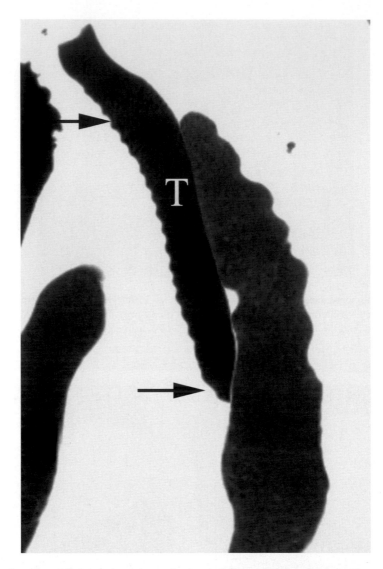

Fig. 5. Normal trachea. Minimum intensity projection (minIP) sagittal multiplanar reformation image shows normal course of the trachea (T). Note change in position from anterior location of proximal extrathoracic trachea (superior arrow) to more posterior location (inferior arrow) at the level of carina.

Tracheal length averages 10–11 cm in adults, including both the extrathoracic (2–4 cm) and intrathoracic (6–9 cm) portions *(2)*. Tracheal length is dynamic, changing with respiration and neck flexion and extension *(2)*. For example, the carina can change in position up to 3 cm between inspiration and expiration *(2)*. Tracheal diameter in men averages 19.5 mm and ranges from 13 to 25 mm in the coronal plane and 13 to 27 mm in the sagittal plane *(2,4–6)*. In women, tracheal diameter averages 17.5 mm and ranges from 10 to 21 mm in the coronal dimension and 10 to 23 mm in the sagittal dimension *(2,4–6)*. Tracheomegaly is defined in women as tracheal diameter >21 mm in the coronal dimension and 23 mm in the sagittal dimension, and in men as tracheal diameter >25 mm in the coronal dimension and 27 mm in the sagittal dimension *(7)*.

On axial CT images, the normal tracheal lumen most commonly demonstrates an oval, round, or horseshoe shape *(4)*. Less commonly, it may appear as a square or inverted pear (bulbous, rounded anterior wall with smaller, rounded posterior wall contour resembling an upside-down pear) *(4)*.

The tracheal index can be calculated by dividing the coronal diameter (mm) by the sagittal diameter (mm). The normal value is approximately 1 *(2,4–6)*. A "saber-sheath" trachea refers to a configuration in which there is marked coronal narrowing and accentuation of the sagittal diameter (sagittal : coronal ratio >2) (Fig. 6) *(8,9)*. This finding is frequently associated with chronic obstructive lung disease. By contrast, a "lunate" trachea refers to accentuation of the coronal diameter with a relative narrowing of the sagittal diameter (coronal : sagittal ratio >1) (Fig. 7) *(10)*. This finding is frequently associated with malacia (excessive expiratory collapsibility of the airway lumen).

The tracheal wall is comprised of several layers, including an inner mucosa layer, followed by submucosa, cartilage or muscle, and an outer adventitia layer *(11)*. On axial CT images, the tracheal wall is usually visible as a 1- to 3-mm soft-tissue density stripe, demarcated internally by the air-filled tracheal lumen and externally by the adjacent fat-density of the mediastinum (Fig. 8) *(11)*. The posterior wall is typically thinner than the anterior and lateral walls. Cartilage within the tracheal wall may normally appear slightly denser than surrounding soft tissue and fat *(11)*. Calcification of cartilage may be observed in older patients, especially women (Fig. 9) *(11)*. Calcified thickening of the tracheal wall is also associated with tracheal pathology, particularly relapsing polychondritis (Fig. 10). A similar pattern may be observed in the main bronchi (Fig. 11).

Thickening of the airway wall (with or without calcification) is an important sign of tracheal pathology. Importantly, axial images are the reference standard for assessing tracheal wall thickening, a finding that may be overlooked at conventional bronchoscopy and 3-D reconstruction images. The distribution of wall thickening can be helpful in limiting the differential diagnosis of the various causes of tracheal stenosis. For example, disorders of cartilage, such as relapsing polychondritis and

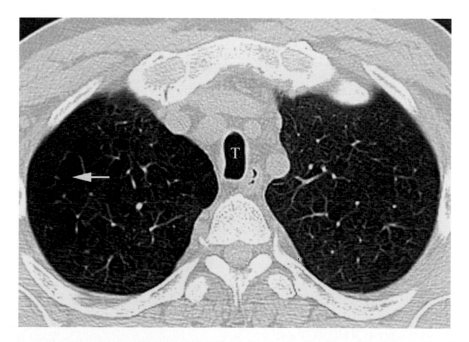

Fig. 6. Saber sheath trachea. Axial CT image demonstrates marked coronal narrowing and accentuation of sagittal diameter of trachea (T), referred to as a "saber sheath" configuration. Note the presence of emphysema (arrow)

A)

B)

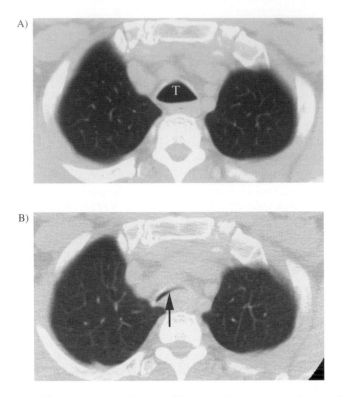

Fig. 7. Lunate trachea. (**A**) Axial end-inspiratory CT image demonstrates elongated coronal diameter of trachea (T) with relative decrease in sagittal dimension, referred to as a lunate configuration. (**B**) Dynamic expiratory CT image shows near complete expiratory tracheal collapse (arrow), consistent with airway malacia

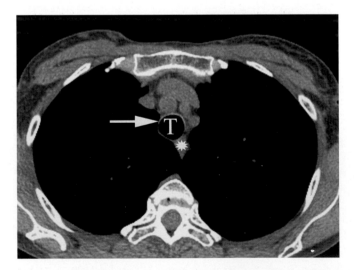

Fig. 8. Normal tracheal wall. Axial CT image at level of brachiocephalic vessels demonstrates normal thin stripe (arrow) of tracheal wall. The wall is slightly thicker anteriorly and laterally than along the posterior membranous wall. Also note relative location of trachea to brachiocephalic vessels anteriorly and esophagus (asterisk) posteriorly

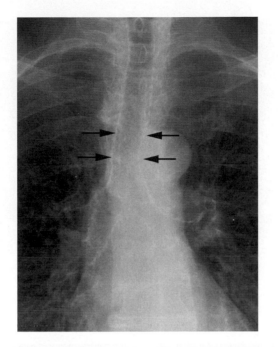

Fig. 9. Calcification of tracheal wall. Coned-down view of frontal chest radiograph demonstrates calcifications of tracheal wall (arrows), an incidental finding frequently observed in older women

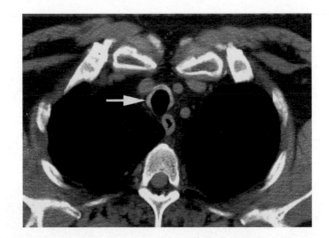

Fig. 10. Calcified tracheal wall thickening due to relapsing polychondritis. Axial CT image of proximal thoracic trachea demonstrates calcified thickening of wall of trachea (arrow) with characteristic sparing of the posterior membranous wall

tracheobronchopathia osteochondroplastica, will spare the posterior membranous wall of the trachea, whereas other disorders generally result in circumferential thickening.

In addition to depicting the anatomy of the airway lumen and wall, CT also demonstrates the relationship of the trachea to adjacent structures, including the thyroid gland (lateral to cervical trachea), vascular structures (anterior to intrathoracic trachea), esophagus (posterior or lateral to the

A)

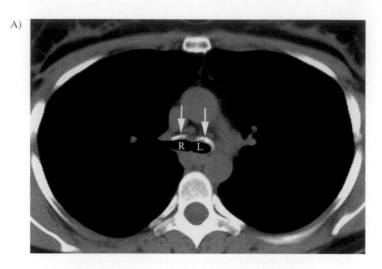

B)

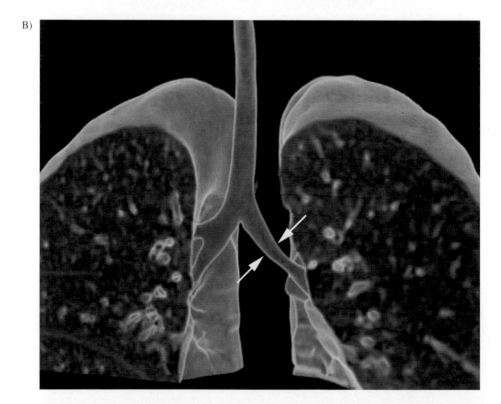

Fig. 11. Main bronchi. (**A**) Axial image below the carina demonstrates right (R) and left (L) main bronchi, which course obliquely to the axial plane. Note marked anterior calcified wall thickening due to relapsing polychondritis. (**B**) 3-D volumetric external rendering of airway of same patient shows symmetrical tapered narrowing of left main bronchus due to polychondritis. Narrowing was better depicted on 3-D image than on the axial image

trachea), and chest wall structures (Fig. 8). Abnormalities of these various structures may result in compression, displacement, or invasion of the trachea. For example, thyroid enlargement is a common cause of tracheal compression and displacement (Fig. 12).

3. MAIN BRONCHI

The main bronchi arise from the trachea at the level of the carina and course obliquely to the axial plane. The right main bronchus is relatively short, usually about 1.1 cm (range 0–2.9 cm), compared with 5 cm for the left main bronchus *(12)*. The left main bronchial diameter is typically clliptical. The smallest diameter of the left main bronchus is about 70% of the transverse tracheal diameter in men, and 65% in women *(13)*. These facts are important because the left main bronchus is typically used for placement of a double lumen tube during thoracic surgery: selection of a tube that is too small could lead to distal migration of the tube, whereas selection of an over-large tube could lead to bronchial rupture. Because of the elliptical shape of the left main bronchus, its diameters cannot be accurately measured from chest radiographs or axial chest CT images. For this reason, a recent paper recommended the use of multiplanar reconstructions to accurately measure left main

A)

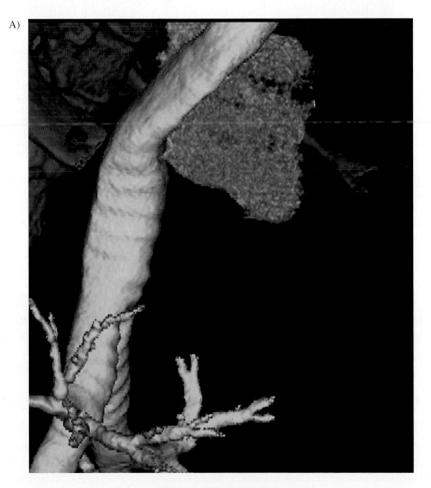

Fig. 12. *(Continued)*

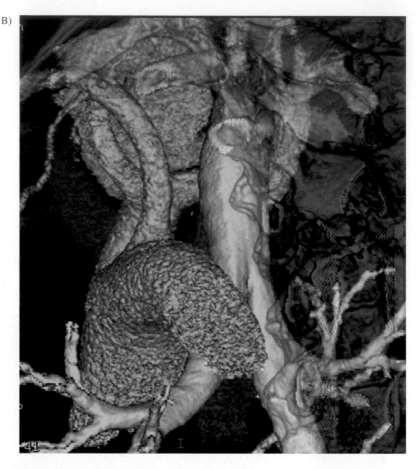

Fig. 12. Tracheal compression from adjacent thyroid malignancy. (**A**) Sagittal oblique 3-D segmentation reconstruction demonstrates compression of trachea (blue) at the level of thoracic inlet from adjacent thyroid mass (green). (**B**) Posterior oblique 3-D segmentation reconstruction shows relationship between thyroid mass (green), vascular structures (arterial structures in gold and venous structures in red), and trachea (blue). [Images courtesy of Shezhang Lin, MD, BIDMC, Boston, MA]

bronchial diameter and assist selection of double-lumen tube size for those in whom thoracic surgery is planned *(13)*. 3-D reconstruction images are also helpful for displaying stenoses of the main bronchi (Fig. 11b).

4. SEGMENTAL AND SUBSEGMENTAL BRONCHI

Segmental bronchial anatomy can be readily identified on axial and multiplanar CT (Figs 13, 14, and 15). Subsegmental bronchi can typically be followed out to the peripheral one-third of lung. Identification of the segmental and subsegmental bronchial pathway can be important for the bronchoscopist, and there are now several automated CT-based methods for planning a bronchoscopic pathway toward a lesion for biopsy *(13–16)*.

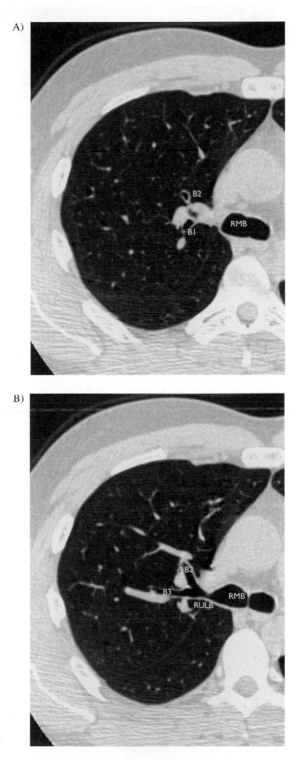

Fig. 13. *(Continued)*

C)

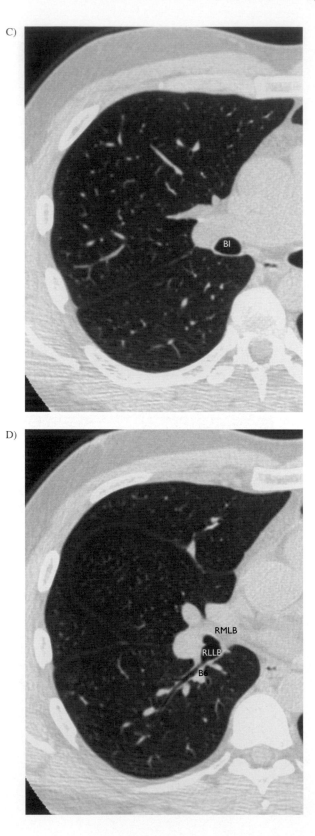

D)

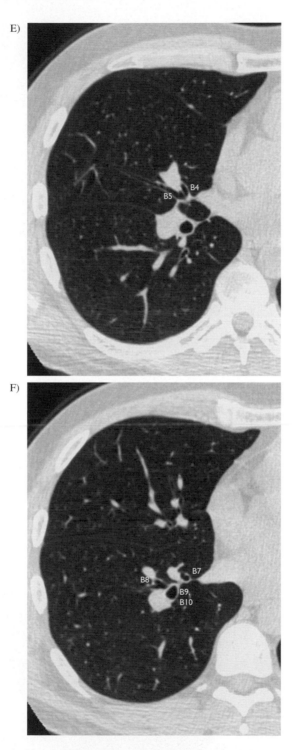

Fig. 13. (**A–F**) Right sided bronchial anatomy, illustrated using Boyden's numbering system (*see* Table 1 of Chapter 1). Selected axial images through the right bronchial tree demonstrate the right main bronchus (RMB), right upper lobe bronchus (RULB), apical (B1), anterior (B2), and posterior (B3) segmental bronchi of right upper lobe; bronchus intermedius (BI); right middle lobe bronchus (RMLB); medial (B4) and lateral (B5) segments of right middle lobe, superior (B6); and the medial basal (B7), anterior basal (B8), lateral basal (B9), and posterior basal (B10) segments of right lower lobe

A)

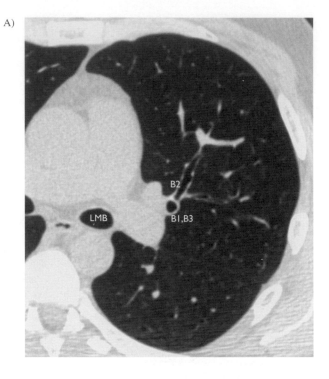

B)

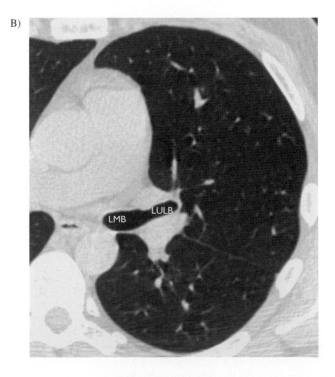

C)

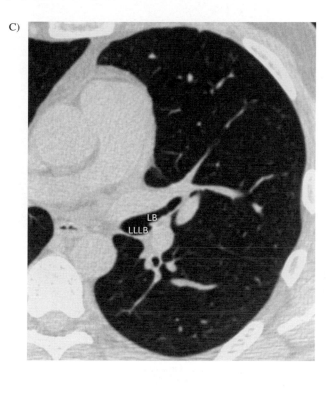

D)

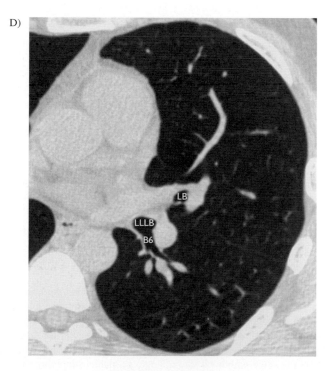

Fig. 14. *(Continued)*

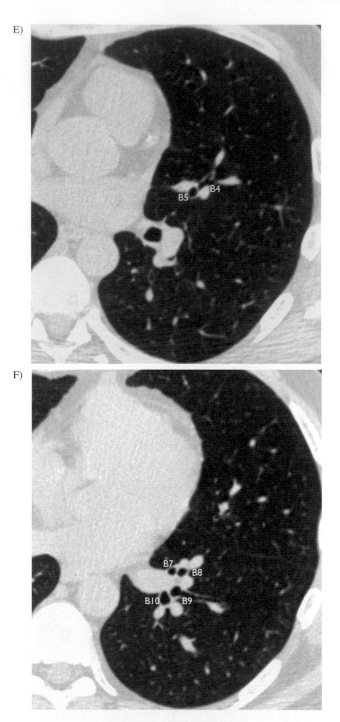

Fig. 14. (**A–F**) Left sided bronchial anatomy, illustrated using Boyden's numbering system (*see* Table 1 of Chapter 1). Selected axial images through the left bronchial tree demonstrate the left main bronchus (LMB), left upper lobe bronchus (LULB), apical (B1), anterior (B2), and posterior (B3) segmental bronchi of left upper lobe; lingular bronchus (LB) superior (B4) and inferior (B5) segments of lingula; left lower lobe bronchus (LLLB); superior (B6), medial basal (B7), anterior basal (B8), lateral basal (B9), and posterior basal (B10) segments of left lower lobe. B7 and B8 are often combined into a single bronchus supplying the anteromedial segment of left lower lobe.

A)

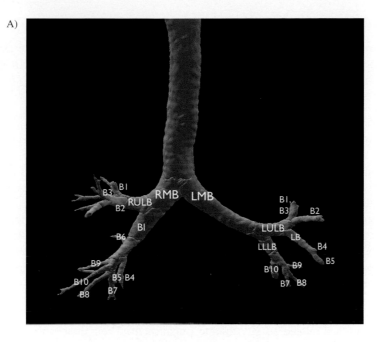

B)

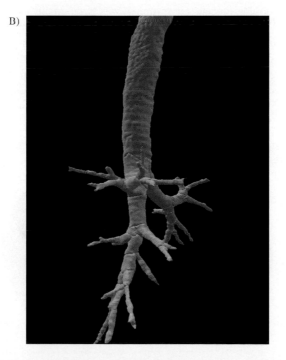

Fig. 15. (**A**) Three-dimensional segmentation of the tracheobronchial tree, viewed in frontal projection, allows identification of main, lobar, and segmental bronchi, labeled using the same abbreviations as in Figs 13 and 14. (**B**) Lateral projection of the same reconstruction

5. SMALL BRONCHI AND BRONCHIOLES

Airways are not normally visible in the peripheral one-third of the lung. In the extreme subpleural region, the bronchiole is not visible, but the accompanying pulmonary arteriole may be visible as a tiny nodular or branching structure 4–10 mm from the pleural surface (Fig. 16) *(17)*.

6. NORMAL FINDINGS ON EXPIRATORY CT

The degree of air trapping that may be identified by CT in normal subjects is controversial. Detection of air trapping in normal subjects depends on the expiratory maneuver used: for example, heterogenous lung attenuation may be normally seen during dynamic imaging of a forced exhalation *(18)*. In a widely used classification, Mastora et al. classified the extent of air trapping as lobular (small areas of hypoattenuation corresponding to fewer than three adjacent secondary pulmonary lobules), segmental (contiguous area of hypoattenuation more than three lobules but less than a segment), and lobar (area of hypoattenuation greater than a segment) *(19)*. In their study of 250 volunteers, with CT scans obtained at end-expiration, air trapping was identified in 62% (lobular in 47%, segmental in 14%, and lobar in 1%). However, most of the individuals in their study were current or former smokers, and 66% of them (predominantly the current smokers) had symptoms of dyspnea. Lobular air trapping was commonly seen in nonsmokers, but segmental and lobar air trapping was more common in current or former smokers (particularly heavy smokers) than in nonsmokers. The presence of air trapping was not related to physiologic impairment. Their conclusion was that lobular air trapping did not reflect small airways disease but that segmental or lobular air trapping did reflect small airways disease.

In a study by Tanaka et al. of 50 asymptomatic subjects (including 24 current or former smokers) with normal pulmonary function and normal inspiratory high-resolution CT, lobular air trapping was identified in 20%, multilobular mosaic air trapping was seen in 28%, and segmental or lobar air trapping was seen in 16% *(20)*. Semi-quantitative assessment of air trapping correlated weakly with FEV1/FVC ratio. In a study by Lee et al of 82 asymptomatic subjects (including 27 smokers), the prevalence of air trapping appeared to increase with age, with air trapping being seen in 76% of subjects aged 61 years or older *(21)*. Although physiologic evaluation was normal in all of those evaluated, the degree of air trapping correlated with the FEV1/FVC ratio.

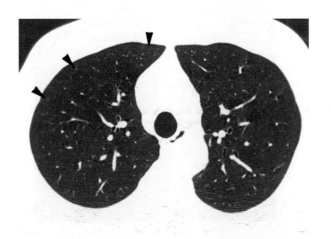

Fig. 16. Normal anatomy on high-resolution CT. In a normal subject, a few centrilobular structures (arrowheads) may be visible as dots or short branching structures 4–10 mm from the pleural surface

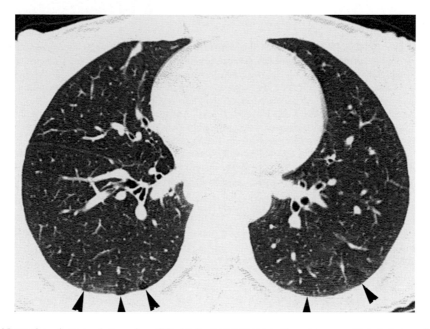

Fig. 17. Normal expiratory air trapping. CT obtained at end-expiration shows multiple lobules of air trapping (arrowheads)

Because these papers indicate that air trapping may be found on expiratory CT in normal subjects (Fig. 17), clinical interpretation of air trapping found on CT must consider the extent of abnormality, associated CT findings of mosaic attenuation or bronchial abnormalities, and physiologic evidence of obstruction.

ACKNOWLEDGMENT

The authors gratefully acknowledge Dr. Robert C. Gilkeson for his outstanding illustrations and descriptions of upper airway anatomy.

REFERENCES

1. Boiselle PM, Gilkeson RC. State-of-the-art airway imaging (Part 2). *J Respir Dis* 2006;12:266–273.
2. Holbert JM, Strollo DC. Imaging of the normal trachea. *J Thorac Imaging* 1995;10:171–179.
3. Stern EJ, Graham CM, Webb WR, Gamsu G. Normal trachea during forced expiration: dynamic CT measurements. *Radiology* 1993;187(1):27–31.
4. Gamsu G, Webb WR. Computed tomography of the trachea: normal and abnormal. *AJR Am J Roentgenol* 1982;139: 321–326.
5. Vock P, Spiegel T, Fram EK, Effmann EL. CT assessment of the adult intrathoracic cross section of the trachea. *J Comput Assist Tomogr* 1984;8:1076–1082.
6. Breatnach E, Abbott GC, Fraser RG. Dimensions of the normal human trachea. *AJR Am J Roentgenol* 1983;141:903–906.
7. Woodring JH, Howard RS, Rehn SR. Congenital tracheobronchomegaly (Mounier-Kuhn) syndrome: a report of 10 cases and review of the literature. *J Thorac Imaging* 1991;6:1–10.
8. Greene R, Lechner GL. "Saber-sheath" trachea: a clinical and functional study of marked coronal narrowing of the intrathoracic trachea. *Radiology* 1975;115:265–268.
9. Trigaux JP, Hermes G, Dubois P, Van Beers B, Delaunois L, Jamart J. CT of saber-sheath trachea: correlation with clinical, chest radiographic and functional findings. *Acta Radiol* 1994;35:247–250.
10. Webb EM, Elicker BM, Webb WR. Using CT to diagnose nonneoplastic tracheal abnormalities. Appearance of the tracheal wall. *AJR Am J Roentgenol* 2000;174:1315–1321.

11. Robinson CL, Muller NL, Essery C. Clinical significance and measurement of the length of the right main bronchus. *Can J Surg* 1989;32:27–28.
12. Olivier P, Hayon-Sonsino D, Convard JP, Laloe PA, Fischler M. Measurement of left mainstem bronchus using multiplane CT reconstructions and relationship between patient characteristics or tracheal diameters and left bronchial diameters. *Chest* 2006;130:101–107.
13. Hautmann H, Schneider A, Pinkau T, Peltz F, Feussner H. Electromagnetic catheter navigation during bronchoscopy: validation of a novel method by conventional fluoroscopy. *Chest* 2005;128:382–387.
14. Mori K, Ema S, Kitasaka T, Mekada Y, Ide I, Murase H, et al. Automated nomenclature of bronchial branches extracted from CT images and its application to biopsy path planning in virtual bronchoscopy. *Med Image Comput Comput Assist Interv Int Conf Med Image Comput Comput Assist Interv* 2005;8:854–861.
15. Schwarz Y, Greif J, Becker HD, Ernst A, Mehta A. Real-time electromagnetic navigation bronchoscopy to peripheral lung lesions using overlaid CT images: the first human study. *Chest* 2006;129:988–994.
16. Webb W, Stein M, Finkbeiner W, Im J-G, Lynch D, Gamsu G. Normal and diseased isolated lungs: high resolution CT. *Radiology* 1988;166:81–87.
17. Webb WR, Stern EJ, Kanth N, Gamsu G. Dynamic pulmonary CT: findings in healthy adult men. *Radiology* 1993;186:117–124.
18. Mastora I, Remy-Jardin M, Sobaszek A, Boulenguez C, Remy J, Edme JL. Thin-section CT finding in 250 volunteers: assessment of the relationship of CT findings with smoking history and pulmonary function test results. *Radiology* 2001;218:695–702.
19. Tanaka N, Matsumoto T, Miura G, Emoto T, Matsunaga N, Ueda K, et al. Air trapping at CT: high prevalence in asymptomatic subjects with normal pulmonary function. *Radiology* 2003;227:776–785.
20. Lee KW, Chung SY, Yang I, Lee Y, Ko EY, Park MJ. Correlation of aging and smoking with air trapping at thin-section CT of the lung in asymptomatic subjects. *Radiology* 2000;214:831–836.
21. Lomasney L, Bergin CJ, Lomasney J, Roggli V, Foster W. CT appearance of lunate trachea. *J Comput Assist Tomogr* 1989;13:520–522.

3

Pathology of the Airways

Chih-Wei Wang and Thomas V. Colby

Summary

The pathology of the bronchi and bronchioles is reviewed and illustrated.

   Key Words: Bronchitis; bronchiolitis; follicular bronchiolitis; constrictive bronchiolitis; panbronchiolitis; organzing pneumonia; Boop.

1. LARGE AIRWAYS

1.1. Introduction

The large airways include trachea and bronchi. Non-neoplastic diseases of the large airways often require a team of clinician, radiologist, and pathologist for thorough evaluation and diagnosis. For some, such as bronchiectasis, diagnosis is achieved with confidence by high-resolution computed tomography (HRCT) and clinical correlation alone. Some of the conditions described in this section are primarily pathologic descriptors [e.g., bronchocentric granulomatosis (BCG)] applied in many clinical disorders.

1.2. Tracheomalacia and Tracheobronchomalacia

Tracheomalacia and tracheobronchomalacia are clinical disorders associated with softening of the cartilage and loss of structural integrity of the trachea and upper bronchi. Both primary and secondary etiologies are recognized. In pediatric patients, prematurity or prolonged mechanical ventilation is often implicated (1). In adults, many cases are posttraumatic or postinflammatory with or without complicating infections (1). Pathologically, the tracheal and bronchial cartilage shows destruction and loss, with associated acute and chronic inflammation and replacement of cartilage by fibrosis. Granulomatous inflammation can be seen in cases associated with Wegener's granulomatosis and granulomatous infections.

1.3. Tracheobronchopathia Osteochondroplastica

Tracheobronchopathia osteochondroplastica is a rare disease of unknown etiology. It is most commonly seen in adult males (2). The disease is characterized by multiple submucosal metaplastic cartilaginous and osseous nodules throughout the large airways (Fig. 1). They appear as firm/hard nonulcerated protruding nodules with fiberoptic bronchoscopy.

1.4. Tracheobronchomegaly

Tracheobronchomegaly (also termed *Mounier–Kuhn syndrome*) is a rare lung disease associated with markedly dilated large airways, leading to recurrent infections (3–8). It usually presents in the

From: *Contemporary Medical Imaging: CT of the Airways*
Edited by: P. M. Boiselle and D. A. Lynch © Humana Press, Totowa, NJ

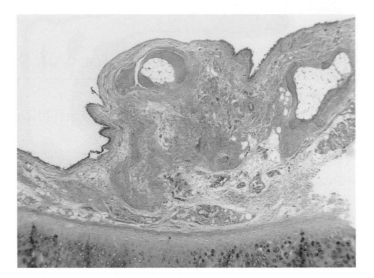

Fig. 1. Tracheobronchopathia osteochondroplastica. A protruding submucosal nodule of bone with fibrosis is noted in the tracheal wall.

third and the fourth decades of life although a few congenital cases have been reported *(3–5)*. The cause is unknown.

Pathologically, atrophy of bronchial cartilage and smooth muscle leads to tracheal and bronchial enlargement and secondary infection and inflammation (Fig. 2). Some cases become indistinguishable from bronchiectasis.

1.5. Infectious Bronchitis

Bronchi are susceptible to many infectious organisms. The pathologic changes are usually acute and/or chronic inflammation or granulomatous inflammation depending on the causative microorganism. Mucosa necrosis, metaplastic changes, and submucosal fibrosis may also occur. The causative organism may (or may not) be recognized with special stains or on the basis of identifiable viral inclusions.

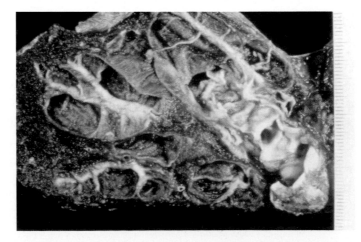

Fig. 2. Tracheobronchomegaly. The bronchi are markedly dilated. (Used with permission of the American Registry of Pathology; originally published as Fig. 9–59, page 425 in: *Non-Neoplastic Disorders of the Lower Respiratory Tract*, Travis WD et al. American Registry of Pathology, Washington, DC, 2002)

1.6. Bronchiectasis

Bronchiectasis is defined as permanent abnormal dilatation of the bronchi, often accompanied by acute and chronic inflammation, although practically speaking most cases are now diagnosed radiologically *(9–14)*. Bronchiectasis has various causes such as postinfectious bronchial damage, cystic fibrosis, ciliary dyskinesia, and collagen vascular diseases (Table 1) *(8, 12, 15–17)*.

Historically, the classification of bronchiectasis has included (i) saccular (cystic) type, in which there is progressive bronchial dilatation from central to peripheral; (ii) varicose type, in which there is both irregular dilatation and constriction of the bronchi; and (iii) cylindrical type, in which there is uniform and cylindrical dilatation of bronchi without normal tapering to the distal end *(15–17)*. This classification is primarily based on bronchography and pathology. Since the advent of HRCT scanning *(11,14,16,18)*, HRCT has become the diagnostic procedure of choice for bronchiectasis, and the above classification is employed less often although the terms may be used descriptively.

Grossly, the bronchi are dilated with or without mucopurulent secretions filling the lumens (Fig. 3). Microscopically, the bronchial wall shows minimal to severe acute and chronic inflammation and fibrosis (Fig. 4) *(13,17,19,20)*. Sometimes, there is total destruction of the bronchial wall. The

Table 1
Causes of Bronchiectasis

Congenital/Genetic
  Cystic fibrosis
  α-1 protease inhibitor deficiency
  Tracheobronchomegaly
  Congenital cartilage deficiency
  Pulmonary sequestration
  Ciliary dyskinesia (Kartagener's syndrome, etc.)
Postinfectious
  Bacterial, fungal, and viral infections
Systemic diseases
  Collagen vascular diseases
  Sarcoidosis
  Amyloidosis
  Inflammatory bowel disease
  Celiac disease
  Yellow nail syndrome
Bronchial obstruction
  COPD
  Tumor
  Foreign body
Immune deficiency disorders
  Complement deficiency, post-chemotherapy, etc.
  Human Immunodeficiency virus infection
Idiopathic
Others
  Asthma
  Middle lobe syndrome
  Post-transplantation
  Diffuse panbronchiolitis
  Idiopathic pulmonary fibrosis

COPD, chronic obstructive pulmonary disease.

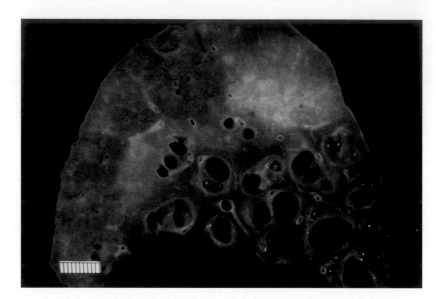

Fig. 3. Bronchiectasis. The lower lobe shows bronchiectasis with markedly dilated bronchi. (Used with permission of the American Registry of Pathology; originally published as Fig. 9–5, page 387 in: *Non-Neoplastic Disorders of the Lower Respiratory Tract*, Travis WD et al. American Registry of Pathology, Washington, DC, 2002)

distal bronchioles may also be affected with partial or complete luminal obstruction and associated inflammation, i.e., changes of constrictive bronchiolitis (*see* Section 3.5). Secondary changes are also seen in the alveolar parenchyma: acute bronchopneumonia, organizing pneumonia, and scarring and obstructive changes may all be seen.

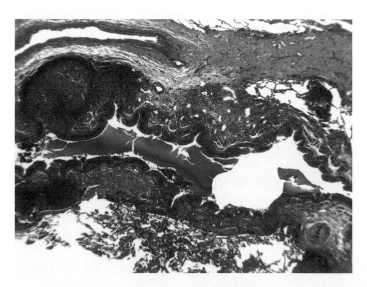

Fig. 4. Bronchiectasis. The bronchus is dilated with chronic inflammation, fibrosis, and reactive lymphoid follicles.

1.7. Cystic Fibrosis

Cystic fibrosis is a hereditary disease that primarily affects the sweat glands, respiratory, digestive, and male reproductive systems. The transport of chloride and sodium across epithelial cells is impaired, resulting in thick and viscid secretions. In the respiratory tract, the retention of mucus causes recurrent pulmonary infections and nearly always leads to bronchiectasis *(21–28)*.

Grossly, the lung shows severe and widespread bronchiectasis with mucus plugs in the bronchi (Fig. 5). Other complications of infection such as pleuritis and adhesion, pneumonia, and lung abscesses may also develop. Microscopically, bronchiectasis with mucous plugging and purulent secretion is a characteristic finding (Fig. 6). Small airways show acute and chronic bronchiolitis and often constrictive changes (see Section 3.5). The pulmonary parenchyma and pleura may show acute and chronic inflammation and eventually fibrotic changes.

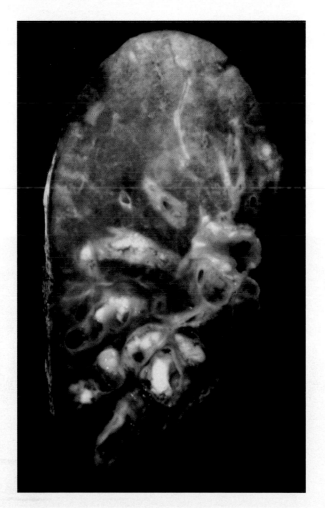

Fig. 5. Cystic fibrosis. In this case of cystic fibrosis, marked bronchiectasis with whitish mucous plugging is noted. (Used with permission of the American Registry of Pathology; originally published as Fig. 9–17, page 396 in: *Non-Neoplastic Disorders of the Lower Respiratory Tract*, Travis WD et al. American Registry of Pathology, Washington, DC, 2002)

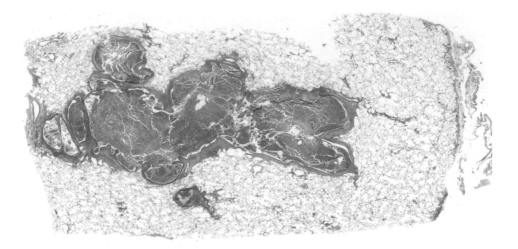

Fig. 6. Cystic fibrosis. Bronchiolectasis with dense mucous plugging is marked.

1.8. Mucoid Impaction of Bronchi

Mucoid impaction of bronchi is a distinctive clinicopathologic syndrome characterized by "allergic mucin" plugs in dilated bronchi *(29–33)*. Thus, mucoid impaction of bronchi is pathologically differently from simple mucus plugging in which there is mucus accumulation in the airways, and it lacks the distinctive morphologic features described below. From the pathologic perspective, mucoid impaction of bronchi and mucus plugging are not synonymous. Patients with mucoid impaction of bronchi usually have underlying allergic disease, typically asthma with allergic bronchopulmonary aspergillosis *(29–32)*.

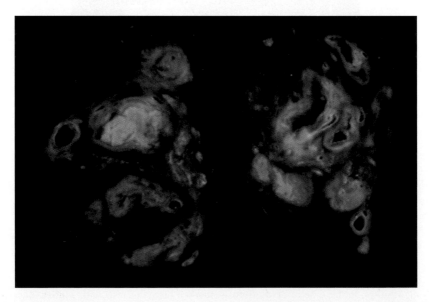

Fig. 7. Mucoid impact of bronchi. The dilated bronchi are filled with mucus plugs. (Used with permission of the American Registry of Pathology; originally published as Fig. 9–40, page 413 in: *Non-Neoplastic Disorders of the Lower Respiratory Tract*, Travis WD et al. American Registry of Pathology, Washington, DC, 2002)

Grossly, the dilated bronchi contain rubbery and brownish to greenish mucus plugs (Fig. 7) *(29–32)*. Microscopically, "allergic mucin" has a laminated appearance with abundant eosinophil debris and Charcot–Leyden crystals (Fig. 8) *(29,31,32,34)*. Charcot–Leyden crystals are long, hexagonal, and bright eosinophilic crystals. In allergic bronchopulmonary fungal disease (ABFD), fungal hyphae may be found in the allergic mucin with the appropriate stains (e.g., methenamine silver stain). Microscopic changes of asthma may also be seen in the airway walls.

1.9. Bronchocentric Granulomatosis

BCG is defined as a bronchocentric and/or bronchiolocentric necrotizing granulomatous inflammation that involves the airway wall, ultimately destroying and replacing it *(33,35–37)*. It is a pathologic

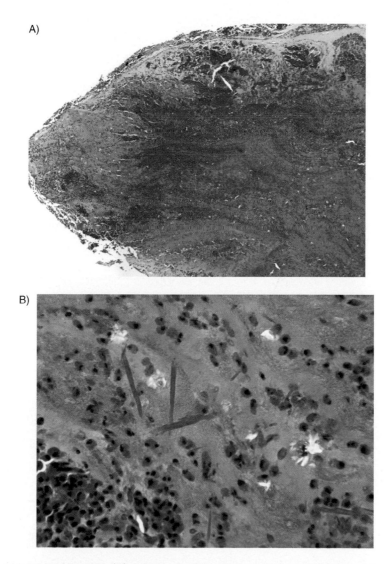

A)

B)

Fig. 8. Mucoid impact of bronchi. (**A**) Allergic mucin is characterized by laminated mucin with eosinophilic debris. This patient had allergic bronchopulmonary fungal disease (ABFD). (**B**) Higher magnification shows many eosinophils and Charcot–Leyden crystals (in the center of the picture) within the allergic mucin.

Table 2
Causes of Bronchocentric Granulomatosis

Infectious etiologies
      Mycobacterial infection
      Fungal infection
      Parasitic infection
Non-infectious etiologies
      Allergic bronchopulmonary fungal disease
      Rheumatoid arthritis
      Wegener's granulomatosis
      Necrotizing sarcoidosis

descriptive term that has infectious or non-infectious etiologies (Table 2) *(15,33,35–37)*. Many cases occur in lung tissue distal to mucoid impaction.

Microscopically, the bronchi and bronchioles are replaced by palisaded histiocytes with central necrotic debris (Fig. 9). Eosinophils are numerous in BCG associated with allergic bronchopulmonary aspergillosis and coccidioidomycosis. The surrounding lung parenchyma usually shows acute and chronic inflammation and sometimes changes of obstructive or eosinophilic pneumonia. When confronted with BCG, one should exclude infection with appropriate cultures and special stains for mycobacterium and fungi should be performed. Wegener's granulomatosis and necrotizing sarcoidosis may be bronchocentric and also enter the differential diagnosis. Foreign body aspiration may show granulomas around the airways, and a careful search for foreign debris such as vegetable debris is suggested. In patients with a clinical history of asthma, allergic bronchopulmonary aspergillosis should be the prime consideration and this is discussed below *(33,35,36)*.

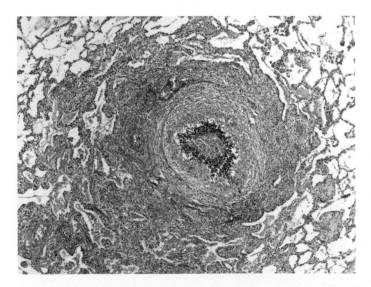

Fig. 9. Bronchocentric granulomatosis. The bronchiole is destroyed and replaced by palisading histiocytes with necrotic debris in the lumen. The bronchiolar nature is recognized by the remaining rim of smooth muscle and the adjacent pulmonary artery. This is a case of allergic bronchopulmonary aspergillosis.

1.10. Allergic Bronchopulmonary Fungal Disease

ABFD is a clinical syndrome typically found in chronic asthmatic patients who have been colonized by Aspergillus (typically *Aspergillus fumigatus*) and developed hypersensitivity to it *(32,33,38–43)*. *Curvularia lunata, Drechslera hawaiiensis*, Helminthosporium, *Torulopsis glabrata, Candida albicans, Bipolaris sp, Pseudoallescheria boydii*, and *Fusarium vasinfectum* are also occasionally implicated in this disease *(32)*.

The lung tissue typically shows combinations of mucoid impaction of bronchi, BCG (Fig. 9), eosinophilic pneumonia (lung tissue predominately infiltrated by eosinophils), and asthmatic changes. When the pathologic and clinical features are suggestive of ABFD, the allergic mucin should be carefully searched for hyphae fragments and cultures and special stains for fungi should be performed.

1.11. Middle Lobe Syndrome

Middle lobe syndrome (MLS) is defined as a recurrent or fixed atelectasis of the right middle lobe or lingula *(44–50)*. It is a clinical syndrome that may result in bronchiectasis, bronchitis, bronchiolitis, and acute or chronic parenchymal inflammatory changes in the affected lung tissue. Initially, MLS was described as obstructive atelectasis of the right middle lobe due to compression of the proximal bronchi by enlarged tuberculous lymph nodes *(45,48)*. Now other neoplastic and non-neoplastic obstructive etiologies are recognized. Benign or malignant neoplasms may obstruct the airway as an endobronchial mass or by external compression. Esophageal diverticula, foreign bodies, endobronchial sarcoidosis, mucous plugs, and conditions of bronchial inflammation leading to granulation tissue formation, submucosal edema, and fibrosis may also be implicated.

There are still a number of cases (perhaps the majority seen currently) with no recognizable cause of obstruction *(48)*: poor drainage of the middle lobe and lingula with transient obstruction and relative anatomic isolation with decreased collateral ventilation and the effects of emphysema elsewhere in the lung may be factors in these cases *(45,48,49)*.

The term "Lady Windermere syndrome" has been used for MLS in middle-aged nonsmoking women with pulmonary *Mycobacterium avium-intracellulare* infection of the middle lobe and/or the lingula *(48,51)*. In one recent study, one fourth of the cases of MLS undergoing lobectomy showed granulomatous inflammation consistent with atypical mycobacterial infection *(48)*.

The pathologic findings of MLS reflect the various infectious and non-infectious causes and complications of bronchial obstruction: bronchiectasis, follicular bronchiolitis, florid lymphoid hyperplasia, broncholithiasis, atelectasis, acute or organizing pneumonia, abscess, granulomatous inflammation, hemosiderosis, interstitial fibrosis, and pleural fibrosis (Fig. 10) *(48)*.

1.12. Relapsing Polychondritis

Relapsing polychondritis (*polychondritis, polychondropathy*) is a rare chronic disorder characterized by recurrent inflammation of the cartilage of the ears, joints, nose, eyes, respiratory tract, and cardiovascular system *(52–55)*. Structural integrity of the cartilage is lost, leading to secondary inflammatory changes. Coexistent connective tissue disease such as adult or juvenile rheumatoid arthritis, Sjogren's syndrome, systemic lupus erythematosus, Reiter's disease, psoriatic arthritis, and ankylosing spondylitis are found in 25% of patients *(53)*.

Microscopically, the cartilage is destroyed by acute and chronic inflammatory infiltrate (Fig. 11) *(52)*. This histology is not specific and cartilaginous destruction in the bronchi is also seen in many infectious and other non-infectious diseases. Secondary inflammatory changes are also found in the distal small airways and lung parenchyma.

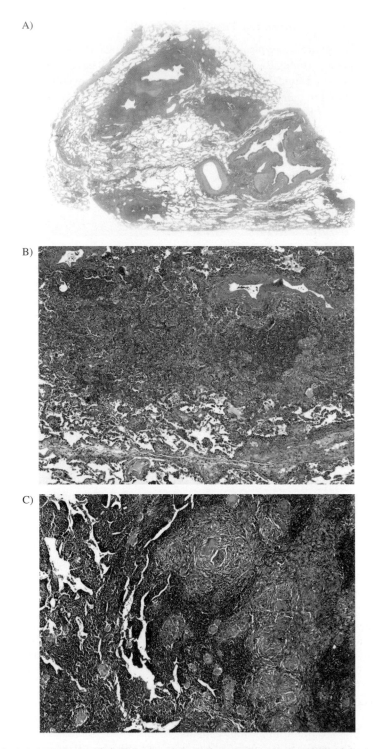

Fig. 10. Middle lobe syndrome. (**A**) Bronchiectasis is frequently seen in middle lobe syndrome. Airway-centered inflammation is prominent. (**B**) Bronchopneumonia of acute inflammatory cells in and surrounding bronchioles is quite common. (**C**) Non-necrotizing granulomas in middle lobe syndrome often correlate with *Mycobacterium avium-intracellulare* infection.

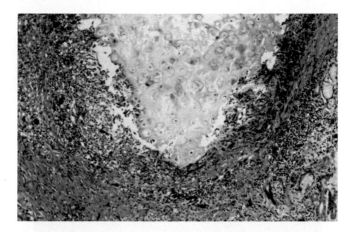

Fig. 11. Relapsing polychondritis. The lung cartilage is destroyed and surrounded by inflammatory cells. (Used with permission of the American Registry of Pathology; originally published as Fig. 9–57 left, page 423 in: *Non-Neoplastic Disorders of the Lower Respiratory Tract*, Travis WD et al. American Registry of Pathology, Washington, DC, 2002)

1.13. Broncholithiasis

Broncholithiasis is a condition in which calcified lymph nodes distort and erode into the tracheobronchial tree and patients may expectorate or aspirate the calcified material *(56–58)*. It is usually a late complication of granulomatous infection by mycobacterial infection or histoplasmosis. Grossly, the airway is fibrotic distorted and the erosion by calcified lymph nodes may be apparent (Fig. 12) *(56)*. Microscopically, the lymph nodes show calcified old granulomas with fibrosis and chronic inflammation (Fig. 13). The eroded airway shows variable acute, chronic, or granulomatous inflammation. Special stains may reveal the causative organisms within the granulomas (Fig. 13B).

2. SMALL AIRWAYS

The small airways include primarily the bronchioles. They are the bridges between large airways and lung parenchyma. Small airway pathology is appreciated by pathologists when abnormalities center on the bronchioles and alveolar ducts at scanning magnification. Scanning of the small airways by power microscopy often correlates with lobular anatomy as recognized on HRCT scans.

Some diseases primarily affect the small airways. However, large airway or lung parenchymal diseases may also show secondary changes in small airways. In practice, there are several pathologic patterns of small airway injury that can be seen. In the following, we will describe the common pathologic patterns of bronchiolitis and some of the associated clinical disorders.

3. PATHOLOGIC PATTERNS OF BRONCHIOLITIS

3.1. Cellular Bronchiolitis

Cellular bronchiolitis or inflammatory bronchiolitis is primarily a cellular reaction centering on the bronchioles. It can be acute or chronic or both depending on the cellular infiltrate presented (Fig. 14). It is quite common and often combined with other pathologic patterns described below. Cellular infiltrates along small airways may be sufficiently dense to be visible on HRCT.

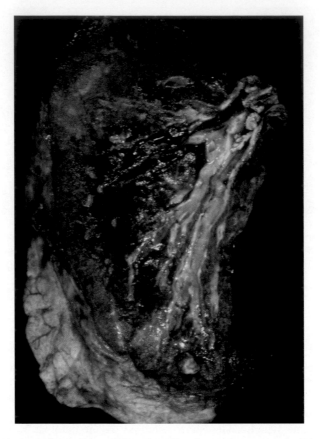

Fig. 12. Broncholithiasis. Broncholiths within the hilar bronchi are noted. (Used with permission of the American Registry of Pathology; originally published as Fig. 9-61 left, page 427 in: *Non-Neoplastic Disorders of the Lower Respiratory Tract*, Travis WD et al. American Registry of Pathology, Washington, DC, 2002)

A)
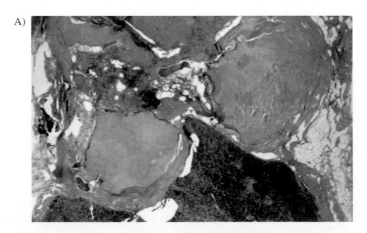

Fig. 13. *(Continued)*

B)

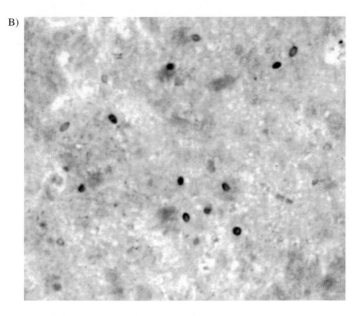

Fig. 13. Broncholithiasis. (**A**) The broncholiths are derived from calcified old granulomas in peribronchial lymph nodes. (**B**) Fungal yeasts of Histoplasma are sometimes found within the broncholiths. (Used with permission of the American Registry of Pathology; originally published as Fig. 9–62 left and right, page 427 in: *Non-Neoplastic Disorders of the Lower Respiratory Tract*, Travis WD et al. American Registry of Pathology, Washington, DC, 2002)

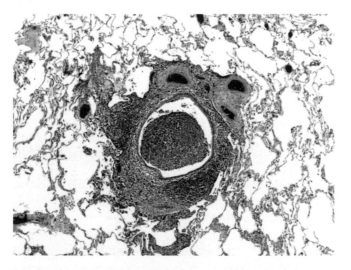

Fig. 14. Cellular bronchiolitis. The bronchiole is surrounded and infiltrated by chronic inflammatory cells with inflammatory debris in the lumen. This is a case of inflammatory bowel disease-related chronic bronchiolitis.

Table 3
Clinical Disorders Associated with Cellular Bronchiolitis

Acute cellular bronchiolitis (with acute inflammation)
      Infection: bacterial and viral
      Acute aspiration
      Wegerner's granulomatosis
      Fume injury
      Toxic exposure
Acute and chronic cellular bronchiolitis
      Infection: bacterial, viral, fungal, mycoplasma
      Allergic reaction (e.g., hypersensitivity pneumonitis or asthma)
      Inflammatory bowel disease-associated pulmonary manifestation
      Changes distal to bronchiectasis
      Collagen vascular diseases
      Diffuse panbronchiolitis
      Post-transplantation
      Wegerner's granulomatosis
      Aspiration
      Idiopathic
Chronic cellular bronchiolitis (primarily chronic inflammatory cells)
      Allergic reaction (e.g., hypersensitivity pneumonitis or asthma)
      Inflammatory bowel disease-associated pulmonary manifestation
      Changes distal to bronchiectasis
      Collagen vascular diseases
      Diffuse panbronchiolitis
      Post-transplantation
      Chronic aspiration
      Langerhans' cell histiocytosis
      Lymphoproliferative disorders
      Idiopathic

There are many clinical disorders associated with cellular bronchiolitis. Most are listed in Table 3 *(59,60)*. Cellular bronchiolitis with acute inflammatory cells is often a clue to an infectious process.

3.2. Follicular Bronchiolitis

Follicular bronchiolitis is a distinct subtype of chronic cellular bronchiolitis. Pathologically, one sees reactive lymphoid follicles and accompanying chronic inflammatory cells around the bronchioles (Fig. 15). It is thought to be due to hyperplasia of mucosa-associated lymphoid tissue along the airways (BALT or bronchus associated lymphoid tissue). Follicular bronchiolitis may be seen as centrilobular nodules on HRCT.

Widespread follicular bronchiolitis has relatively short differential diagnoses and sometimes can be used as a clue for diagnosis. The associated clinical disorders are listed in Table 4 *(59,60)*. There is overlap with lymphoid interstitial pneumonia.

3.3. Respiratory Bronchiolitis

Respiratory bronchiolitis (RB) is viewed as histologic evidence of cigarette smoking and is seen in virtually all cigarette smokers. Mild RB is common in the lung specimens (especially resections for lung carcinoma), and it usually does not cause clinical symptoms by itself. When it is the sole pathologic finding in patients with radiologic and clinical evidence of diffuse interstitial lung disease,

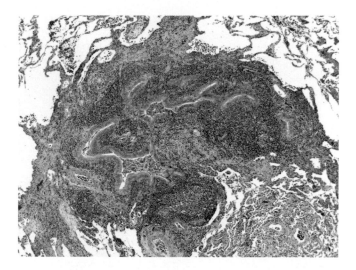

Fig. 15. Follicular bronchiolitis. The bronchiolar wall is infiltrated by chronic inflammatory cells, and there are two surrounding lymphoid follicles with reactive germinal centers.

the term respiratory bronchiolitis–interstitial lung disease (RB-ILD) is appropriate. RB, RB-ILD, and desquamative interstitial pneumonia (DIP) are considered part of a spectrum of smoking-related disease. DIP is characterized by diffuse and marked alveolar macrophages distributed uniformly in the alveolar spaces.

Pathologically, there is mild chronic inflammatory infiltrate involving the respiratory bronchioles with extension to the adjacent alveoli and variable numbers of lightly pigmented ("smokers") macrophages in the lumens of the respiratory bronchioles (Fig. 16). Mild fibrosis of the respiratory bronchioles and adjacent alveoli and emphysema may also be present.

3.4. Bronchiolitis Obliterans with Intraluminal Polyps (BOOP or OP pattern)

Bronchiolitis obliterans with intraluminal polyps is discussed here because there are bronchiolar changes, although most cases showing this pattern are not "airway diseases." Pathologically, there are intrabronchiolar polypoid plugs of loose connective tissue (Fig. 17). Bronchiolitis obliterans with intraluminal polyps usually occurs in combination with similar intraluminal changes in the

Table 4
Clinical Disorders Associated with Follicular Bronchiolitis

Collagen vascular disease
Middle lobe syndrome
Diffuse panbronchiolitis
Immunodeficiency (congenital or acquired; e.g., HIV infection)
Hypersensitivity reaction
Changes distal to bronchiectasis
Lymphoproliferative disease (especially MALT lymphoma)
Lymphoid hyperplasia
Lymphocytic interstitial pneumonia
Idiopathic

MALT, mucosa-associated lymphoid tissue.

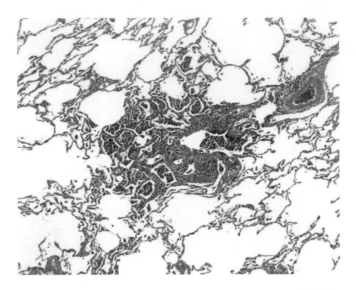

Fig. 16. Respiratory bronchiolitis. There are lightly pigmented macrophages in the lumen of the respiratory bronchiole and the immediately adjacent alveolar spaces.

alveolar ducts and alveolar spaces, and the entire histologic spectrum has been termed bronchiolitis obliterans organizing pneumonia (BOOP). Recently, the American Thoracic Society/European Respiratory Society (ATS/ERS) classification of idiopathic interstitial pneumonias suggests using the term "organizing pneumonia pattern" for BOOP *(61,62)*.

Bronchiolitis obliterans with intraluminal polyps (BOOP/organizing pneumonia pattern) is viewed as a subacute repair reaction to diffuse or localized lung injury which includes some pathology in the small airways as well as distal parenchyma *(59,63)*. It can be either major or minor pathologic change. Table 5 lists the clinical disorders in which bronchiolitis obliterans with intraluminal polyps (organizing pneumonia pattern) can be seen *(60)*. The term cryptogenic organizing pneumonia is applied to cases of interstitial lung disease of unknown cause showing a BOOP pattern.

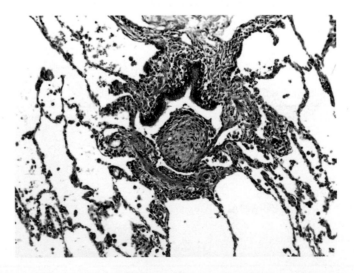

Fig. 17. Bronchiolitis obliterans with intraluminal polyps. A polypoid plug of loose connective tissue is seen within the bronchiolar lumen.

Table 5
Clinical Disorders Associated with Bronchiolitis Obliterans with Intraluminal Polyps (Organizing Pneumonia Pattern)

Diffuse alveolar damage
Infection
Aspiration pneumonia
Drug or toxic exposure
Collagen vascular disease
Changes distal to obstruction
Hypersensitivity pneumonitis
Eosinophilic pneumonia
Chronic bronchiolitis
Bronchiectasis
Post-lung transplantation
Graft versus host disease
Idiopathic (cryptogenic organizing pneumonia)

3.5. Constrictive Bronchiolitis

Constrictive bronchiolitis can be applied to a constellation of histologic changes including narrowed bronchiolar lumens due to submucosal scarring, hypertrophy of bronchiolar smooth muscle, mucus stasis, adventitial scarring, and often cellular infiltrates (Fig. 18). Only a minority of the small airways show complete luminal obliteration. Constrictive bronchiolitis is one of the patterns for which the term "bronchiolitis obliterans" has been used. Clinically, patients with widespread constrictive bronchiolitis present with mild to severe obstructive pulmonary deficits and characteristic radiologic findings (mosaic hypoperfusion pattern, etc.). Table 6 lists some clinical disorders associated with constrictive bronchiolitis *(59,60)*. It may be viewed as a form of repair process to various forms of airway injury although idiopathic cases (cryptogenic constrictive bronchiolitis) are encountered.

A)

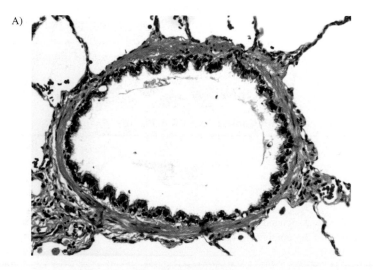

Fig. 18. *(Continued)*

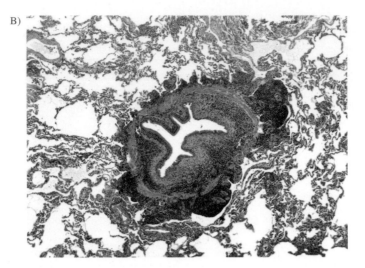

Fig. 18. Constrictive bronchiolitis. (**A**) This normal bronchiole is for comparison. Note the bronchiolar lumen is not narrowed. The submucosal space is thin. There is no medial hypertrophy, nor adventitial scarring. (**B**) In constrictive bronchiolitis, the lumen of bronchiole is compromised because of varying degrees of submucosal inflammatory scarring, medial hypertrophy, adventitial fibrosis, and chronic inflammation. This is a case of rheumatoid associated constrictive bronchiolitis.

3.6. Peribronchiolar Metaplasia (Bronchiolarization)

Peribronchiolar metaplasia, also called bronchiolarization, presents as metaplastic growth of bronchiolar epithelium involving the peribronchiolar alveoli (Fig. 19). It is presumed to be a late manifestation of bronchiolar injury and thus a nonspecific finding. Table 7 lists some of the clinical disorders in which peribronchiolar metaplasia can be seen *(59,60)*. Peribronchiolar metaplasia primarily manifests as interstitial lung disease and not as obstructive airway disease.

3.7. Bronchiolocentric Nodules

Some conditions present as bronchiolocentric nodules grossly or at scanning magnification; these result from nodular aggregates of cells, granulomas, and/or associated fibrosis (Fig. 20). The cells composing of these nodules can be inflammatory or neoplastic. Bronchiolocentric nodules are recognized as centrilobular nodules on HRCT and are more likely to be considered interstitial diseases, clinically,

Table 6
Clinical Disorders Associated with Constrictive Bronchiolitis

Post-infection
Fume or toxin
Collagen vascular disease
Post-transplantation
Drug
Inflammatory bowel disease-associated pulmonary manifestation
Asthma (usually severe with the component of irreversible obstruction)
Idiopathic

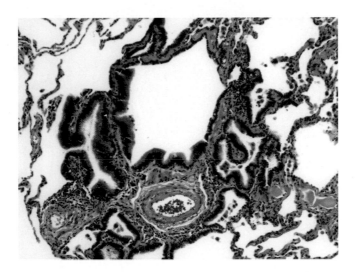

Fig. 19. Peribronchiolar metaplasia. The alveolar walls surrounding the bronchiole are lined by metaplastic bronchiolar epithelium.

Table 7
Clinical Disorders Associated with Peribronchiolar Metaplasia

Healed bronchiolar injury (many causes)
Chronic hypersensitivity pneumonitis
Changes distal to bronchiectasis
Incidental finding, including in diffuse lung diseases
Idiopathic

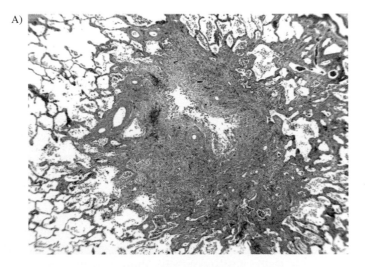

Fig. 20. *(Continued)*

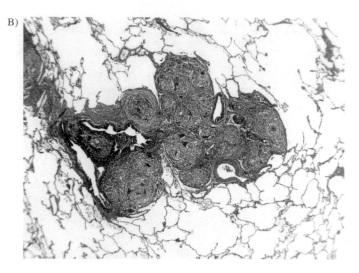

Fig. 20. Bronchiolocentric nodules. (**A**) Langerhans cell histiocytosis. This is a case of Langerhans cell histiocytosis illustrating bronchiolocentric nodules. The Langerhans cells aggregate around the bronchiole, appearing as a bronchiolocentric nodule. The bronchiolar wall is destroyed but the adjacent pulmonary artery is still recognizable. (**B**) Sarcoidosis. This case of sarcoidosis shows bronchiolocentric nodules. Non-necrotizing granulomas coalesce along the bronchiolovascular bundle.

Table 8
Lesions that may Present Bronchiolocentric Nodules Pathologically

Cellular bronchiolitis
Follicular bronchiolitis
Respiratory bronchiolitis
Hypersensitivity pneumonitis
Diffuse panbronchiolitis
Organizing pneumonia (many causes)
Pulmonary Langerhans' cell histiocytosis
Pneumoconioses
Bronchocentric granulomatosis (*see* Table 2)
Sarcoidosis
Lymphangitic/bronchiolocentric neoplasms
Diffuse idiopathic pulmonary neuroendocrine cell hyperplasia/tumorlets

rather than airway diseases. Table 8 lists the common clinical disorders presenting as bronchiolocentric nodules *(59,60)*. Some of the previously described patterns of bronchiolitis are also included because they are also bronchiolocentric under the scanning power of microscope.

4. AIRWAY PATHOLOGY IN SELECTED CLINICOPATHOLOGIC ENTITIES

4.1. Asthma

Asthma is a distinct chronic inflammatory airway disorder with recurrent and reversible episodes of airflow obstruction *(64)*. The pathologic changes are more prominent in small bronchi but are also seen in bronchioles. Classically, involved airways show epithelial shedding, goblet cell hyperplasia, thickened mucosal basement membrane, edema, smooth muscle hyperplasia, submucosal mucous

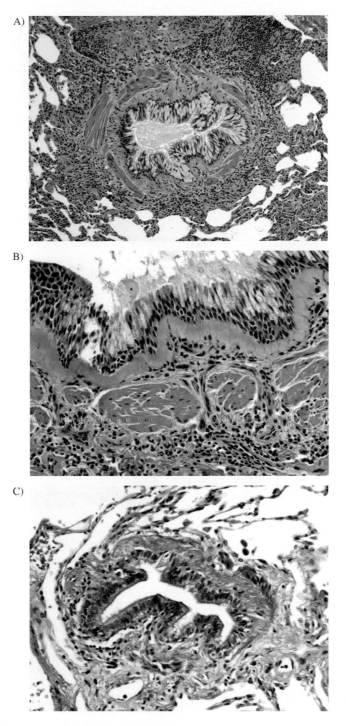

Fig. 21. Asthma. (**A**) The bronchiole shows mucus stasis, marked goblet cell hyperplasia, submucosal edema, smooth muscle hyperplasia, and cellular bronchiolitis. (**B**) At high-power magnification, thickened mucosal basement membrane and infiltration of eosinophils are seen. (**C**) In this case of chronic asthma, the trichrome stain for collagen shows scarring in the submucosa and adventitia, indicative of the changes of constrictive bronchiolitis, and this often correlates with irreversible airflow obstruction.

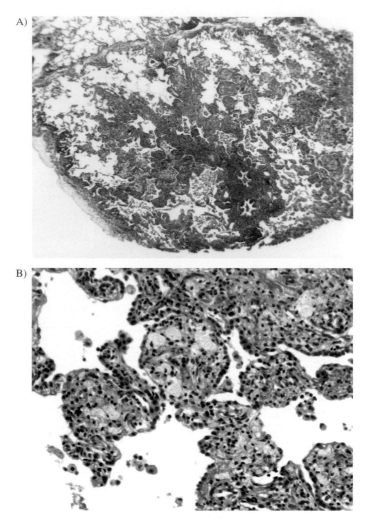

Fig. 22. Diffuse panbronchiolitis. (**A**) At scanning magnification, this is an acute and chronic cellular bronchiolitis with mild extension to the alveolar ducts and alveolar septa. (**B**) At high magnification, the presence of interstitial foam cells is a key feature of diffuse panbronchiolitis.

gland hyperplasia, and infiltration of inflammatory cells rich in eosinophils (Fig. 21) *(59,65)*. Mucus plugs with Charcot–Leyden crystals, Curschmann's spirals, and Creola bodies are seen within the bronchial lumen. Other manifestations such as mucoid impaction of bronchi, ABFD, and BCG may also occur. Airway pathology of asthma may be subtle especially in patients with mild disease or between attacks: the changes described above are muted and some airways may appear normal. Chronic and late bronchiolar changes of asthma include chronic cellular bronchiolitis, peribronchiolar metaplasia, and constrictive bronchiolitis. These may correlate with the development of "fixed obstruction" in asthmatics.

4.2. Diffuse Panbronchiolitis

Diffuse panbronchiolitis is a distinctive disorder with characteristic clinical, radiologic, and pathologic features. It was first described by Yamanaka et al., and most reported cases come from Japan with rare

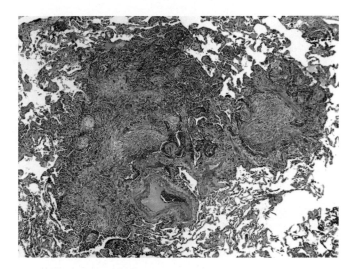

Fig. 23. Fume-related bronchiolar injury. In the subacute phase, organizing connective tissue fills the bronchiolar lumen.

cases identified in non-Asian populations *(66–69)*. The age at presentation is between 40 and 70 years with clinical symptoms of dyspnea, wheezing, and chronic productive cough. Chronic sinusitis is seen in 80% of patients.

Grossly, the lungs are hyperinflated with yellowish bronchiolocentric nodules. Microscopically, early disease is primarily confined to the bronchioles with relative sparing of alveoli. Acute and chronic cellular bronchiolitis with distinctive foamy histiocytes in the interstitium of the respiratory bronchioles, alveolar ducts, and some alveolar septa are noted (Fig. 22) *(70)*. Bronchiectasis and bronchiolectasis may develop over time.

4.3. Fume-Related Bronchiolar Injury

Inhalation of toxic fumes or gases can lead to direct injury of bronchioles. In the acute phase, there is mucosal necrosis with acute cellular bronchiolitis *(71)*. In some cases, there is coexisting pulmonary edema and diffuse alveolar damage. During the subacute phase, intraluminal organization/BOOP-like changes may be seen (Fig. 23). In most cases, there is complete recovery without sequelae. Late constrictive bronchiolitis with persistent obstructive findings occasionally occurs *(71)*.

REFERENCES

1. Carden KA, Boiselle PM, Waltz DA, Ernst A. Tracheomalacia and tracheobronchomalacia in children and adults: an in-depth review. *Chest* 2005;127:984–1005.
2. Prakash UB. Tracheobronchopathia osteochondroplastica. *Semin Respir Crit Care Med* 2002;23:167–75.
3. Bateson EM, Woo-Ming M. Tracheobronchomegaly. *Clin Radiol* 1973;24:354–8.
4. Johnston RF, Green RA, Tracheobronchomegaly. Report of 5 cases and demonstration of familial occurrence. *Am Rev Respir Dis* 1965:91:35–50.
5. Katz I, Levine M, Herman P. Tracheobronchomegaly. The Mounier-Kuhn Syndrome. *AJR Am J Roentgenol* 1962;88:1084–94.
6. Landing BH, Dixon LG. Congenital malformation and genetic disorders of the respiratory tract. *Am Rev Respir Dis* 1979;120:151–85.
7. Stocker JT. Congenital and developmental disease. In: Dail DH, Hammar SP, eds. *Pulmonary Pathology*, 2nd ed. New York: Springer-Verlag; 1994:155–90.
8. Swartz, MN. Bronchiectasis. In: Fishman AP, ed. *Fishmans Pulmonary Diseases and Disorders*, 3rd ed. New York: McGraw Hill; 1998:2045–70.

9. Annest LS, Kratz JM, Crawford FA. Current results of treatment of bronchiectasis. *J Thorac Cardiovasc Surg* 1982;83: 546–50.
10. Cohen M, Sahn SA. Bronchiectasis in systemic diseases. *Chest* 1999;116:1063–74.
11. Grenier P, Maurice F, Musset D. Bronchiectasis: assessment by thin-section CT. *Radiology* 1986;161:95–9.
12. Hansell DM. Bronchiectasis. *Radiol Clin North Am* 1998;36:107–28.
13. Heard BE, Khatchatourov V, Otto H, Putov NV, Sobin L. The Morphology of emphysema, chronic bronchitis, and bronchiectasis: definition, nomenclature and classification. *J Clin Pathol* 1979;32:882–92.
14. Kang EY, Miller RR, Muller NL. Bronchiectasis: comparison of preoperative thin-section CT and pathologic findings in resected specimens. *Radiology* 1995;195:649–54.
15. Colby TV. Bronchial disorders. In: Travis WD, Colby TV, Koss MN, Rosado-de-Christenson ML, Muller NL, King TE Jr, eds. *Atlas of Nontumor Pathology, Fascicle 2. Non-Neoplastic Disorders of the Lower Respiratory Tract.* Washington, DC: American Registry of Pathology and the Armed Forces Institute of Pathology; 2002 pp 381–434.
16. Kim JS, Muller NL, Park CS. Cylindrical bronchiectasis: diagnostic findings on thin-section CT. *AJR Am J Roentgenol* 1997;168:751–4.
17. Saito K, Cagle P, Berend N, Thurlbeck WM. The "destructive index" in nonemphysematous and emphysematous lungs. Morphologic observations and correlation with function. *Am Rev Respir Dis* 1989;139:308–12.
18. Young K, Aspestrand F, Kolbenstvedt A. High-resolution CT and bronchography in the assessment of bronchiectasis. *Acta Radiol* 1991;32:439–41.
19. Thurlbeck WM. Chronic airflow obstruction. In: Thurlbeck WM, Churg AM, eds. *Pathology of the Lung*, 2nd ed. New York: Thieme; 1995:739–826.
20. Whitwill F. A study of the pathology and pathogenesis of bronchiectasis. *Thorax* 1952;7:213–39.
21. Bedrossian CW, Greenberg SD, Singer DB, Hansen JJ, Rosenberg HS. The lung in cystic fibrosis. A quantitative study including prevalence of pathologic findings among different age groups. *Hum Pathol* 1976;7:195–204.
22. Boat TF. Cystic fibrosis. In: Nelson WE, ed. *Nelson Textbook of Pediatrics*, 15th ed. Philadelphia: WB Saunders; 1996:1239–51.
23. Elborn JS, Shale DJ. Lung injury in cystic fibrosis. *Thorax* 1990;45:970–3.
24. Esterly JR, Oppenheimer EH. Observations in cystic fibrosis of the pancreas. 3. Pulmonary lesions. *Johns Hopkins Med J* 1968;122:94–101.
25. Friedman PJ, Harwood IR, Ellenbogen PH. Pulmonary cystic fibrosis in the adult: early and late radiologic findings with pathologic correlation. *AJR Am J Roentgenol* 1981;136:1131–44.
26. Geddes DM, Alton ER. The CF gene: 10 years on. *Thorax* 1999;54:1052–4.
27. Hunt B, Geddes DM. Newly diagnosed cystic fibrosis in middle and later life. *Thorax* 1985;40:23–6.
28. Schwiebert EM, Benos DJ, Fuller CM. Cystic fibrosis: a multiple exocrinopathy caused by dysfunctions in a multifunctional transport protein. *Am J Med* 1998;104:576–90.
29. Hutcheson JB, Shawrr RR, Paulson DL, Kee JL. Mucoid impaction of the bronchi. *Am J Clin Pathol* 1960;33:427–32.
30. Irwin RS, Thomas HM. Mucoid impaction of the bronchus. Diagnosis and treatment. *Am Rev Respir Dis* 1973;108:955–9.
31. Jelihovsky T. The structure of bronchial plugs in mucoid impaction, bronchocentric granulomatosis and asthma. *Histopathology* 1983;7:153–67.
32. Katzenstein AL, ed. Immunologic lung disease. In: *Katzenstein and Askin's Surgical Pathology of Non-Neoplastic Lung Disease*, 3rd ed. Philadelphia: WB Saunders; 1997:138–67.
33. Katzenstein AL, Liebow AA, Friedman PJ. Bronchocentric granulomatosis, mucoid impaction, and hypersensitivity reactions to fungi. *Am Rev Respir Dis* 1975;111:497–537.
34. Aubry MC, Fraser R. The role of bronchial biopsy and washing in the diagnosis of allergic bronchopulmonary aspergillosis. *Mod Pathol* 1998;11:607–11.
35. Katzenstein AL, ed. Angiitis and granulomatosis. In: *Katzenstein and Askin's Surgical Pathology of Non-Neoplastic Lung Disease*, 3rd ed. Philadelphia: WB Saunders; 1997:193–222.
36. Koss M, Robinson R, Hochholzer L. Bronchocentric granulomatosis. *Hum Pathol* 1981;12:632–8.
37. Myers JL, Katzenstein AL. Granulomatous infection mimicking bronchocentric granulomatosis. *Am J Surg Pathol* 1986;10:317–22.
38. Bosken CH, Myers JL, Greenberger PA, Katzenstein AL. Pathologic features of allergic bronchopulmonary aspergillosis. *Am J Surg Pathol* 1988;12:216–22.
39. Cockrill BA, Hales CA. Allergic bronchopulmonary aspergillosis. *Annu Rev Med* 1999;50:303–16.
40. Fink JN. Allergic bronchopulmonary aspergillosis. *Chest* 1985;87:81S–4S.
41. Glimp RA, Bayer AS. Fungal pneumonias. Part 3. Allergic bronchopulmonary aspergillosis. *Chest* 1981;80:85–94.
42. Greenberger PA, Patterson R. Allergic bronchopulmonary aspergillosis. Model of bronchopulmonary disease with defined serologic, radiologic, pathologic and clinical findings from asthma to fatal destructive lung disease. *Chest* 1987;91: 165S–71S.
43. Ricketti AJ, Greenberger PA, Mintzer RA, Patterson R. Allergic bronchopulmonary aspergillosis. *Chest* 1984;86:773–8.

44. Bertelsen S, Struve-Christensen E, Aasted A, Sparup J. Isolated middle lobe atelectasis: aetiology, pathogenesis, and treatment of the so-called middle lobe syndrome. *Thorax* 1980;35:449–52.
45. Culner MM. The right middle lobe syndrome, a non-obstructive complex. *Dis Chest* 1966;50:57–66.
46. Dees SC, Spock A. Right middle lobe syndrome in children. *JAMA* 1966;197:78–84.
47. Eskenasy A, Eana-Iorgulescu L. Pathology of the middle lobe syndromes. A histopathologic and pathogenetic analysis of sixty surgically-cured cases. *Med Interne* 1982;20:73–80.
48. Kwon KY, Myers JL, Swensen SJ, Colby TV. Middle lobe syndrome: a clinicopathological study of 21 patients. *Hum Pathol* 1995;26:302–7.
49. Rosenbloom SA, Ravin CE, Putman CE, et al. Peripheral middle lobe syndrome. *Radiology* 1983;149:17–21.
50. Saha SP, May OP, Long GA, Mcelvein RB. Middle lobe syndrome: diagnosis and management. *Ann Thorac Surg* 1982;33:28–31.
51. Wagner RB, Johnston MR. Middle lobe syndrome. *Ann Thorac Surg* 1983;35:679–86.
52. Gardner DL. Pathologic basis of the connective tissue diseases. Philadelphia: Lea & Febiger; 1992:711–5.
53. King TE Jr. Connective tissue disease. In: Schwarz MI, King TE Jr, eds. *Interstitial Lung Diseases*. Hamilton: BC Decker, 1998:451–505.
54. Tillie-Leblond I, Wallaert B, Leblond D, et al. Respiratory involvement in relapsing polychondritis. Clinical, functional, endoscopic, and radiographic evaluations. *Medicine* 1998;77:168–76.
55. Wiedemann HP, Matthay RA. Pulmonary manifestations of the collagen vascular diseases. *Clin Chest Med* 1989;10: 677–722.
56. Arrigoni MG, Bernatz PE, Donoghue FE. Broncholithiasis. *J Thorac Cardiovasc Surg* 1971;62:231–7.
57. Conces DJ, Tarver RD, Vix VA. Broncholithiasis: CT features in 15 patients. *AJR Am J Roentgenol* 1991;157:249–53.
58. Olson EJ, Utz JP, Prakash UB. Therapeutic bronchoscopy in broncholithiasis. *Am J Respir Crit Care Med* 1999;160:766–70.
59. Colby TV, Leslie KO. Small airway lesions. In: Cagle PT, ed. *Diagnostic Pulmonary Pathology*. New York: Marcel Dekker; 2000:231–49.
60. Colby TV. Bronchiolar disorders. In: Travis WD, Colby TV, Koss MN, Rosado-de-Christenson ML, Muller NL, King TE Jr, eds. *Atlas of Nontumor Pathology, Fascicle 2. Non-Neoplastic Disorders of the Lower Respiratory Tract*. Washington, DC: American Registry of Pathology and the Armed Forces Institute of Pathology; 2002 pp 351–380.
61. Colby TV, Myers JL. Clinical and histologic spectrum of bronchiolitis obliterans organizing pneumonia. *Semin Respir Med* 1992;13:113–9.
62. Travis WD, King TE, Bateman ED, et al. ATS/ERS international multidisciplinary consensus classification of idiopathic interstitial pneumonia. *Am J Respir Crit Care Med* 2002;165:277–304.
63. King TE Jr. Bronchiolitis. In: Schwartz MI, King TE Jr, eds. *Interstitial Lung Disease*, 3rd ed. London: BC Decker; 1998:645–84.
64. National Heart, Lung and Blood institute. *Expert Panel Report 2: Guidelines for the Diagnosis and Management of Asthma*. Bethesda, MD: NIH publication No. 97–4051, 1997.
65. Colby TV. Bronchiolar pathology. In: Epler GR, ed. *Diseases of the Bronchioles*. New York: Raven Press; 1994:77–100.
66. Yamanaka A, Saiki S, Tamura S, Saito K. Problems in chronic obstructive bronchial disease, with special reference to diffuse panbronchiolitis. *Naika* 1969;23:442–51.
67. Homma H, Yamanaka A, Tanimoto S, et al. Diffuse panbronchiolitis: a disease of the transitional zone of the lung. *Chest* 1983;83:63–9.
68. Poletti V, Patelli M, Poletti G, Bertanti T, Spiga L. Diffuse panbronchiolitis observed in an Italian [Letter]. *Chest* 1990;98:515–6.
69. Randhawa P, Hoagland MH, Yousem SA. Diffuse panbronchiolitis in North America. Report of three cases and review of the literature. *Am J Surg Pathol* 1991;15:43–7.
70. Kitachi M, Nishimura K, Izumi T. Diffuse panbronchiolitis. In: Sharma OP, ed. *Lung Disease in the Tropics*. New York: Marcel Dekker; 1991:479–509.
71. Douglas WW, Colby TV. Fume-related bronchiolitis obliterans. In: Epler GR, ed. *Diseases of the Bronchioles*. New York: Raven Press; 1994:187–214.

4

Anatomical Airway Imaging Methods

Phillip M. Boiselle and David A. Lynch

Summary

Recent advances in CT technology have revolutionized non-invasive imaging of the airways *(1–3)*. It is now possible to image the entire airway tree in a few seconds and to create elegant 3-D CT reconstructions of the airways in only a few minutes (Fig. 1) *(1–3)*. Fast scanning techniques also allow for volumetric acquisition of CT data during expiratory maneuvers, revolutionizing the non-invasive assessment of tracheobronchomalacia and small airway disorders. This chapter reviews recent advances in CT imaging techniques and describes currently available CT imaging methods for imaging the large and small airway disorders.

Key Words: Trachea; bronchi; bronchioles; CT; high-resolution CT; 3-D reconstructions; multiplanar reformations.

1. HELICAL AND MULTIDETECTOR-ROW CT TECHNOLOGY

The clinical introduction of helical CT in 1991 dramatically improved the quality of CT images of the airway and other thoracic structures *(4)*. Compared with conventional "stop and shoot" CT scanners, which used a long scan time and acquired a series of individual axial slices with repeated breath holds, helical CT has a short scan time and results in a single volumetric data set in one breath hold. Helical CT eliminated respiratory misregistration, reduced respiratory and cardiac motion, and markedly improved the quality of 2-D and 3-D reformation images *(4)*. However, this technology was still limited by relatively long breath-holding requirements of 25–30 s for routine thick slices and even longer scanning times for thin slice images.

More recently, multidetector CT (MDCT) scanners have been introduced *(5–8)*. Compared with standard helical CT scanners, which employ only a single row of detectors, these newer CT scanners use multiple rows of detectors, allowing for simultaneous registration of multiple channels of information with each gantry rotation *(4–8)*. On the basis of the configuration of the scanner, MDCT scanners currently allow for up to a 64-fold increase in the capacity to register slices compared with single-row helical CT scanners. The speed of scanning with MDCT is further enhanced by fast gantry rotation times, which are <0.5 s with state-of-the-art scanners.

With MDCT scanners, thin-section images of the entire central airways can be obtained in only a few seconds, creating an isotropic data set in which the resolution is the same in the axial, coronal, and sagittal planes *(5)*. Compared with standard helical CT scanners, MDCT scanners provide higher spatial resolution, faster speed, greater anatomic coverage, and higher quality multiplanar reformation and 3-D reconstruction images. Together, these features have combined to revolutionize CT imaging of the large airways.

From: *Contemporary Medical Imaging: CT of the Airways*
Edited by: P. M. Boiselle and D. A. Lynch © Humana Press, Totowa, NJ

A)

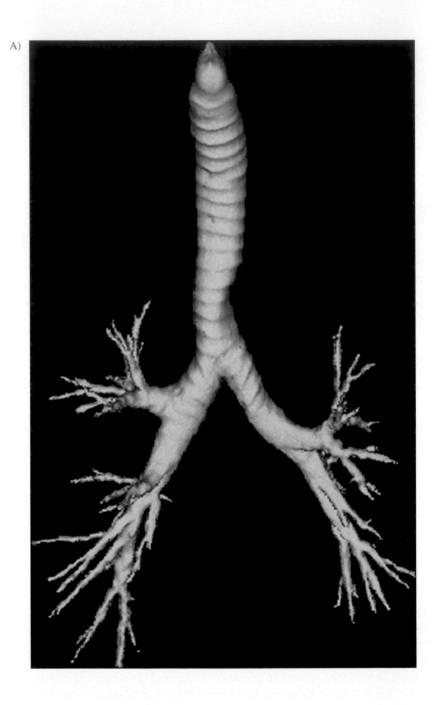

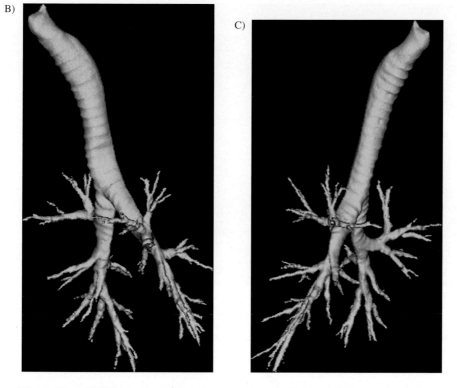

Fig. 1. Normal 3-D segmentation of central airways obtained from axial multidetector CT (MDCT) data set. 3-D segmentation images shown in anterior (**A**) and bilateral oblique (**B, C**) projections provide a continuous anatomical display of the airways from the central trachea and bronchi distally beyond segmental level.

2. AXIAL CT IMAGES

Axial CT images provide anatomical information regarding the airway lumen, airway wall, and adjacent mediastinal and lung structures (Fig. 2). Although axial CT images are considered the reference standard for airway imaging, it is important to be aware of the limitations of the axial plane for assessing the airways, including limited ability to detect subtle airway stenoses; underestimation of the craniocaudal extent of disease; difficulty displaying complex 3-D relationships of the airway; and inadequate representation of airways oriented obliquely to the axial plane *(1,2,9–14)*. These limitations have important implications for the assessment of certain airway disorders such as airway stenoses and complex, congenital airway abnormalities.

3. ALTERNATIVE CT DISPLAY METHODS: MULTIPLANAR AND 3-D RECONSTRUCTIONS

Multiplanar and 3-D reconstruction images help to overcome the limitations of axial images by providing a more anatomically meaningful display of complex structures such as the airways *(1,2,9–15)*. These images have been shown to enhance the detection of airway stenoses (Fig. 3), to aid the assessment of the craniocaudal extent of stenoses, and to clarify complex, congenital airway abnormalities (Fig. 4) *(12)*. They have also been shown to improve diagnostic confidence of

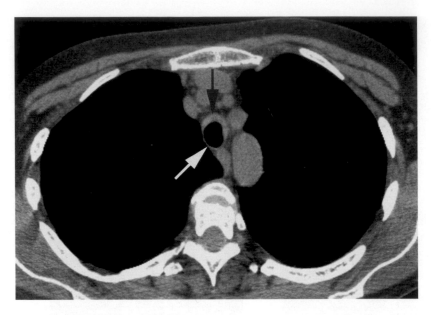

Fig. 2. Axial CT image of patient with relapsing polychondritis. Axial 1.0-mm collimation CT image (soft tissue windows) depicts normal "paper-thin" appearance of posterior membranous tracheal wall (white arrow). Anterior (black arrow) and lateral walls are markedly thickened because of involvement by relapsing polychondritis, an inflammatory condition of the cartilage.

interpretation, enhance pre-procedural planning for bronchoscopy and surgery, and improve communication among radiologists, clinicians, and patients (*1,2,9*). Because multiplanar and 3-D images effectively reduce large CT data sets to a considerably smaller number of images, these methods also facilitate an efficient review of pertinent findings between radiologists and referring clinicians.

Although multiplanar and 3-D reconstruction images do not actually create new data, they provide an alternative method of viewing CT data that is often more visually accessible and anatomically meaningful. Importantly, however, the axial images provide a more comprehensive review of the entirety of the thoracic structures and also serve as an important point of reference for optimal interpretation of multiplanar and 3-D images. Thus, it is essential that the radiologist review the traditional axial images in addition to the alternative display images when interpreting a CT study of the central airways.

4. IMAGING TECHNIQUE: OPTIMIZING IMAGE QUALITY

Although multiplanar and 3-D images can be created from data obtained with any type of helical CT scanners, MDCT scanners are preferred over single-detector helical scanners because of their faster speed and improved resolution. In order to enhance the quality of multiplanar and 3-D images, the use of narrow (<3 mm) collimation is recommended (*1–3,10,15,16*). The use of overlapping reconstruction intervals (50%) is also suggested unless very narrow collimation (0.5–1 mm) is employed (*17*). Such thin collimation results in an isotropic data set, in which spatial resolution is the same regardless of whether images are viewed in the axial, coronal, or sagittal planes, and avoids the need for overlapping reconstruction intervals.

Airway studies are ideally prospectively planned and tailored to the area of interest. However, an advantage of MDCT is the ability to retrospectively change slice thickness, thus allowing one to obtain high-quality reconstruction images from routine CT studies. This feature allows for routine cases

A)

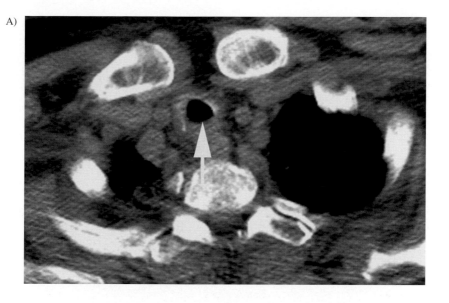

B)

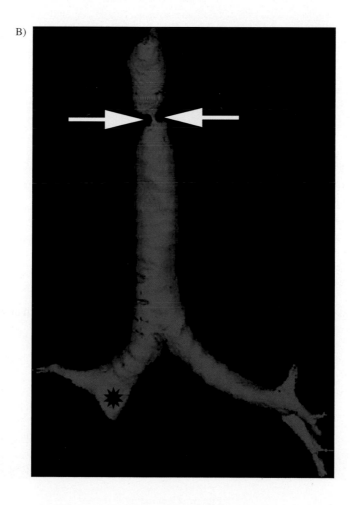

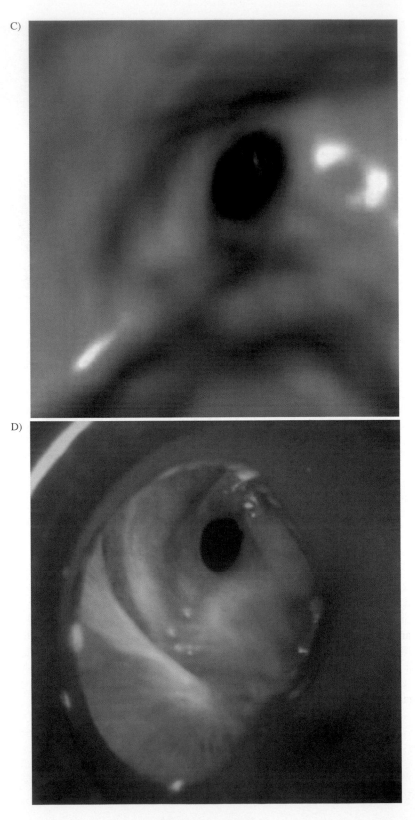

Fig. 3. *(Continued)*

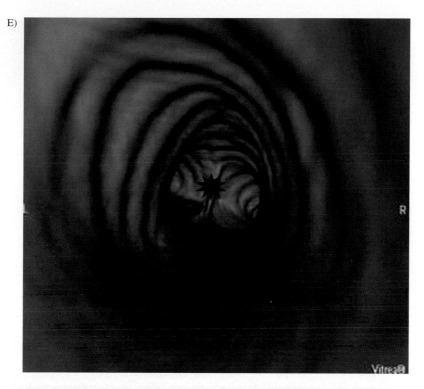

Fig. 3. Focal tracheal stenosis due to airway injury from traumatic intubation. (**A**) Axial 5.0-mm collimation CT image (soft tissue window) demonstrates mild narrowing of proximal trachea (arrow). (**B**) 3-D airway segmentation image depicts focal high-grade tracheal stenosis (arrows), which was markedly underestimated on axial CT image (A) due to partial volume averaging. Apparent cut-off of bronchus intermedius (asterisk) was shown to be due to retained secretions on axial CT (not shown). Thus, 3-D and axial images are complementary. (**C**) 3-D virtual bronchoscopic image shows high-grade narrowing from an intraluminal perspective. (**D**) Conventional bronchoscopy confirmed a high-grade stenosis but could not assess airways beyond stenosis. (**E**) Virtual bronchoscopy allowed assessment of airways distal to lesion, showing normal caliber of trachea through the level of carina (asterisk).

to benefit from the creation of multiplanar and 3-D reconstructions without the need for additional imaging of the patient.

Intravenous contrast is not routinely employed for benign airway disorders such as malacia and post-intubation stenoses. However, it is recommended for evaluation of airway involvement by malignancy and in the setting of extrinsic airway compression by enlarged lymph nodes, vascular anomaly, or thyroid mass. Intravenous contrast is also recommended for the assessment of lobar collapse, as it helps to distinguish an obstructing mass from the adjacent collapsed lung.

Airway imaging is routinely performed at end-inspiration during a single breath hold. State-of-the-art scanners allow the entire central airways to be imaged in a few seconds *(3)*. Such speed is of particular benefit when imaging patients with airway disorders, because many of these patients cannot tolerate longer breath-holding periods. It also aids assessment of young children who may not be able to understand breathing instructions. With fast scanners, such children can be successfully imaged during quiet breathing, without the need for sedation. Quiet breathing can also be employed for severely dyspneic adult patients who may not be able to cooperate with suspended-inspiration breath holding.

A)

B)

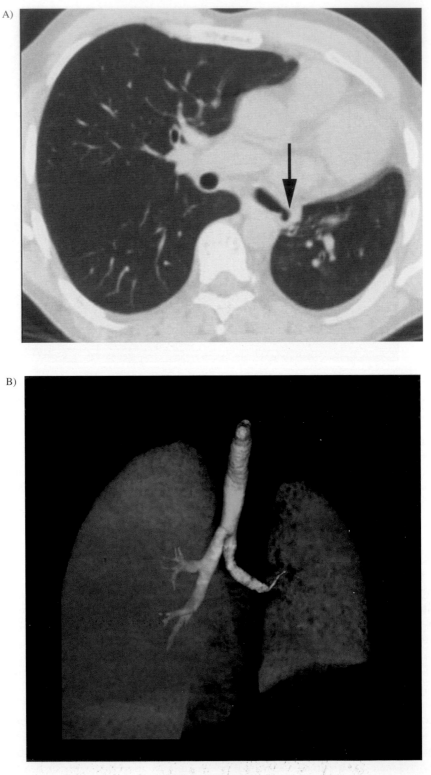

Fig. 4. *(Continued)*

C)

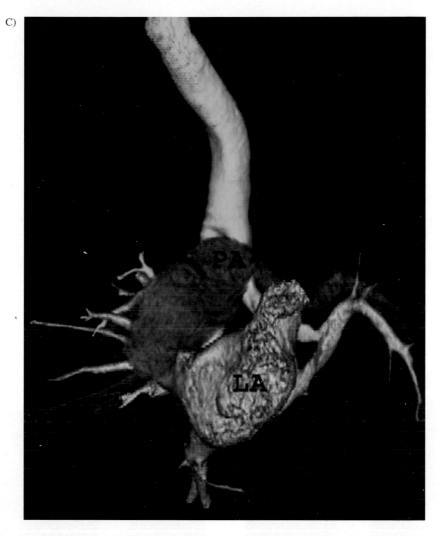

Fig. 4. Enhanced display of congenital thoracic abnormality by 3-D reconstruction images. (**A**) Axial 5-mm collimation CT image (lung window) shows narrowing of distal left main bronchus (arrow) and absence of usual branching pattern into left upper and lower lobe divisions. Also note small left lung with leftward shift of mediastinum. Blurring of left cardiac contour is due to motion artifact. (**B**) 3-D segmentation of airway demonstrates a hypoplastic single bronchus to the diminutive left lung. (**C**) 3-D segmentation of airways (blue), arteries (red), and veins (gold) shows single artery and vein to hypoplastic left lung. LA, left atrium; PA, main pulmonary artery. [Images courtesy of Shezhang Lin, MD, and Diana Litmanovich, MD, BIDMC, Boston, MA]

5. CT RECONSTRUCTION AND REFORMATION METHODS

5.1. 3-D Reconstruction Methods

3-D reconstructions generally require transfer of data to a separate workstation, which allows for interactive display of 3-D images in real time. Fortunately, such workstations are becoming increasingly commonplace in a variety of inpatient and outpatient radiology department settings. Moreover, the newest thin client systems allow for better integration with picture archive communication systems (PACS), so that reconstructions can be created and interpreted during "real time" interpretation of scans.

Most commercially available workstations provide a menu of options comprised of various pre-set reconstruction algorithms, including dedicated airway techniques. The use of clip-editing planes (also referred to as trimming or extraction functions) precludes the need for tracing regions of interest and significantly enhances the efficiency with which one can obtain 3-D images *(2,18)*. Using this method, a trained technologist or radiologist can complete a series of reconstructions in only a few minutes. There are two basic types of 3-D images, external rendering and internal rendering *(9–12,15)*.

External 3-D rendering of the airways depicts the external surface of the airway and its relationship to adjacent structures (Fig. 4) *(11,12)*. In recognition of its similarity to conventional bronchographic images, this technique also been referred to as "CT bronchography." External 3-D rendered images have been shown to improve the detection of subtle airway stenoses (Fig. 3B) and to help illustrate complex airway abnormalities *(11,12)*. 3-D segmentation techniques provide an anatomical map of the airways and can also be used to calculate quantitative estimates of airway volume at end-inspiration and end-expiration (Fig. 5).

Internal rendering of the airways combines helical CT data and virtual reality computing techniques to allow the viewer to navigate through the internal lumen of the airways in a fashion similar to that of conventional bronchoscopy *(17–29)*. Because this method produces images (Fig. 3C and E) that closely correlate with conventional bronchoscopic images, it has been coined "virtual bronchoscopy."

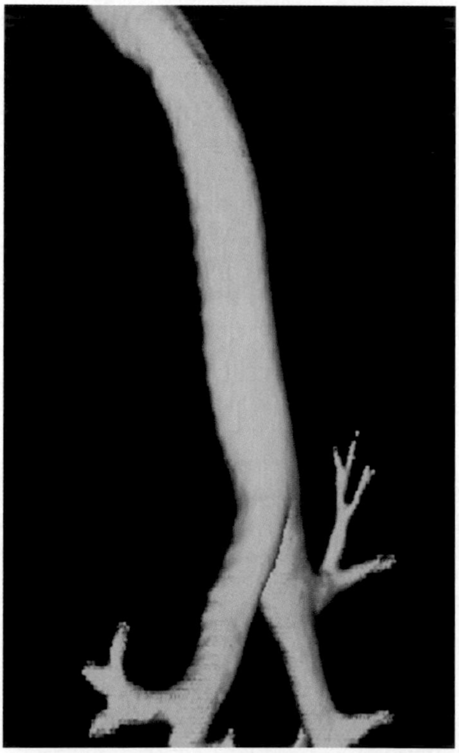

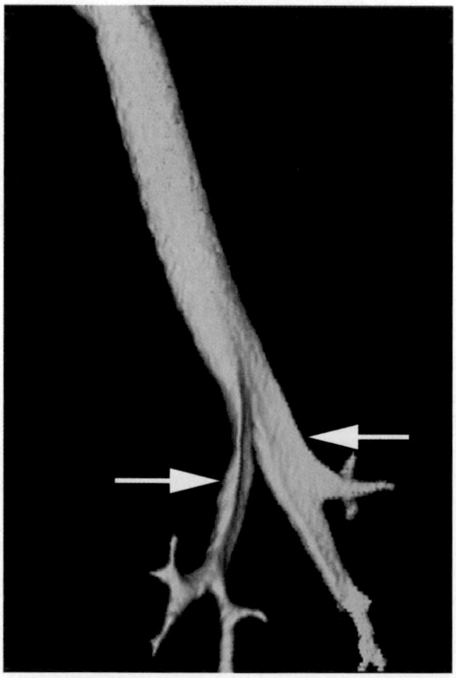

Fig. 5. 3-D segmentation of airways at end-inspiration and dynamic expiration. (**A**) End-inspiratory 3-D image of trachea and bronchi displayed in lateral projection is normal. (**B**) Dynamic expiration 3-D image demonstrates marked expiratory decrease in volume of main bronchi (arrows) consistent with bronchomalacia, a finding confirmed by conventional bronchoscopy.

Virtual bronchoscopy is primarily still an investigational tool *(15)*. Potential applications include the assessment of airway stenoses, guiding transbronchial biopsy procedures, and lung cancer screening *(1,2)*. One of the most promising applications for virtual bronchoscopy is its ability to evaluate the airways distal to a high-grade stenosis, beyond which a conventional bronchoscope cannot pass (Fig. 3) *(27)*.

Recently, virtual bronchoscopy has also been used in conjunction with electromagnetic guidance systems to guide bronchoscopic biopsy of lung nodules *(30)*. This innovative technique has the potential to improve the diagnostic accuracy of bronchoscopic biopsy of lung nodules and also offers the possibility of providing guidance for administering targeted therapy via bronchoscopy. During the procedure, the patient is placed in a low-frequency magnetic field, which is generated by a board below the mattress of the endoscopy table. Sensors are placed on the torso of the patient and on the endoscopy probe. Feedback regarding the position (*x*, *y*, and *z* axes) and movement of the probe is displayed in real time on a monitor. Coupled with data from a previously acquired CT, this creates a virtual environment for guiding biopsy.

5.2. 2-D Multiplanar Reformation Methods

2-D reformation methods include *multiplanar reformations* and *multiplanar volume reformations* *(10,15)*. These images are easy to generate and can be interactively performed in real-time at the CT console, as well as at a dedicated workstation.

Multiplanar reformation images are single-voxel thick sections that may be displayed in coronal and sagittal planes or in a curved fashion along the axis of the airway. Multiplanar volume reformation images comprise a thick slab of adjacent thin slices and represent a block of contiguous images (Fig. 6). The thickness of such blocks or slabs varies, but usually ranges from 5 to 10 mm. Multiplanar

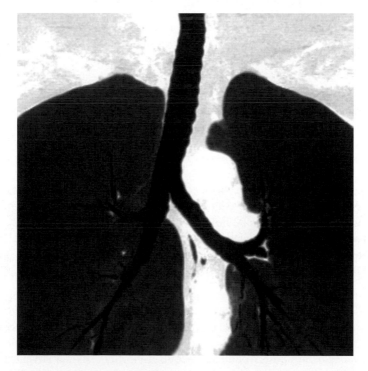

Fig. 6. Normal multiplanar reformation image of the airways. Use of curved oblique plane allows for inclusion of entire central airways on single image. Note use of minimum intensity projection, which highlights low-attenuation voxels.

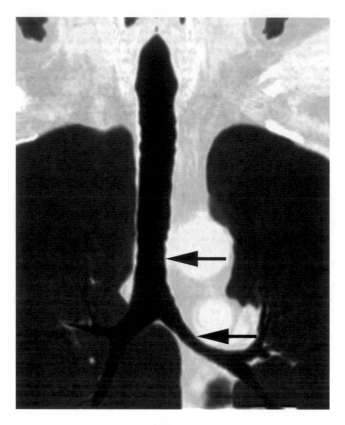

Fig. 7. Multiplanar reformation of tracheobronchial stenosis. Multiplanar reformation image displayed in minimum intensity projection demonstrates diffuse tracheobronchial stenosis most marked in the mid to distal trachea and left main bronchus (arrows).

volume reformation images thus combine the spatial resolution of multiplanar reformation images with the anatomical display of thick slices *(9)*. The use of minimum intensity projection, which highlights low-attenuation voxels, enhances the visibility of airways within lung parenchyma and can be useful for displaying central airway disorders such as stenoses (Fig. 6, 7).

Multiplanar reformation images aid the assessment of airway stenoses, airway stents, tracheomalacia, and extrinsic airway compression. With regard to the assessment of airway stenoses, these methods aid in the depiction of mild stenoses, determining the length of stenoses, and identifying horizontal webs *(13,15,31,32)*. Review of multiplanar images has also been shown to aid pre-procedural planning prior to stent placement or surgery *(32)*.

6. TECHNIQUES FOR DETECTION OF SMALL AIRWAY ABNORMALITY

For detection of small airway abnormality, inspiratory and expiratory high-resolution CT (HRCT) images should be obtained, using thin collimation. The inspiratory high-resolution images may be either obtained as non-contiguous images acquired at intervals of 1 or 2 cm or reconstructed from a volumetric spiral acquisition. Although non-contiguous thin collimation images are associated with a substantially lower radiation dose, volumetric acquisition offers several advantages, including the ability to evaluate the larger airways for associated bronchiectasis, and the possibility of reconstructing multiplanar or post-processed images to facilitate detection and characterization of airway-related

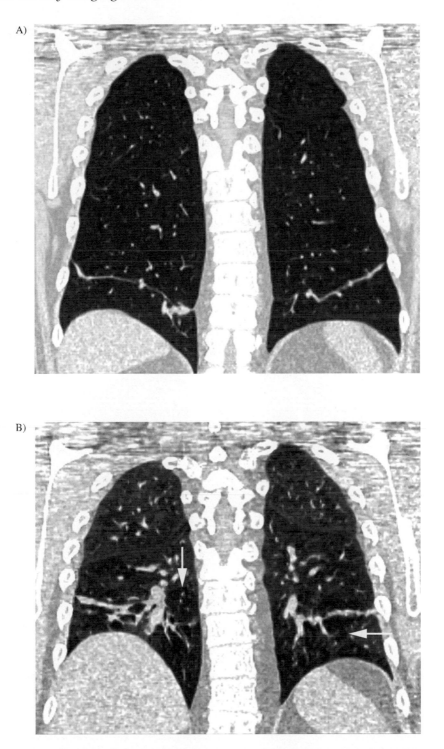

Fig. 8. Volumetric inspiratory and expiratory CT in asthma. (**A**) Inspiratory coronal CT reformation demonstrates homogeneous lung attenuation with superimposed areas of discoid atelectasis in the lower lobes. (**B**) End-expiratory coronal CT reformation image demonstrates inhomogeneous lung attenuation, with lobular areas of low attenuation (arrows), consistent with air trapping.

A)

B)

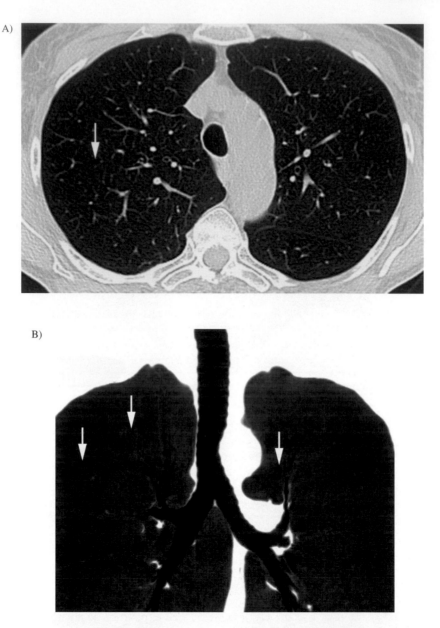

Fig. 9. Minimum intensity projection enhances detection of low-attenuation foci of lung attenuation. (**A**) Axial CT image (2.5-mm collimation, lung algorithm) at the level of aortic arch demonstrates a minimum focus of emphysema (arrow), which could be easily overlooked. (**B**) By enhancing the depiction of the lowest attenuation voxels, the coronal minimum intensity projection (minIP) CT image shows a greater number of foci of centrilobular emphysema (arrows) than routine CT algorithm (A). The same principle applies to depiction of air trapping (Fig. 10).

abnormalities (Fig. 8) *(33)*. In particular, maximum intensity projection images may facilitate the recognition of centrilobular nodules: on thin-section images, it is often difficult to determine whether such nodules are truly centrilobular.

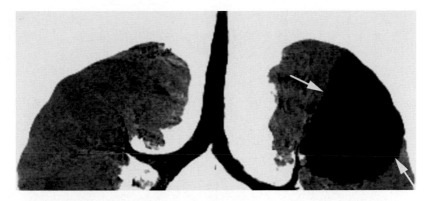

Fig. 10. Minimum intensity projection depiction of air trapping in bronchial atresia. Expiratory coronal reformation minimum intensity projection (minIP) image demonstrates a wedge-shaped area of air trapping in the left upper lobe (arrows) due to bronchial atresia.

6.1. Expiratory CT

There is no clear consensus on the optimal expiratory maneuver for expiratory CT. The majority of studies acquire images at the end of a deep expiration, presumably close to residual volume *(34–36)*. However, others have used an acquisition at the end of a forceful expiration *(37)*. Continuous acquisition of images during a forced or slow expiratory maneuver *(38–42)* (dynamic expiratory CT) may be more sensitive for detection of air trapping, but also leads to detection of air trapping in normal individuals *(39)*. Spirometric confirmation of the level of expiration *(43,44)* is not usually obtained, presumably because spirometric control is quite cumbersome and technically complex. However, in the absence of a spirometric tracing, it can be difficult to determine whether an adequate expiratory effort has been made. In the upper thorax, observation of flattening or concavity of the posterior tracheal membrane can confirm the presence of an appropriate expiratory level, but in the lower lungs it may be difficult to confirm that the expiratory effort is adequate.

Acquiring expiratory CT images in children to document air trapping is challenging. Bilateral decubitus CT allows detection of air trapping in the dependent lung *(45)*. Controlled ventilation in sedated infants allows image acquisition at suspended end-expiration, facilitating detection of air trapping *(46)*. Most recently, cine acquisition during quiet breathing, with a temporal resolution of 0.3 s, has been used to detect air trapping *(47)*.

The number of expiratory CT images acquired in studies of small airway disease is quite variable. Most sites obtain non-contiguous expiratory images in the upper, mid, and lower lungs, as part of their routine HRCT acquisition. The number of scans obtained ranges from 3 *(48)* to 10 *(49)*. However, at other institutions a complete volumetric end-expiratory acquisition is obtained *(50)*, using relatively low dose techniques *(51)*. A further potential technique is the use of short volumetric acquisitions at two or more levels *(52,53)*. The advantage of volumetric acquisition is that it allows multiplanar reconstructions and volume rendering, facilitating recognition of air trapping (Fig. 8) *(51)*. In particular, the use of minimum intensity projections appears to enhance the visual detectability of air trapping (Figs. 9, 10) *(52)*. The use of a density mask technique with expiratory images may facilitate recognition and quantification of air trapping (Fig. 11).

7. DUAL ENERGY CT

Dual source CT scanners were initially designed to increase the temporal resolution of CT. Recently, however, exciting new CT imaging options have become available with this technology by concurrently running two orthogonal tubes at different energy levels (80 and 140 kVp) *(54)*.

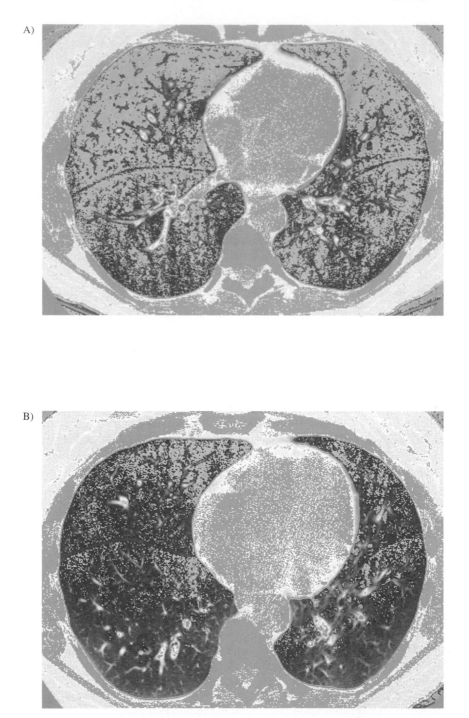

Fig. 11. Density mask image processing in asthma. (**A**) Expiratory axial CT processed using density mask. CT attenuation values less than −856 HU are shown in yellow and represent 56.6% of the total lung area. (Image courtesy of John D Newell, MD, National Jewish Medical and Research Center). (**B**) Expiratory axial CT on same patient, imaged following inhalation of bronchodilator, shows substantial decrease in extent of air trapping, now involving only 14.3% of the lung area. (Image courtesy of John D Newell, MD, National Jewish Medical and Research Center).

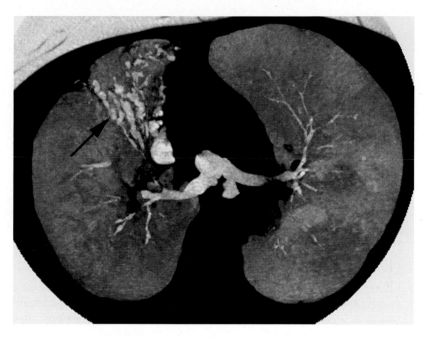

Fig. 12. Isolation of airways using dual energy CT in patient with bronchiectasis. Axial 25-mm-thick maximal intensity projection image displays airways as tubular structures of high density in isolation from vascular structures. Note bronchiectasis anteriorly in right lung (arrow) (Image courtesy of Dr. Ioannis "Johnny" Vlahos, NYU Department of Radiology).

This imaging method is also referred to as "dual energy" CT. By exploiting differences in the mass attenuation coefficients of different materials as a function of energy, this technique provides enhanced discrimination and quantification between different tissue elements, providing greater tissue characterization than traditional CT techniques *(54)*. Because the 80- and 140-kVp data sets are acquired simultaneously, there is no misregistration between the data sets. This allows for precise subtraction or fusion of the data sets that may be utilized to highlight specific substances or anatomy (Fig. 12). At the time of this writing, the potential applications for this exciting new technology are only beginning to be explored. We anticipate that it will play an important role in airway imaging in the near future.

8. CONCLUSION

Recent advances in CT technology have revolutionized the non-invasive assessment of the airway. Although axial CT images provide exquisite anatomic detail of the airway lumen and airway wall, there are important limitations of axial images for assessing the airways. Alternative CT display methods help to overcome these limitations by more accurately depicting the craniocaudal extent of airway abnormalities, detecting subtle areas of stenosis, and defining complex anatomical relationships. The addition of dynamic expiratory images allows for the assessment of airway malacia. For small airway disease, the use of inspiratory and end-expiratory high-resolution images is critical. In all forms of airway disease, the optimal use of CT requires tailoring of technique to the clinical problem being evaluated. Table 1 provides some recommended acquisition and reconstruction techniques for common airway problems (the optimal techniques for evaluation of tracheobronchomalacia, bronchiectasis, and pediatric small airway disease are discussed in Chapters 8, 9, and 16, respectively). Future advances in CT technology, data processing, and image display, as well as increased clinical experience with

Table 1
CT Imaging of Airway Disease: Recommended Techniques

Indication	Phase of respiration	CT acquisition technique	Reconstructions	Optional additional acquisitions or reconstructions
Large airway anatomical imaging	End-inspiration	Volumetric acquisition through central airways on inspiration	Contiguous axial, coronal, and sagittal multiplanar reconstructions	CT bronchography, virtual bronchoscopy, Minimum intensity projection
Tracheobron-chomalacia	During forced expiration	Volumetric acquisition through central airways during forced expiration, using low-dose technique (40 mAs)	Axial	Cine CT acquisition during coughing (with 64-detector scanner)
Bronchiectasis	End-inspiration	Volumetric acquisition through thorax during inspiration	Contiguous 2.5–5 mm axial images, 1–1.5 mm axial images spaced at 10 mm intervals	Multiplanar reformations in coronal and sagittal planes or along axis of airway of interest; paddlewheel reconstruction through central airways
Bronchiolitis	(a) End-inspiration	High-resolution images, acquired either as non-contiguous images or during a volumetric acquisition	1–1.5 mm axial images, spaced at 10–20 mm intervals	Maximum intensity projection (if volumetric acquisition is obtained)
	(b) End-expiration	High-resolution images acquired either as non-contiguous images or during a volumetric acquisition	3–10 axial images, obtained at spaced intervals through the chest	Minimum intensity projection (if volumetric acquisition is obtained); Density mask for quantification of air trapping; Coronal and sagittal multiplanar reformations from volumetric CT data

advanced imaging reconstruction methods, will likely further expand the role of multiplanar and 3-D reconstruction images in the assessment of a wide variety of disorders of the central airways in the near future.

REFERENCES

1. Boiselle PM, Ernst A. Recent advances in central airway imaging. *Chest* 2002;121:1651–1660.
2. Boiselle PM, Reynolds KF, Ernst A. Multiplanar and three-dimensional imaging of the central airways with multidetector CT. *AJR Am J Roentgenol* 2002;179:301–308.
3. Boiselle PM, Lee KS, Ernst A. Multidetector CT of the central airways. *J Thorac Imaging* 2005;20:186–195.
4. Leung AN. Spiral CT of the thorax in daily practice: optimization of technique. *J Thorac Imaging* 1997;12:2–10.

5. Choi RJ, Boiselle PM. Multidetector helical computed tomography. In: Boiselle PM, White CS, Eds. *New Techniques in Thoracic Imaging*. Marcel Dekker: New York; 2001; pp. 71–90.

6. Hu H, He HD, Foley WD, Fox SH. Four multidetector-row helical CT: image quality and volume coverage speed. *Radiology* 2000;215:55–62.

7. Klingenbeck-Regn K, Schaller S, Flohr T, Ohnesorge B, Kopp AF, Baum U. Subsecond multi-slice computed tomography: basics and applications. *Eur J Radiol* 1999;31:110–124.

8. Rydberg J, Buckwalter KA, Caldemeyer KS, et al. Multislice CT: scanning techniques and clinical applications. *Radiographics* 2000;20:1787–1806.

9. Salvolini L, Secchi EB, Costarelli L, De Nicola M. Clinical applications of 2D and 3D CT imaging of the airways—a review. *Eur J Radiol* 2000;34:9–25.

10. Naidich DP, Gruden JF, McGuiness GM, McCauley DI, Bhalla M. Volumetric (helical/spiral) CT (VCT) of the airways. *J Thorac Imaging* 1997;12:11–28.

11. Remy-Jardin M, Remy J, Artaud D, Fribourg M, Naili A. Tracheobronchial tree: assessment with volume rendering-technical aspects. *Radiology* 1998;208:393–398.

12. Remy-Jardin M, Remy J, Artaud D, Fribourg M, Duhamel A. Volume rendering of the tracheobronchial tree: clinical evaluation of bronchographic images. *Radiology* 1998;208:761–770.

13. Remy-Jardin M, Remy J, Deschildre F, Artaud D, Ramon P, Edme JL. Obstructive lesions of the central airways: evaluation by using spiral CT with multiplanar and three-dimensional reformations. *Eur Radiol* 1996;6:807–816.

14. Rubin GD. Data explosion: the challenge of multidetector-row CT. *Eur J Radiol* 2000;36:74–80.

15. Ravenel JG, McAdams HP, Remy-Jardin M, Remy J. Multidimensional imaging of the thorax: practical applications. *J Thorac Imaging* 2001;16:269–281.

16. Rubin GD, Beailieu CF, Argiro V, et al. Perspective volume rendering of CT and MR images: applications for endoscopic imaging. *Radiology* 1996;199:321–330.

17. Higgins WE, Ramaswamy K, Swift RD, McLennan G, Hoffman EA. Virtual bronchoscopy for three-dimensional pulmonary image assessment: state of the art and future needs. *Radiographics* 1998;18:761–778.

18. Lawler LP, Fishman EK. Multi-detector row CT of thoracic disease with emphasis on 3D volume rendering and CT angiography. *Radiographics* 2001;21:1257–1273.

19. Honda O, Johkoh T, Yamamoto S, et al. Comparison of quality of multiplanar reconstructions and direct coronal multidetector CT scans of the lung. *AJR Am J Roentgenol* 2002;79:875–879.

20. Haponik EF, Aquino SL, Vining DJ. Virtual bronchoscopy. *Clin Chest Med* 1999;20:201–217.

21. Hopper KD, Iyriboz AT, Wise SW, Neuman JD, Mauger DT, Kasales CJ. Mucosal detail at CT virtual reality: surface versus volume rendering. *Radiology* 2000;214:517–522.

22. Kauczor HU, Woicke B, Fischer B, Mildenberger P, Lorenz J, Thelen M. Three-dimensional helical CT of the tracheobronchial tree: evaluation of imaging protocols and assessment of suspect stenoses with bronchoscopy correlation. *AJR Am J Roentgenol* 1996,167.419–424.

23. Boiselle PM, Patz EF Jr, Vining DJ, Weissleder R, Shepard JA, McLoud TC. Imaging of mediastinal lymph nodes: CT, MR, and FDG PET. *Radiographics* 1998;18:1061–1069.

24. McAdams HP, Goodman PC, Kussin P. Virtual bronchoscopy for directing transbronchial needle aspiration of hilar and mediastinal lymph nodes: a pilot study. *AJR Am J Roentgenol* 1998;170:1361 1364.

25. Rodenwaldt J, Kopka L, Roedel R, Margas A, Grabbe E. 3D virtual endoscopy of the upper airway: optimization of the scan parameters in a cadaver phantom and clinical assessment. *J Comput Assist Tomogr* 1997;21:405–411.

26. Fleiter T, Merkle EM, Aschoff AJ, et al. Comparison of real-time virtual and fiberoptic bronchoscopy in patients with bronchial carcinoma: opportunities and limitations. *AJR Am J Roentgenol* 1997;169:1591–1595.

27. Summers RM, Selbie WS, Malley JD, et al. Polypoid lesions of airways: early experience with computer-assisted detection by using virtual bronchoscopy and surface curvature. *Radiology* 1998;208:331–337.

28. Summers RM, Shaw DJ, Shelhamer JH. CT virtual bronchoscopy of simulated endobronchial lesions: effect of scanning, reconstruction, and display settings and potential pitfalls. *AJR Am J Roentgenol* 1998;170:947–950.

29. Vining DJ, Liu K, Choplin RH, Haponik EF. Virtual bronchoscopy: relationships of virtual reality endobronchial simulations to actual bronchoscopic findings. *Chest* 1996;109:549–553.

30. Becker HD, Herth F, Ernst A, et al. Bronchoscopic biopsy of peripheral lung lesions under electromagnetic guidance. *J Bronchol* 2005;12:9–13.

31. Quint LE, Whyte RI, Kazerooni EA, et al. Stenosis of the central airways: evaluation by using helical CT with multiplanar reconstructions. *Radiology* 1995;194:871–877.

32. LoCicero J, Costello P, Campos CT, et al. Spiral CT with multiplanar and 3-D reconstructions accurately predicts tracheobronchial pathology. *Ann Thorac Surg* 1996;62:811–817.

33. Beigelman-Aubry C, Hill C, Guibal A, Savatovsky J, Grenier PA. Multi-detector row CT and postprocessing techniques in the assessment of diffuse lung disease. *Radiographics* 2005;25:1639–1652.

34. Spaggiari E, Zompatori M, Verduri A, et al. Early smoking-induced lung lesions in asymptomatic subjects. Correlations between high resolution dynamic CT and pulmonary function testing. *Radiol Med (Torino)* 2005;109:27–39.

35. Kauczor HU, Hast J, Heussel CP, Schlegel J, Mildenberger P, Thelen M. Focal airtrapping at expiratory high-resolution CT: comparison with pulmonary function tests. *Eur Radiol* 2000;10:1539–1546.
36. Leung AN, Fisher K, Valentine V, et al. Bronchiolitis obliterans after lung transplantation: detection using expiratory HRCT. *Chest* 1998;113:365–370.
37. Lee ES, Gotway MB, Reddy GP, Golden JA, Keith FM, Webb WR. Early bronchiolitis obliterans following lung transplantation: accuracy of expiratory thin-section CT for diagnosis. *Radiology* 2000;216:472–477.
38. Stern EJ, Webb WR. Dynamic imaging of lung morphology with ultrafast high-resolution computed tomography. *J Thorac Imaging* 1993;8:273–282.
39. Webb WR, Stern EJ, Kanth N, Gamsu G. Dynamic pulmonary CT: findings in healthy adult men. *Radiology* 1993;186:117–124.
40. Stern EJ, Webb WR, Gamsu G. Dynamic quantitative computed tomography. A predictor of pulmonary function in obstructive lung diseases. *Invest Radiol* 1994;29:564–569.
41. Gotway MB, Lee ES, Reddy GP, Golden JA, Webb WR. Low-dose, dynamic, expiratory thin-section CT of the lungs using a spiral CT scanner. *J Thorac Imaging* 2000;15:168–172.
42. Zhang J, Hasegawa I, Hatabu H, Feller-Kopman D, Boiselle PM. Frequency and severity of air trapping at dynamic expiratory CT in patients with tracheobronchomalacia. *AJR Am J Roentgenol* 2004;182:81–85.
43. Zeidler MR, Goldin JG, Kleerup EC, et al. Small airways response to naturalistic cat allergen exposure in subjects with asthma. *J Allergy Clin Immunol* 2006;118:1075–1081.
44. Goldin JG, Tashkin DP, Kleerup EC, et al. Comparative effects of hydrofluoroalkane and chlorofluorocarbon beclomethasone dipropionate inhalation on small airways: assessment with functional helical thin-section computed tomography. *J Allergy Clin Immunol* 1999;104:S258–S267.
45. Choi SJ, Choi BK, Kim HJ, et al. Lateral decubitus HRCT: a simple technique to replace expiratory CT in children with air trapping. *Pediatr Radiol* 2002;32:179–182.
46. Long FR, Williams RS, Adler BH, Castile RG. Comparison of quiet breathing and controlled ventilation in the high-resolution CT assessment of airway disease in infants with cystic fibrosis. *Pediatr Radiol* 2005;35:1075–1080.
47. Goo HW, Kim HJ. Detection of air trapping on inspiratory and expiratory phase images obtained by 0.3-second cine CT in the lungs of free-breathing young children. *AJR Am J Roentgenol* 2006;187:1019–1023.
48. Hashimoto M, Tate E, Watarai J, Sasaki M. Air trapping on computed tomography images of healthy individuals: effects of respiration and body mass index. *Clin Radiol* 2006;61:883–887.
49. Chooi WK, Morcos SK. High resolution volume imaging of airways and lung parenchyma with multislice CT. *Br J Radiol* 2004;77 Spec No 1:S98–S105.
50. Mergo PJ, Williams WF, Gonzalez-Rothi R, et al. Three-dimensional volumetric assessment of abnormally low attenuation of the lung from routine helical CT: inspiratory and expiratory quantification. *AJR Am J Roentgenol* 1998;170:1355–1360.
51. Nishino M, Hatabu H. Volumetric expiratory HRCT imaging with MSCT. *J Thorac Imaging* 2005;20:176–185.
52. Berstad AE, Aalokken TM, Kolbenstvedt A, Bjortuft O. Performance of long-term CT monitoring in diagnosing bronchiolitis obliterans after lung transplantation. *Eur J Radiol* 2006;58:124–131.
53. Wittram C, Batt J, Rappaport DC, Hutcheon MA. Inspiratory and expiratory helical CT of normal adults: comparison of thin section scans and minimum intensity projection images. *J Thorac Imaging* 2002;17:47–52.
54. Kalender W. Dual energy CT: Is there escape from the Hounsfield unit cage? In: Glazer GM, Rubin GD, Eds. Stanford Radiology 8th Annual International Symposium on Multidetector-Row CT Syllabus, 2006, Stanford University School of Medicine, Palo Alto, CA; pp. 27–28.

5

Functional Airway Imaging Methods

Jonathan G. Goldin

Summary

The techniques for CT evaluation of the airway are directed at improving both the detection and measurement of structural changes as well as providing quantitative measures of function. With the introduction of the latest generation of sub-half-second multidetector computed tomography (MDCT) scanners, scanning the entire lung at a static lung volume, as well as dynamic imaging during a breathing maneuver, is now possible. In order for quantitative image analysis to be clinically useful, it must be easy to perform reproducible, observer independent, and valid measurement of disease presence and extent. Furthermore, imaging protocols must be tailored to ensure the validity and reproducibility of the quantitative measures. The accuracy and reproducibility of all functional imaging measurements are dependent on both subject- and scanner-related image acquisition and reconstruction features. The quantitative information obtained with high-resolution CT (HRCT) can advance our understanding of pulmonary pathophysiology and offer insight into the potential mechanisms involved in the progression of lung disease. Prior to quantitation, accurate and valid segmentation of the thoracic anatomy, including the lungs, lobes and segments, and airways from the trachea to the segmental airways, must be performed. The advances in functional imaging of the airways have become clinically useful, and most likely these techniques will become increasingly utilized, complementing and potentially replacing conventional lung function tests. Unlike conventional lung function tests, these techniques very powerful and useful because of the ability of CT measures of airway structure function to assess not only individual lungs but also individual lung segments and even smaller regions.

Key Words: Computed tomography; function; lung; airways; segmentation; computer-aided diagnosis.

1. INTRODUCTION

The techniques for CT evaluation of the airway are directed at improving both the detection and measurement of structural changes as well as providing quantitative measures of function. It is important to distinguish the static and dynamic abnormalities as well as assess regional (segmental) variations. The ability to characterize regional function offers the potential to detect the early onset of airway disease before the onset of visible structural changes on conventional CT imaging or detection by global conventional lung function tests. Furthermore, these techniques offer the possibility to monitor efficacy of new airway-targeted therapies better.

With the introduction of the latest generation of sub-half-second multidetector computed tomography (MDCT) scanners, scanning the entire lung at a static lung volume [including total lung capacity (TLC), functional reserve capacity (FRC), and residual volume (RV)], as well as dynamic imaging during a breathing maneuver, is now possible. This has enabled more precise evaluation of both the structure and function of the airways. Multiplanar reconstructions of the data sets allow for visualization and measurement of the airways and quantitation of regional lung attenuation

From: *Contemporary Medical Imaging: CT of the Airways*
Edited by: P. M. Boiselle and D. A. Lynch © Humana Press, Totowa, NJ

changes indicative of air trapping *(1–3)*. Using minimum intensity projection reconstructions, air trapping on these multi-slice studies can be further visualized *(2–6)*. Combined with the development of sophisticated image analysis software, reproducible and accurate quantitative measures can be obtained.

In order for quantitative image analysis to be clinically useful, it must be easy to perform reproducible, observer independent, and valid measurement of disease presence and extent *(7)*. Furthermore, imaging protocols need to be tailored to ensure the validity and reproducibility of the quantitative measures. The purpose of this chapter is to offer practical guidelines for performing the functional CT imaging examinations and computer-aided measurements of the airways.

2. IMAGING PROTOCOLS

With rapidly changing CT technology, the best imaging protocol for assessing the airways is in constant evolution *(8–11)*. Current MDCT scanners with 16 or more channels can now rapidly acquire image volumes through the entire lungs in less than 8 s. These data sets allow for sub-millimeter reconstruction of isotropic voxels along any axis, which in turn enables 3-D volume rendering of the airways to be performed. This has improved the accuracy of measurements of airway dimensions by allowing multiplanar reconstructions to assess the different airway generations using planes perpendicular to the long axis of the airway *(12)*.

There has also been an improvement in the lower limit to spatial resolution, dependent on pixels size and the intrinsic point spread function, of current generation CT scanners to a pixel size of 0.25×0.25 mm. The smallest visible normal airways on which reasonably accurate measurements of the diameter and wall thickness can be made are in the range of 1.5–2 mm in diameter (with corresponding wall thickness of 0.2–0.3 mm), which corresponds to the seventh to ninth generation of small airways *(13–18)*. An additional benefit of full lung volume scanning is that it allows data to be acquired through broad regions of interest (ROIs) during different phases of respiration or under different physiologic and pharmacologic conditions, providing further insights into the relationships between structure and function *(19–21)*.

It is important that the CT machines are calibrated correctly and close attention is paid to all aspects of image acquisition and reconstruction to ensure repeatable valid measurements. In functional imaging, the CT scanner is used as a densitometer to make quantitative measures and, akin to all medical devices used for lung function measurements (e.g., spirometer) *(22)*, requires precise calibration and standardization of acquisition and interpretation techniques. To date, no such guidelines, such as those that exist for conventional lung function testing, exist for functional CT imaging although some progress has been made to address standardization in the setting of clinical trials *(23–26)*.

A typical static functional imaging protocol (acquired at a suspended lung volume) to assess the airways is summarized in Table 1. The most often used imaging protocols are obtained at suspended inspiration (which can be called static-volume triggered scans) at either TLC or RV. Sometimes, scanning at FRC rather than TLC is performed. All scans should be performed in the supine position, without intravenous contrast and with careful attention given to the breath-hold instructions provided along with the faithful execution of the required breath-hold by the patient. The automatic voice instructions should never be utilized.

In contrast to the acquisition of images at static suspended lung volumes, dynamic functional studies can now be performed during different breathing maneuvers. Dynamic expiratory high-resolution CT (HRCT) can be acquired during a forced expiration. A typical sequence is summarized in Table 2. Dynamic CT acquisition requires image acquisition times between 50 and 200 ms in order to acquire a sufficient number of images during a respiratory maneuver *(14,16,27–32)*. The necessary technical parameters will vary according to the specific application, degree of resolution

Table 1
Typical Imaging Protocol for Static End-Inspiratory
and End-Expiratory Volume Assessment

CT protocol	Static static
Optimum CT platform	MDCT 64 detector CT
Minimum CT requirement	MDCT 16 detectors
Series 1	TLC scout
Series 2	TLC full chest
Breathing instructions	Take a full and deep breath in until lungs are completely full
kVp, mAs	120, 80–100
Collimation	16 × 0.75
Table feed	18 mm (1.5)
Rotation speed	≤0.5 s
Reconstruction	0.6–2 mm no overlap
Kernel	Smooth, no edge enhancement
Breath-hold	4–10 s
Dose	
Series 3	RV scout
Series 4	RV full chest
Breathing instructions	After deep breath in blow all air out until lungs feel completely empty
kVp, mAs	120, 80–100
Collimation	16 × 0.75
Table feed	18 mm (1.5)
Rotation speed	≤0.5 s
Reconstruction	1.5 mm/1 mm overlap
Kernel	B 30 f
Breath-hold	7–10 s
Dose	

MDCT, multidetector computed tomography; TLC, total lung capacity; RV, residual volume.

required, and anatomic region under examination. ECG gating may also be used to study the lower lobes without the presence of cardiac motion artifacts *(33)*. Dose is an important consideration given the number of images acquired during a dynamic acquisition series, and low-dose techniques are recommended *(34)*.

New methods for acquiring rapid volumetric images during multiple respiratory cycles are currently under development *(35)*. This is similar to the approach used for cardiac CT acquisitions where retrospective gating is used to build up images at multiple phases from the portions of successive heartbeats. Adaptation of this technique for respiratory dynamic image acquisition is more challenging given the greater length of the respiratory cycle and marked cycle-to-cycle variations in a respiration (as compared with the cardiac cycle). For most pulmonary functional applications, sequences acquired through the upper, middle, and lower lungs provide an adequate sample of the lungs. By integrating the spirometric and imaging data, changes in lung attenuation for isolated ROIs can be measured as a function of time, airflow, and lung volume.

The accuracy and reproducibility of all functional imaging measurements are dependent on both subject- and scanner-related image acquisition and reconstruction features. Subject-related image

Table 2
CT Protocol Dynamic Volume

Airflow protocol	Dynamic dynamic
Series 5	Dynamic
Breathing instructions	After deep breath in blow air out as hard and fast as possible
kVp, mAs	120, 80–100
Collimation	16 × 0.75
Table feed	0 (no feed)
Rotation speed	≤0.5 s
Image sequence	5 q 1 s and 5 q 3 s5 scans every 1 s followed by 5 scans every 3 s
Reconstruction	3 mm contiguous
Kernel	B 30 f
Scan duration	20 s
Dose	

quality determinants include immobility and breath-hold reproducibility. The volume at which the lung is imaged is the most important factor influencing both visual and computer-aided quantitative assessment of the airways (36,37). This is due to the fact that the normal airway dimensions change during the respiratory cycle, thus affecting direct measurements of airway size and wall thickness. Secondly, an important indirect CT measure of air trapping is based on the pixel density (CT attenuation density) of the lungs, which is directly proportional to volume at which it is measured.

A standardization of the lung volume to TLC, RV, or a known lung volume in between the two at the time of scan acquisition is critical to ensure both the validity of quantitative measures and reproducibility of measures on repeated studies. This is most accurately achieved with spirometric gating in which the CT scan is triggered and airflow is mechanically inhibited at a predetermined user-selected level of breath-hold (1,36,38,39). The availability of commercial apparatus or spirometric gating or triggering is scarce, and thus, most quantitative studies are performed without such methods. It is possible with volume acquisition techniques to confirm lung volume reproducibility without the need for spirometric gating (40,41). Good reproducibility of lung volumes within 10% of baseline volume has been achieved in multicenter studies without gating (23).

Several scanner-related hardware and software features [e.g., collimation, kilovolt peak (kVp), milliampere per second (mAs), reconstruction algorithm] can also affect the accuracy, reproducibility, and validity of quantitative assessment of functional CT image data (42–46). There has been a dramatic increase in the rate of evolution of CT scanner technology. The improvement in technology has, in fact, lead to increased accuracy and precision in the quantitation of lung disease. This has been achieved through improvements in spatial resolution, temporal resolution, signal-to-noise ratio, and better reconstruction techniques. As CT technology evolves, there will be significant need to create imaging protocols that preserve the fundamental characteristics. Beam hardening causes artifactual variations in brightness or grayscale non-uniformities that are particularly evident in the vicinity of anatomic structures, such as the bony thorax and heart, and will affect image quality and, subsequently, measurement accuracy and validity. The radiographic tissue attenuation inside of a single volume element (pixel area X slice thickness) is represented by a single Hounsfield number [Hounsfield Unit (HU)]. Partial volume errors due to the finite image slice thickness and, to a lesser extent, the finite area of a pixel will cause the largest errors in the assessment of air trapping, which are based on measuring the percentage of air in each voxel. Finally, the reconstruction algorithm or kernel creates the digital image from the raw scan data measured at the x-ray detectors. CT scanners have several choices of reconstruction kernel, and manufacturers differ in their naming and interpretation of the optimum kernel to be used for lung imaging.

Several studies have examined the effects of technical parameter variability on quantitative CT results, such as that of Kemerink et al. *(47)*, which has focused on the reproducibility of average HU values in homogeneous media or over large ROIs in heterogeneous media *(42,47)*. Boedeker et al. *(44)* studied the effect of different reconstruction kernels on the assessment of CT attenuation for the assessment of lung attenuation in a multicenter study of emphysema patients. Using the data acquired in one acquisition (one exposure), these subjects had their data reconstructed first with a standard filter (defined in the table such as GE standard) and then with a smoothing filter and/or a sharpening filter (e.g., GE Bone) and/or an over-enhancing filter (e.g., GE Lung), where the filter type was defined by its characteristics on the modulation transfer function (MTF) curve described in Fig. 1. The attenuation mask score was calculated for each reconstructed data set. Then, for each subject, the difference in density mask score between the reference reconstruction algorithm (i.e., standard) and

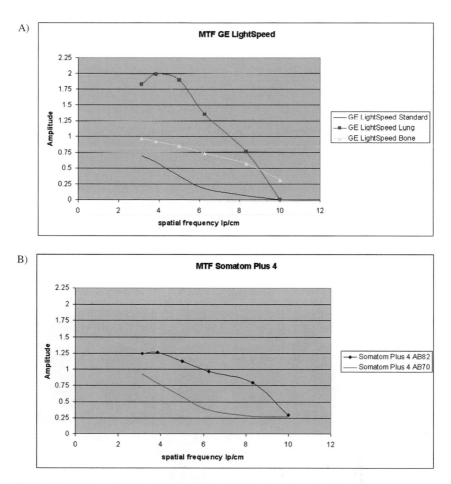

Fig. 1. (A) Modulation transfer function (MTF) curve (a plot of spatial frequency vs. amplitude) for GE LightSpeed reconstruction algorithms. *y*-Axis is modulation value, *x*-axis is spatial frequency. **(B)** MTF curve for Siemens Somatom Plus 4 reconstruction algorithms. *y*-Axis is modulation value, *x*-axis is spatial frequency.

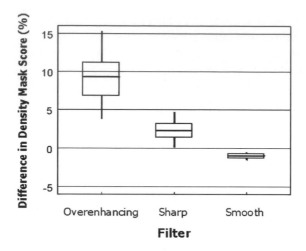

Fig. 2. Box plot of the change in density mask score (compared with standard filter) as a function of reconstruction filter category. Note that over-enhancing filter can differ from standard by as much as 15% (average of 9% for the category).

the alternative algorithm (smooth or sharp or over-enhancing) was calculated. Figure 2 demonstrates that the use of an over-enhancing filter [such as GE Lung (GE Medical Systems, Milwaukee, USA)] can yield results that are as much as 15% higher than the same data set reconstructed with a standard filter, illustrating the magnitude of the effects of kernel alone in these relevant quantitative measures. The effect of kernel on follow-up quantitative measures is well demonstrated in Fig. 3, which illustrates a subject with emphysema who was scanned on two occasions with good reproduction of lung volumes but incorrect kernel use in the reconstruction of the 6-month visit scan. This leads to an apparent increase in density mask score (from 16.2 to 29.5%) for the 6-month follow-up study. If the subject was on a treatment regimen during this period, the effects of the reconstruction kernel would mask any improvement due to the therapy. The importance of attention to detail at the time of scan acquisition cannot be overstated.

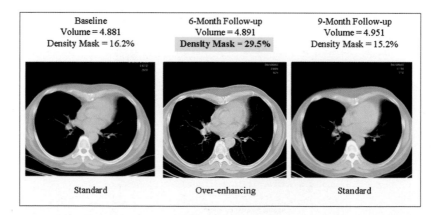

Fig. 3. CT images and density mask measurements for one patient over three visits where the 6-month follow-up (middle visit) images were reconstructed with an over-enhancing filter and the other visits were reconstructed with a standard filter. The density mask value artificially increases from 16.2 to 29.5% due primarily to reconstruction filter effects.

3. TECHNIQUES FOR CT QUANTITATIVE MEASURE OF AIRWAY STRUCTURE AND FUNCTION

The quantitative information obtained with HRCT can advance our understanding of pulmonary pathophysiology and offer insights into the potential mechanisms involved *(15,16,48–65)*. Prior to quantitation, accurate and valid segmentation of the thoracic anatomy, including the lungs, lobes, and segments as well as the airways from the trachea to the segmental airways, must be performed. These techniques are demonstrated in Figs 4 and 5. There has been a proliferation in investigations to provide quantitative structural and functional information from digitally acquired image data. These methods include visual quantitation scoring systems, image display (such as multiplanar reformations, surface shading for 3-D, and volume rendering) *(66–69)*, anatomic image quantitation (e.g., area and volume of airways and lungs) *(38,50,54,55,70–78)*, and regional characterization of lung tissue (analyzing attenuation, changes in attenuation, and texture patterns in the imaged lung) *(11,34,79–82)*. QIA can also be used as a measure of the efficacy of novel therapeutic techniques due to their ability to detect subtle regional variations *(83)*.

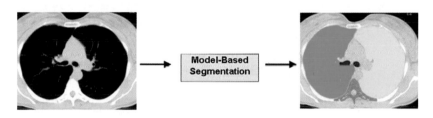

Fig. 4. Model-based segmentation of the thorax: spine (orange), main stem bronchi (red), right lung (green), and left lung (yellow).

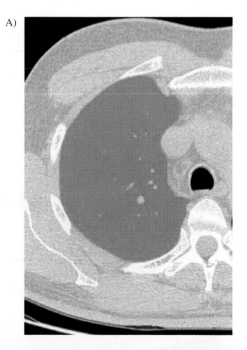

Fig. 5. *(Continued)*

B)

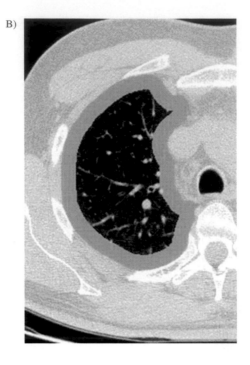

C)

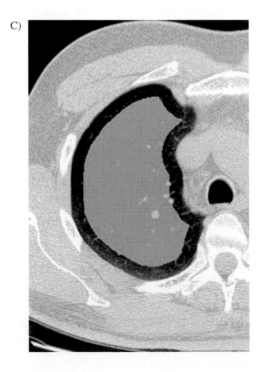

D)

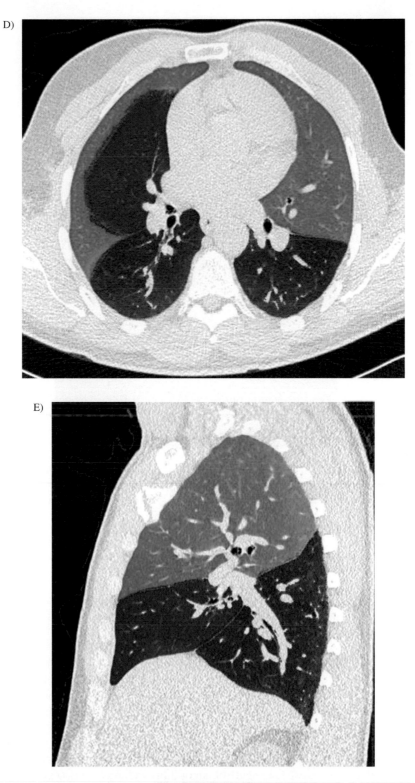

Fig. 5. *(Continued)*

F)

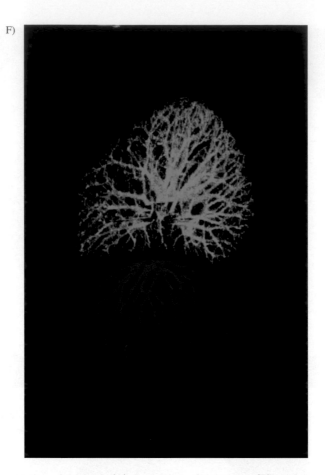

Fig. 5. Regional segmentation of the lung: (**A**) single slice of right lung; (**B**) axial component; (**C**) peripheral (outer 1 cm) component; and (**D**) lobar segmentation of the right lung into upper (green), middle (red), and lower (purple lobes) in axial (**E**) and coronal planes and (**F**) 3-D reconstruction of volumetric segmentation of airways in each lobe.

Two basic types of QIA measurements are made to evaluate airway disease. The first category is direct measures of airway dimensions (including lumen size, wall thickness). The second category consists of measurements of lung volumes and indirect measures of air trapping in the lung based on attenuation statistics within the lung region supplied by the airway generation being evaluated.

3.1. Airway Measurements

Quantitative analysis of the structure and function of the human airway tree is important for comprehensive diagnosis and assessment of various lung diseases, particularly obstructive diseases such as asthma, bronchiectasis, and emphysema. While CT has been used to obtain information about airway structure, methods to extract this information in an automated fashion have been limited in terms of robustness and the extent of the airway tree that has been successfully segmented. Although current segmentation methods have made an important contribution to lung imaging research, they use limited knowledge of the airways in heuristic algorithms and, thus, only segment a small fraction of the airways beyond the fourth and fifth generations *(74,84–91)*. Even with multidetector CT technology, airway walls that turn and run parallel to the scan plane are difficult for current systems to detect because of partial volume averaging and lack of continuity in 3-D. Because the majority of airways run oblique to scan plane at some point, intelligent image segmentation methods are required.

Airway segmentation is a challenging task for several reasons. When a single voxel contains a mixture of tissues of different attenuation, the resulting attenuation will be an intermediate value due to partial volume. This is a significant cause of artifact when attempting to segment small airways. Although an airway would be expected to have an attenuation in the lumen of −1000 HU surrounded by a wall of soft tissue attenuation, partial volume averaging means that voxels in the lumen will typically have values well above −1000 HU and the airway walls will have much lower attenuation than soft tissue; thus, the contrast between the lumen and wall is low, making attenuation-based thresholding an unreliable technique for airway segmentation (Fig. 6). The difficulty is even greater

A)

B)

C)

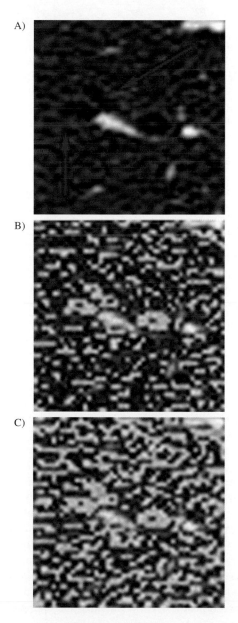

Fig. 6. *(Continued)*

D)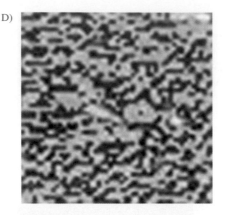

Fig. 6. Difficulties in segmenting airways in CT-based attenuation threshold. (**A**) Original image with airways branching oblique to scan plane shown with red arrows. (**B**) Thresholding below –970 HU with incomplete segmentation of airways. (**C**) Thresholding below –930 HU with segmentation of airways still incomplete but more background parenchymal pixels incorrectly included. (**D**) Thresholding below –900 HU with complete airway segmentation but contiguous "leakage" into background pixels.

for airways running parallel to the scan plane. Given these challenges, a number of algorithms have been developed that have made significant contributions to the problem.

Tschirren developed a method for automated segmentation of human airway tree, its skeletonization, and identification of branch points *(84)*. Airway segmentation occurs through seeded region growing. The focus of this work was branch point intra- and inter-subject airway branch point matching. Wood also applied thresholding and region-growing to segment the airway tree *(86)*. Branch points were determined automatically to enable measurement of branch length and segment diameter. They validated these measurements in a plexiglass phantom as well as applying the technique to human image data. They noted that with simple thresholding and region-growing, there are leaks into nearby structures with similar intensities and manual editing is required. They found that simple thresholding could not resolve airways smaller than 2 mm that were oriented close to the scan plane. Aykac added a low-pass filtering step to remove noise and a grayscale morphological operation to identify 2-D candidate airways on CT slices and then reconstruct a connected 3-D airway tree *(85)*. Kiraly combined adaptive region-growing with 2-D morphological operations with structuring elements of various sizes to generate airway candidates *(87)*. The system requires user intervention to select a filter to be applied to the image data prior to segmentation, and editing may be needed to remove segmentation leakages through partial volume averaged airway walls.

Park used a rule-based representation of knowledge about airways in the segmentation process *(90)*. They included rules relating to brightness of airways and vessels, the adjacency of these structures, and the degree of wall existence around airways. These rules were applied to 2-D image candidates to classify them as airways, vessels, or neither. Uncertainty in the rules and classification was handled using fuzzy logic. Fetita used similar domain knowledge but formulated the problem as a 3-D controlled growth (energy minimization) approach *(88)*. Chiplunkar used a priori information on how lung airways branch and adaptively determined thresholds to segment airway trees *(89)*. Reinhardt et al. *(92)* focused their airway segmentation work on improving the accuracy of lumen diameter and wall thickness measurements. A simple model of the scanning process for an ideal airway was developed. The model predicts the shape of the gray-level profiles along rays cast from the airway centroid and uses a maximum-likelihood method to estimate airway inner and outer radius. An optimization technique is used to adjust the model parameters and minimize differences between the predicted and the actual observed profiles. They validated the approach using a plexiglass phantom.

Current techniques perform reasonably well given the challenges associated with airway segmentation. The technique described by Wood showed a 20% overestimation of full airway diameters larger than 2 mm in diameter *(86)*. An alternative technique proposed by Amirav *(93)* utilizing the full width at half maximum principal achieved a coefficient of variation of 4.4% for airways approximately 6 mm in diameter. However, for airways of around 1 mm, this technique was less accurate, achieving a coefficient of variation of about 16.6%. More sophisticated model-based methods for accurate detection and measurements of the airway walls have been shown to be more accurate over a wide range of airway sizes between 1 and 15 mm in diameter. Reinhardt et al. *(92)* published an automated segmentation algorithm of the first five to six airway generations. This program can apparently match airway trees with 150–200 branch points very rapidly. This has been validated with phantom and in vivo scans. An alternate approach allowing for automated segmentation to a similar generation of airways was recently published by Yuen et al. (Fig. 7) *(94)*. Both these methods allow for automatic labeling of the airway tree and for measuring airway dimensions. It can be anticipated that these or similar algorithms will be useful analysis techniques for assessing airway dimensions in the future.

3.2. Lung Attenuation

For purposes of lung attenuation measurements, the lung is considered to be made up of structures equal in attenuation to either air or water. Lung attenuation curves (LACs) are x-ray attenuation (HU) histograms that plot the frequency of occurrence of voxels of individual HU values within the

A)

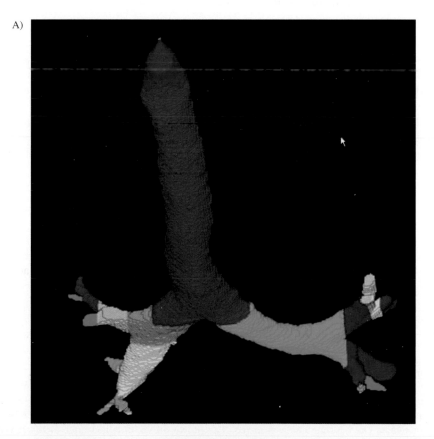

Fig. 7. *(Continued)*

B)

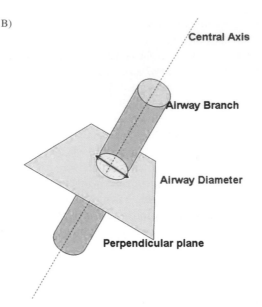

Fig. 7. (A) Automated segmentation of the airway demonstrating trachea main stem bronchi and segmental airways using an automated knowledge-based software program and **(B)** demonstration of the importance of measurement of the airway perpendicular to its course.

lung parenchyma. The distribution of an LAC reflects the tissue/air ratio within the parenchyma. The greater the leftward shift of the LAC (e.g., reflecting a greater proportion of low attenuation), the more extensive the lung destruction due to emphysema and/or expiratory airflow obstruction (Fig. 8). The attenuation statistics are derived from the attenuation histogram. These include mean, median, 5th percentile, regional histogram, and standard deviation. The changes in the regional lung attenuation at various phases of inspiration can be used as a measure of ventilation, and attenuation changes from inspiration to expiration as measures of gas trapping. Several objective measures of attenuation have been used including (i) mean attenuation of voxels *(95)*; (ii) a calculation summarizing pixels

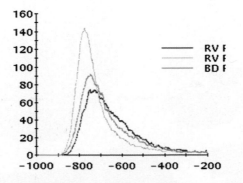

Fig. 8. Lung attenuation curves (LACs) depict the frequency distribution of attenuation (HU) within the ROI. The greater the leftward shift of the LAC (reflecting a greater proportion of low attenuation), the more extensive the emphysema and/or expiratory airflow obstruction. A rightward shift of the curve (to a greater proportion of high attenuation) reflects an increase either in blood flow or in the interstitial, cellular, or fluid content of the lung parenchyma. The baseline curve is in red. The brown curve, obtained after methacholine challenge, demonstrates leftward shift, followed by a return to baseline distribution post bronchodilator (green curve).

with attenuation above or below the specified critical values *(96)*; (iii) frequency and cumulative histograms of the distribution of attenuation values *(50,97)*; (iv) the percentage of pixels below a certain attenuation value, which can also be expressed as a "density mask" highlighting regions below the predetermined attenuation *(53,98)*; (v) mean attenuation and expiratory/inspiratory ratios *(99)*; and (vi) the rate of change of lung attenuation expressed as HU/time *(28,100)*. Attenuation values derived at other lung volumes (e.g., end-expiration) or based on differences between pre- and post-bronchial provocation can also provide useful additional information *(50,80)*.

From images acquired at a single anatomical level during an expiratory maneuver, plots of median attenuation (HU) and cross-sectional area versus time (HU/*t* and Area/*t* curves) during the expiratory maneuver in a ROI can be calculated *(28,29,81)*. Figure 9 shows that patients with the same severity of parenchyma destruction by emphysema (density mask) can have very different regional airflow (HU/*t* curve) function both between lungs in the same patient and between subjects. Thus, QIA is able to provide comparative information about the individual lungs that is not possible with conventional pulmonary function tests (PFTs) that provide only global measures of lung function. Furthermore, this technique is robust and may offer further insights into the pathophysiology of subjects with chronic obstructive pulmonary disease (COPD) as well as better stratify subjects in future treatment trials into those with predominant parenchymal destruction versus predominant airflow limitation versus combined parenchyma and airflow limitation subgroups.

3.3. Lung Volume Analysis

Various automated lung segmentation software packages are available which can extract the lung parenchyma to accurately and reproducibly measure whole lung and regional lung volumes *(82,101)*. The correlation between CT lung volume and plethysmography-determined lung volumes is excellent, with Pearson correlation coefficients (*r* values) of the order 0.85–0.95 (Fig. 10). However, CT volume measurements typically overestimate TLC and underestimate RV measurements made by conventional plethysmography *(17,101)*.

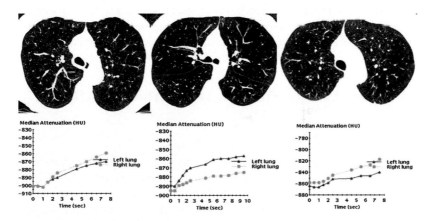

Fig. 9. Selected segmented images from three subjects with same emphysema severity score. The graphs below each image show the change in median lung attenuation over time during a dynamic expiratory acquisition. The patient on the left shows moderate impairment of airflow bilaterally. The patient in the middle shows good expiratory airflow in the left lung, but marked air trapping on the right. The patient on the right shows marked air trapping on the left and moderate air trapping on the right.

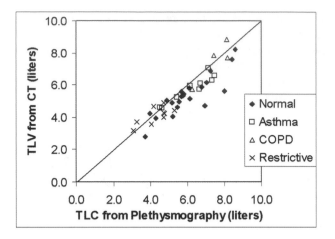

Fig. 10. Plot of total lung volume (TLV) calculated from CT against total lung capacity (TLC) from body plethysmography. The plot shows that volumes from the two methods are well correlated. The normal subjects have a range of lung volumes, while the three lung disease groups tend to be separated, as would be expected. The correlation line between CT TLV and plethysmography measured TLC is excellent as shown ($R = 0.92$).

4. NOVEL CT VENTILATION TECHNIQUES

Several CT contrast agents for ventilation have been studied, including aerosolized, iodinated contrast, fluorine containing FS 36 and xenon gas *(102–105)*. Xenon has a K-edge close to that of iodine and can be detected by its attenuation on CT images *(104,105)*. In animal models, accurate quantitative CT images of region-specific ventilation (ventilation per unit volume air in the lung) can be obtained with multi-slice scanners with temporal resolution less than 400 ms. The distribution of fraction in the lung can be mapped using the pre-xenon gas inhalation CT attenuation values. Following xenon administration, specific ventilation can also be mapped. The potential ability to overlay the functional ventilation maps onto the corresponding high-resolution anatomic displays available from CT makes this a potentially powerful tool. With the additional use of intravenous contrast enhancement, quantitative perfusion scans of the lung can be obtained using CT. Combined with the ventilation assessment of the xenon, the potential for assessing ventilation perfusion relationships may be possible *(106)*. At this stage, these techniques are experimental and are not discussed further in this chapter.

5. CLINICAL CT MEASURES OF THE AIRWAYS AND AIRWAY FUNCTION

5.1. Trachea

The anatomic location and relatively large dimension of the trachea facilitate segmentation and direct measurements of lumen size and wall thickening. The most useful measure is change in tracheal lumen diameter or cross-sectional area from end-inspiration to end-expiration. Although making such measurements from conventional 2-D axial scans is often sufficient, the measurements are optimized by using full-volume thin-section acquisitions and 3-D reconstructions *(107–109)*.

The tracheal cartilages protect the anterior and lateral walls of the intrathoracic trachea from collapse during the expiratory maneuver. The posterior membranous portion is however normally susceptible to the intraluminal pressure changes in normal subjects. A change in tracheal airway surface of up to 35% from full inspiration to end-expiration is seen in normal subjects *(110)*. This is mostly due to bowing of the posterior membranous trachea. In patients with tracheomalacia, the coronal diameter of the trachea is much larger than the sagittal diameter at end-expiration *(111)*.

Dynamic expiratory CT has now become a useful clinical alternative to bronchoscopy for assessing tracheal collapse. In patients with collapse of greater than 75% of the airway lumen, tracheomalacia can be diagnosed with confidence *(12,112)*. In patients with COPD, the high downstream resistance can also result in tracheal caliber changes greater than 50% with expiration despite normal intrinsic tracheal compliance. For this reason, a decrease in the tracheal lumen cross-sectional area of more than 75% should be used to diagnose the tracheomalacia *(110)*.

5.2. Proximal Airways

CT has become a very important diagnostic and investigational tool for the evaluation of the proximal airway function. The techniques allow for measurement of dynamic changes in the airway caliber not possible with conventional lung function and measurements such as airway and lung resistance *(81,113)*. HRCT is capable of directly assessing airway responsiveness in vivo, and this is not possible with other techniques *(20,114–118)*. CT-based measurements include direct measurements of airway lumen size (cross-sectional area and a diameter) and bronchial wall thickness, as well as indirect methods of assessing parenchymal attenuation as a measure of air trapping. CT studies of airway reactivity are providing new insights into the pathophysiology of asthma. The majority of these studies to date are all based on traditional 2-D HRCT methods *(93,118–122)*.

5.3. Peripheral Airways

At this stage, CT cannot directly visualize the distal lung units at the gas exchange level in the lung parenchyma. Changes in air content in the lung result in corresponding changes in volume and CT attenuation in the ROI *(38,123)*. CT studies have measured a change in the regional lung attenuation at various phases of inspiration or pre- and post-treatment to evaluate air trapping as an indirect measure of peripheral small airway function. CT may be useful in asthma to either quantify the extent of air trapping or the degree of airway wall thickening and luminal narrowing, as well as assess novel drug treatment efficacy *(50,80,91,122,124,125)*. These approaches are complementary. Assessment of airway wall changes requires meticulous technique to achieve accurate reproducible measurement. Interpretation of airway wall measures is difficult unless one knows the order of the measured bronchus within the bronchial tree. Measurement of air trapping, though indirect, is a relatively simple and useful method for the quantitation of asthma severity.

The degree of change of lung attenuation at suspended full inspiration compared with suspended end-expiration is now commonly used in clinical practice to assess the severity of asthma *(126–130)*. The change in lung attenuation is often due to air trapping, the hallmark of small airway obstruction (but can also be due to regional abnormality in pulmonary compliance), at end-expiration. The attenuation of normal lung increases because the gas volume is decreased, whereas the lung attenuation may remain unchanged in subjects with air trapping in the presence of small airway disease. Additionally, the volume of normal lung decreases on expiration whereas regions with air trapping remain unchanged in size *(126–130)*.

The most dependent lung regions show the greatest increase in attenuation on expiration in normal lungs *(131)*. In up to 80% of normal subjects with normal lung function tests, end-expiratory CT may show one to three areas of air trapping in the dependent parts of the lower lobes, usually limited to two or three adjacent pulmonary lobules *(132,133)*. There is slight increase in frequency of these findings in older individuals *(112,132,133)*. Air trapping is generally considered abnormal when it involves non-dependent areas of the lung and when the region affected is equal to or greater than a lung segment *(134)*. Air trapping has been demonstrated in a number of pulmonary diseases including constrictive (obliterative) bronchiolitis, asthma, sarcoid, hypersensitivity pneumonitis, bronchitis, bronchiectasis, and emphysema *(4,78,130,135–139)*.

Several studies have demonstrated that additional information relating to air flow limitation can be obtained by analyzing the dynamic series of images in comparison with images obtained at suspended expiration *(140)*. The correlation between CT measures of air trapping has a variable correlation with conventional PFTs, although some studies have shown a reasonable to good correlation with PFTs *(14,96,110,124,130,136,140–144)*. Other studies have not shown a good correlation *(80,96,122,124, 141)*. It is generally accepted that the use of PFT measurements as reference standards is problematic because it may represent the global average measured at the mouth, whereas dynamic CT analysis may show limited focal or multifocal regions of air trapping that may not be sufficiently extensive to alter the global spirometry measurements.

6. CONCLUSION

Functional imaging of the airways has become clinically useful, and these techniques will most likely become increasingly utilized, complementing and potentially replacing conventional lung function tests *(145,146)*. The ability of CT measures of airway structure function to assess not only individual lungs but also individual lung segments and even smaller regions, unlike conventional lung function tests, makes these techniques very powerful and useful. The functional images may allow us to detect lung disease early before structural abnormalities develop. Further regional functional measures may improve the way in which disease progression and treatment efficacy are assessed.

ACKNOWLEDGMENTS

I thank Carole Barrinuevo for her time and assistance with this book chapter.

REFERENCES

1. Kalender WA, Rienmuller R, Seissler W, Behr J, Welke M, Fichte H. Measurement of pulmonary parenchymal attenuation: use of spirometric gating with quantitative CT. *Radiology* 1990; 175:265–268.
2. Fotheringham T, Chabat F, Hansell DM, et al. A comparison of methods for enhancing the detection of areas of decreased attenuation on CT caused by airways disease. *J Comput Assist Tomogr* 1999; 23:385–389.
3. Wittram C, Batt J, Rappaport DC, Hutcheon MA. Inspiratory and expiratory helical CT of normal adults: comparison of thin section scans and minimum intensity projection images. *J Thorac Imaging* 2002; 17:47–52.
4. Bhalla M, Naidich DP, McGuinness G, Gruden JF, Leitman BS, McCauley DI. Diffuse lung disease: assessment with helical CT – preliminary observations of the role of maximum and minimum intensity projection images. *Radiology* 1996; 200:341–347.
5. Yang GZ, Hansell DM. CT image enhancement with wavelet analysis for the detection of small airways disease. *IEEE Trans Med Imaging* 1997; 16:953–961.
6. Remy-Jardin M, Remy J, Gosselin B, Copin MC, Wurtz A, Duhamel A. Sliding thin slab, minimum intensity projection technique in the diagnosis of emphysema: histopathologic-CT correlation. *Radiology* 1996; 200:665–671.
7. Goldin JG. Quantitative CT of the lung. *Radiol Clin North Am* 2002; 40:145–162.
8. Hu H, He HD, Foley WD, Fox SH. Four multidetector-row helical CT: image quality and volume coverage speed. *Radiology* 2000; 215:55–62.
9. Klingenbeck-Regn K, Schaller S, Flohr T, Ohnesorge BM, Kopp AF, Baum U. Subsecond multi-slice computed tomography: basics and applications. *Eur J Radiol* 1999; 31:110–124.
10. Lawler LP, Fishman EK. Multi-detector row CT of thoracic disease with emphasis on 3D volume rendering and CT angiography. *Radiographics* 2001; 21:1257–1273.
11. Rydberg J, Buckwalter KA, Caldemeyer KS, et al. Multisection CT: scanning techniques and clinical applications. *Radiographics* 2000; 20:1787–1806.
12. Grenier PA, Beigelman-Aubry C, Fetita C, Preteux F. Large airways at CT: bronchiectasis, asthma and COPD. In: Kauczor HU, ed. *Functional Imaging of the Chest*. Berlin: Springer, 2004; 39–54.
13. King GG, Muller NL, Pare PD. Evaluation of airways in obstructive pulmonary disease using high resolution computed tomography. *Am J Respir Crit Care Med* 1999; 159:992–1004.
14. Knudson RJ, Standen JR, Kaltenborn WT, et al. Expiratory computed tomography for assessment of suspected pulmonary emphysema. *Chest* 1991; 99:1357–1366.

15. Murata K, Itoh H, Todo G, et al. Centrilobular lesions of the lung: demonstration by high-resolution CT and pathologic correlation. *Radiology* 1986; 161:641–645.

16. Webb WR, Stern EJ, Kanth N, Gamsu G. Dynamic pulmonary CT: findings in healthy adult men. *Radiology* 1993; 186:117–124.

17. Webb WR. High-resolution CT of the lung parenchyma. *Radiol Clin North Am* 1989; 27:1085–1097.

18. Klein J, Gamsu G. High resolution computed tomography of diffuse lung disease. *Invest Radiol* 1989; 24:805–812.

19. Brown RH, Mitzner W, Zerhouni E, Hirschman CA. Direct in vivo visualization of bronchodilation induced by inhalational anesthesia using high-resolution computer tomography. *Anesthesiology* 1993; 78:295–300.

20. Brown RH, Zerhouni EA, Mitzner W. Visualization of airway obstruction in vivo during lung vascular engorgement and edema. *J Appl Physiol* 1995; 78:1070–1078.

21. Herold CJ, Brown RH, Mitzner W, Links JM, Hirshman CA, Zerhouni EA. Assessment of pulmonary airway reactivity with high-resolution CT. *Radiology* 1991; 181:369–374.

22. Standardization of Spirometry, 1994 Update. American Thoracic Society. *Am J Respir Crit Care Med* 1995; 152: 1107–1136.

23. Roth MD, Connett JE, D'Armiento JM, et al. Feasibility of retinoids for the treatment of emphysema study. *Chest* 2006; 130:1334–1345.

24. Pais RC, Brown MS, Shah SK, Qing D, da Costa I, Goldin JG. Web and XML technologies that enable analysis and reporting for a radiology core facility in multicenter clinical trials. In: Radiological Society of North America scientific assembly and annual meeting program 2005; 815.

25. Newell JD, Hogg JC, Snider GL. Report of a workshop: quantitative computed tomography scanning in longitudinal studies of emphysema. *Eur Respir J* 2004; 23:769–775.

26. Cosio MG, Snider GL. Chest computed tomography: is it ready for major studies of chronic obstructive pulmonary disease? *Eur Respir J* 2001; 17:1062–1064.

27. Stern EJ, Webb WR, Golden JA, Gamsu G. Cystic lung disease associated with eosinophilic granuloma and tuberous sclerosis: air trapping at dynamic ultrafast high resolution CT. *Radiology* 1992; 182:325–329.

28. Markstaller K, Arnold M, Dobrich M, et al. A software tool for automatic image-based ventilation analysis using dynamic chest CT-scanning in healthy and in ARDS lungs. *Rofo Fortschr Geb Rontgenstr Neuen Bildgeb Verfahr* 2001; 173:830–835.

29. Gevenois PA, De Vuyst P, Sy M, et al. Pulmonary emphysema: quantitative CT during expiration. *Radiology* 1996; 199:825–829.

30. Im JG, Kim SH, Chung MJ, Koo JM, Han MC. Lobular low attenuation of the lung parenchyma on CT: evaluation of 48 patients. *J Comput Assist Tomogr* 1996; 20:752–762.

31. Johnson JL, Kramer SS, Mahboubi S. Air trapping in children: evaluation with dynamic lung densitometry with spiral CT. *Radiology* 1998; 206:95–101.

32. Lucidarme O, Grenier PA, Cadi M, Mourey-Gerosa I, Benali K, Cluzel P. Evaluation of air trapping at CT: comparison of continuous-versus suspended-expiration CT techniques. *Radiology* 2000; 216:768–772.

33. Okazawa M, Muller N, McNamara AE, Child S, Verburgt L, Pare PD. Human airway narrowing measured using high resolution computed tomography. *Am J Respir Crit Care Med* 1996; 154:1557–1562.

34. Gotway MB, Lee ES, Reddy GP, Golden JA, Webb WR. Low-dose, dynamic, expiratory thin-section CT of the lungs using a spiral CT scanner. *J Thorac Imaging* 2000; 15:168–172.

35. Hoffman EA, Reinhardt JM, Sonka M, et al. Characterization of the interstitial lung diseases via density-based and texture-based analysis of computed tomography images of lung structure and function. *Acad Radiol* 2003; 10:1104–1118.

36. Rienmuller RK, Behr J, Kalender WA, et al. Standardized quantitative high resolution CT in lung diseases. *J Comput Assist Tomogr* 1991; 15:742–749.

37. Kalender WA, Fichte H, Bautz W, Skalej M. Semiautomatic evaluation procedures for quantitative CT of the lung. *J Comput Assist Tomogr* 1991; 15:248–255.

38. Hoffman EA, McLennan G. Assessment of the pulmonary structure-function relationship and clinical outcomes measures: quantitative volumetric CT of the lung. *Acad Radiol* 1997; 4:758–776.

39. Tran BQ, Tajik JK, Chiplunkar RA, et al. E. Lung volume control for quantitative x-ray CT. *J Biomed Eng* 1996; 24:S66.

40. Becker MD, Berkmen YM, Austin JH, et al. Lung volumes before and after lung volume reduction surgery: quantitative CT analysis. *Am J Respir Crit Care Med* 1998; 157:1593–1539.

41. Gierada DS, Yusen RD, Pilgram TK, et al. Repeatability of quantitative CT indexes of emphysema in patients evaluated for lung volume reduction surgery. *Radiology* 2001; 220:448–454.

42. Kemerink GJ, Lamers RJ, Thelissen GR, van Engelshoven JM. CT densitometry of the lungs: scanner performance. *J Comput Assist Tomogr* 1996; 20:24–33.

43. Reinhardt JM, Hoffman EA. Quantitative pulmonary imaging: spatial and temporal considerations in high resolution CT. *Acad Radiol* 1998; 5:539–546.

44. Boedeker KL, McNitt-Gray MF, Rogers SR, et al. Emphysema: effect of reconstruction algorithm on CT imaging measures. *Radiology* 2004; 232:295–301.
45. Kemerink GJ, Kruize HH, Lamers RJ, van Engelshoven JM. CT lung densitometry: dependence of CT number histograms on sample volume and consequences for scan protocol comparability. *J Comput Assist Tomogr* 1997; 21:948–954.
46. Stoel BC, Bakker ME, Stolk J, et al. Comparison of the sensitivities of 5 different computed tomography scanners for the assessment of the progression of pulmonary emphysema: a phantom study. *Invest Radiol* 2004; 39:1–7.
47. Kemerink GJ, Lamers RJ, Thelissen GR, van Engelshoven JM. Scanner conformity in CT densitometry of the lungs. *Radiology* 1995; 197:749–752.
48. Brown MS, Goldin JG, McNitt-Gray MF, et al. Knowledge-based segmentation of thoracic computed tomography images for assessment of split lung function. *Med Phys* 2000; 27:592–598.
49. Goldin JG, Aberle DR. Functional imaging of the airways. *J Thorac Imaging* 1997; 12:29–37.
50. Goldin JG, McNitt-Gray MF, Sorenson SM, et al. Airway hyperreactivity: assessment with helical thin-section CT. *Radiology* 1998; 208:321–329.
51. Kramer SS, Hoffman EA. Physiologic imaging of the lung with volumetric high resolution CT. *J Thorac Imaging* 1995; 10:280–290.
52. Lynch DA, Newell JD, Tschomper BA, Cink TM, Newman LA, Bethel R. Uncomplicated asthma in adults: comparison of CT appearance of the lungs in asthmatic and healthy subjects. *Radiology* 1993; 188:829–833.
53. Muller NL, Staples CA, Miller RR, Abboud RT. "Density mask." An objective method to quantitate emphysema using computed tomography. *Chest* 1988; 94:782–787.
54. Naidich DP, Webb WR, Muller NL. Thoracic computed tomography: current concepts. In: Potchen EJ, Grainger RG, Greene R, eds. *Pulmonary Radiology*. Philadelphia: W.B. Saunders, 1993; 386–404.
55. Naidich DP. Volumetric scan change perceptions in thoracic imaging. *Diagn Imaging* 1993; 15:70–74.
56. Remy-Jardin M, Remy J, Deffontaines C, Duhamel A. Assessment of diffuse infiltrative lung disease: comparison of conventional CT and high resolution CT. *Radiology* 1991; 181:157–162.
57. Swensen SJ, Aughenbaugh GL, Douglas WW, Myers JL. High resolution CT of the lungs: findings in various pulmonary diseases. *AJR Am J Roentgenol* 1992; 158:971–979.
58. Uppaluri R, Mitsa T, Sonka M, Hoffman EA, McLennan G. Quantification of pulmonary emphysema from lung computed tomography images. *Am J Respir Crit Care Med* 1997; 156:248–254.
59. Zagers R, Vrooman HA, Aarts NJM, et al. Quantitative analysis of computed tomography scans of the lungs for the diagnosis of pulmonary emphysema: a validation study of a semiautomated contour detection technique. *Invest Radiol* 1995; 30:552–562.
60. Goldin JG, Brown MS, McNitt-Gray MF, Aberle DR. Automated assessment of split lung function in post lung transplant evaluation. *Proc SPIE* 1998; 3337:14–23.
61. Kaneko M, Ehuchi K, Ono R. Three-dimensional display of bronchial images by helical scanning CT. *Radiology* 1990; 177:174.
62. Remy-Jardin M, Remy J, Marquette CH, Wattinne L, Giraud F, Tonnel AB. Central airways in asthmatics and control subjects: evaluation with spirometric-gated spiral CT. *Radiology* 1992; 185:131.
63. Schaefer CM, Prokop M, Zinh C. Spiral CT of the anastamotic complications after lung transplantation. *Radiology* 1993; 189:263.
64. Uppaluri R, McLennan G, Sonka M, Hoffman EA. Computer-based objective quantitative assessment of pulmonary parenchyma via x-ray CT. *Proc SPIE* 1998; 3337:377–383.
65. Uppaluri R, McLennan G, Enright P, Standen JR, Boyer-Pfersdorf P, Hoffman EA. Adaptive multiple feature method (AMFM) for the early detection of parenchymal pathology in a smoking population. *Proc SPIE* 1998; 3337:8–13.
66. Ney DR, Kuhlman JC, Hruban RH. Three-dimensional CT – volumetric reconstruction and display of the bronchial tree. *Invest Radiol* 1990; 25:736–742.
67. Rubin GD, Dake MD, Semba CP. Current status of three-dimensional spiral CT scanning for imaging the vasculature. *Radiol Clin North Am* 1995; 33:51–70.
68. Rubin GD, Napel S, Leung AN. Volumetric analysis of volume data: achieving a paradigm shift. *Radiology* 1996; 200:312–317.
69. Laws KI. Textured image segmentation. In: USCIPI technical report no. 940. University of Southern California, 1980.
70. Adachi S, Kono M, Takemura T. Evaluation of 3D spiral CT bronchoscopy in patients with lung cancer. *Radiology* 1993; 189:264–269.
71. Archer DC, Coblentz CL, de Kemp R, Nahmias C, Norman G. Automated in vivo quantification of emphysema. *Radiology* 1993; 188:835–838.
72. Bae KT, Sloane RM, Gierada DS, Yusen RD, Cooper JD. Patients with emphysema: quantitative CT analysis before and after lung volume reduction surgery. *Radiology* 1997; 203:705–714.
73. Disler DG, Marr S, Rosenthal DI. Accuracy of volume measurements of computed tomography and magnetic resonance imaging phantoms by three-dimensional reconstruction and preliminary clinical applications. *Invest Radiol* 1994; 29:739–745.

74. Wood SA, Hoford JD, Hoffman EA, Zerhouni EA, Mitzner W. A method for measurement of cross sectional area, segment length, and branching angle of airway tree structures in situ. *Comput Med Imaging Graph* 1995; 19:145–152.
75. Wu M, Chang J, Chiang A, et al. Use of quantitative CT to predict postoperative lung function in patients with lung cancer. *Radiology* 1994; 191:257–262.
76. Brown MS, McNitt-Gray MF, Mankovich NJ, Goldin JG, Aberle DR. Knowledge-based automated technique for measuring total lung weight from CT. *Proc SPIE* 1996; 2709:63–74.
77. Brown MS, McNitt-Gray MF, Goldin JG, Aberle DR. Automated measurement of split and total lung volume from helical CT. *Radiology* 1997; 205:224.
78. Remy-Jardin M, Campistron P, Amara A, et al. Workflow issue with multi-slice CT (MSCT) of the thorax: usefulness of multiplanar reformations in the diagnostic approach of infiltrative lung disease. *Eur Radiol* 2002; 12:134 (abst).
79. Hirose N, Lynch DA, Cherniack RM, Doherty DE. Correlation between high resolution computed tomography and tissue morphometry of the lung bleomycin-induced pulmonary fibrosis in the rabbit. *Am Rev Respir Dis* 1993; 147:730–738.
80. Laurent F, Latrabe V, Raherison C, Marthan R, Tunon-de-Lara JM. Functional significance of air trapping detected in moderate asthma. *Eur Radiol* 2000; 10:1404–1410.
81. Brown RH, Croisille P, Mudge B, Diemer FB, Permutt S, Togias A. Airway narrowing in healthy humans inhaling methacholine without deep inspirations demonstrated by HRCT. *Am J Respir Crit Care Med* 2000; 161:1256–1263.
82. Brown MS, McNitt-Gray MF, Goldin JG, et al. Automated measurement of single and total lung volume from CT. *J Comput Assist Tomogr* 1999; 23:632–640.
83. Goldin JG, Tashkin DP, Kleerup EC, et al. Comparative effects of hydrofluoroalkane and chlorofluorocarbon beclomethasone dipropionate inhalation on small airways: assessment with functional helical thin-section computed tomography. *J Allergy Clin Immunol* 1999; 104:S258–S267.
84. Tschirren J, Palagyi K, Reinhardt JM, Hoffman EA, Sonka M. Segmentation, skeletonization, and branchpoint matching – a fully automated quantitative evaluation of human intrathoracic airway trees. In: MICCAI 5th International Conference. Tokyo, Japan: Springer Berlin/Heidelberg, 2004; 12–19.
85. Aykac D, Hoffman EA, McLennan G, Reinhardt JM. Segmentation and analysis of the human airway tree from three-dimensional x-ray CT images. *IEEE Trans Med Imaging* 2003; 22:940–950.
86. Wood SA, Zerhouni EA, Hoford JD, Hoffman EA, Mitzner W. Measurement of three-dimensional lung tree structures by using computed tomography. *J Appl Physiol* 1995; 79:1687–1697.
87. Kiraly AP, Higgins WE, McLennan G, Hoffman EA, Reinhardt JM. Three-dimensional human airway segmentation methods for clinical virtual bronchoscopy. *Acad Radiol* 2002; 9:1153–1168.
88. Fetita CI, Preteux F. Quantitative 3D CT bronchography. *Proc IEEE Int Symp Biomed Imaging* 2002; 221–224.
89. Chiplunkar RA, Reinhardt JM, Hoffman EA. Segmentation and quantitation of the primary human airway tree. *SPIE Med Imaging* 1997; 3033:403–414.
90. Park W, hoffman EA, Sonka M. Segmentation of intrathoracic airway trees: a fuzzy logic approach. *IEEE Trans Med Imaging* 1998; 17:489–497.
91. Nakano Y, Muro S, Sakai H, et al. Computed tomographic measurements of airway dimensions and emphysema in smokers. Correlation with lung function. *Am J Respir Crit Care Med* 2000; 162:1102–1108.
92. Reinhardt JM, d'Souza ND, Hoffman EA. Accurate measurement of intrathoracic airways. *IEEE Trans Med Imaging* 1997; 16:820–827.
93. Amirav I, Kramer SS, Grunstein MM, Hoffman EA. Assessment of methacholine-induced airway constriction by ultrafast high-resolution computed tomography. *J Appl Physiol* 1993; 75:2239–2250.
94. Yuen S, Brown MS, Shah SK, et al. A probabilistic model for predicting diameters of lung airways. *Proc SPIE* 2005; 5747:704–714.
95. Goddard PR, Nicholson EM, Laszlo G, Watt I. Computed tomography in pulmonary emphysema. *Clin Radiol* 1982; 33:379–387.
96. Newman KB, Lynch DA, Newman LS, Ellegood D, Newell JD, Jr. Quantitative computed tomography detects air trapping due to asthma. *Chest* 1994; 106:105–109.
97. Wegener OH, Koeppe P, Oeser H. Measurement of lung density by computed tomography. *J Comput Assist Tomogr* 1978; 2:263–273.
98. Adams H, Bernard MS, McConnochie K. An appraisal of CT pulmonary density mapping in normal subjects. *Clin Radiol* 1991; 43:238–242.
99. Kubo K, Eda S, Yamamoto H, et al. Expiratory and inspiratory chest computed tomography and pulmonary function tests in cigarette smokers. *Eur Respir J* 1999; 13:252–256.
100. Goldin JG, Szold O, McNitt-Gray MF, Levine MS, Tashkin DP. Use of EBCT in the evaluation of patients post single lung transplantation. *Am J Respir Crit Care Med* 1995; 9:81.
101. Brown MS, Goldin JG, McNitt-Gray MF, et al. Knowledge-based segmentation of thoracic computed tomography images for assessment of split lung function. *Med Phys* 2000; 27:592–598.
102. Thiele J, Kloppel R. [Computerized tomography measurement of lung ventilation by inhalation of Isovist-300]. *Rontgenpraxis* 1995; 48:259–260.

103. Yamaguchi K, Soejima K, Koda E, Sugiyama N. Inhaling gas with different CT densities allows detection of abnormalities in the lung periphery of patients with smoking-induced COPD. *Chest* 2001; 120:1907–1916.

104. Tajik JK, Chon D, Won C, Tran BQ, Hoffman EA. Subsecond multisection CT of regional pulmonary ventilation. *Acad Radiol* 2002; 9:130–146.

105. Simon B, Marcucci C, Fung M, Lele S. Parameter estimation and confidence intervals for Xe-CT ventilation studies: a Monte Carlo approach. *J Appl Physiol* 1998; 84:709–716.

106. Kreck TC, Krueger MA, Altemeier WA, et al. Determination of regional ventilation and perfusion in the lung using xenon and computed tomography. *J Appl Physiol* 2001; 91:1741–1749.

107. Ravenel JG, McAdams HP, Remy-Jardin M, Remy J. Multidimensional imaging of the thorax: practical applications. *J Thorac Imaging* 2001; 16:269–281.

108. Remy-Jardin M, Remy J, Artaud D, Fribourg M, Naili A. Tracheobronchial tree: assessment with volume rendering-technical aspects. *Radiology* 1998; 208:393–398.

109. Boiselle PM, Reynolds KF, Ernst A. Multiplanar and three-dimensional imaging of the central airways with multidetector CT. *AJR Am J Roentgenol* 2002; 179:301–308.

110. Stern EJ, Graham CM, Webb WR, Gamsu G. Normal trachea during forced expiration: dynamic CT measurements. *Radiology* 1993; 187:27–31.

111. Zhang J, Hasegawa I, Feller-Kopman D, Boiselle PM. 2003 AUR Memorial Award. Dynamic expiratory volumetric CT imaging of the central airways: comparison of standard-dose and low-dose techniques. *Acad Radiol* 2003; 10:719–724.

112. Gilkeson RC, Ciancibello LM, Hejal RB, Montenegro HD, Lange P. Tracheobronchomalacia: dynamic airway evaluation with multidetector CT. *AJR Am J Roentgenol* 2001; 176:205–210.

113. Brown RH, Scichilone N, Mudge B, Diemer FB, Permutt S, Togias A. High resolution computed tomographic evaluation of airway distensibility and the effects of lung inflation on airway caliber in healthy subjects and individuals with asthma. *Am J Respir Crit Care Med* 2001; 163:994–1001.

114. Brown RH, Herold CJ, Hirshman CA, Zerhouni EA, Mitzner W. Individual airway constrictor response heterogeneity to histamine assessed by high resolution computed tomography. *J Appl Physiol* 1993; 74:2615–2620.

115. Brown RH, Herold C, Mitzner W, Zerhouni EA. Spontaneous airways constrict during breath holding studied by high resolution computed tomography. *Chest* 1994; 106:920–924.

116. Brown RH, Zerhouni EA, Mitzner W. Variability in the size of individual airways over the course of one year. *Am J Respir Crit Care Med* 1995; 151:1159–1164.

117. Brown RH, Mitzner W. Effect of lung inflation and airway muscle tone on airway diameter in vivo. *J Appl Physiol* 1996; 80:1581–1588.

118. Brown RH, Mitzner W, Bulut Y, Wagner EM. Effect of lung inflation in vivo on airways with smooth muscle tone or edema. *J Appl Physiol* 1997; 82:491–499.

119. King GG, Muller NL, Pare PD. Evaluation of airways in obstructive pulmonary disease using high resolution computed tomography. *Am J Respir Crit Care Med* 1999; 159:992–1004.

120. McNamara AE, Muller NL, Okazawa M, Arntorp J, Wiggs BR, Pare PD. Airway narrowing in excised canine lungs measured by high resolution computed tomography. *J Appl Physiol* 1992; 73:307–316.

121. Brown RH, Georakopoulos I, Mitzner W. Individual canine airways responsiveness to aerosol histamine and methacholine in vivo. *Am J Respir Crit Care Med* 1998; 157:491–497.

122. Beigelman-Aubry C, Capderou A, Grenier PA, et al. Mild intermittent asthma: CT assessment of bronchial cross-sectional area and lung attenuation at controlled lung volume. *Radiology* 2002; 223:181–187.

123. Hoffman EA, Gefter WB, Venegas J. Frontier pulmonary imaging. In: Fishman AP, ed. *Update: Pulmonary Diseases and Disorders*. New York: McGraw-Hill, 1992; 323–340.

124. Lucidarme O, Coche E, Cluzel P, Mourey-Gerosa I, Howarth N, Grenier PA. Expiratory CT scans for chronic airway disease: correlation with pulmonary function test results. *AJR Am J Roentgenol* 1998; 170:301–307.

125. Nakano Y, Muller NL, King GG, et al. Quantitative assessment of airway remodeling using high-resolution CT. *Chest* 2002; 122:271S–275S.

126. Lucidarme O, Coche E, Cluzel P, Mourey-Gerosa I, Howarth N, Grenier P. Expiratory CT scans for chronic airway disease: correlation with pulmonary function test results. *AJR Am J Roentgenol* 1998; 170:301–307.

127. Stern EJ, Frank MS. Small-airway diseases of the lungs: findings at expiratory CT. *AJR Am J Roentgenol* 1994; 163:37–41.

128. Desai SR, Hansell DM. Small airways disease: expiratory computed tomography comes of age. *Clin Radiol* 1997; 52:332–337.

129. Verschakelen JA, Scheinbaum K, Bogaert J, Demedts M, Lacquet LL, Baert AL. Expiratory CT in cigarette smokers: correlation between areas of decreased lung attenuation, pulmonary function tests and smoking history. *Eur Radiol* 1998; 8:1391–1399.

130. Arakawa H, Webb WR. Air trapping on expiratory high resolution CT scans in the absence of inspiratory scan abnormalities: correlation with pulmonary function tests and differential diagnosis. *AJR Am J Roentgenol* 1998; 170:1349–1353.

131. Verschakelen JA, Van Fraeyenhoven L, Laureys G, Demedts M, Baert AL. Difference in CT density between dependent and nondependent portions of the lung: influence of lung volume. *AJR Am J Roentgenol* 1993; 161:713–717.
132. Verschakelen JA, Scheinbaum K, Bogaert J, Demedts M, Lacquet LL, Baert AL. Expiratory CT in cigarette smokers: correlation between areas of decreased lung attenuation, pulmonary function tests and smoking history. *Eur Radiol* 1998; 8:1391–1399.
133. Lee KW, Chung SY, Yang I, Lee Y, Ko EY, Park MJ. Correlation of aging and smoking with air trapping at thin-section CT of the lung in asymptomatic subjects. *Radiology* 2000; 214:831–836.
134. Grenier PA, Beigelman-Aubry C, Fetita C, Preteux F, Brauner MW, Lenoir S. New frontiers in CT imaging of airway disease. *Eur Radiol* 2002; 12:1022–1044.
135. Arakawa H, Webb WR, McCowin M, Katsou G, Lee KN, Seitz RF. Inhomogeneous lung attenuation at thin-section CT: diagnostic value of expiratory scans. *Radiology* 1998; 206:89–94.
136. Gleeson FV, Traill ZC, Hansell DM. Evidence on expiratory CT scans of small airway obstruction in sarcoidosis. *AJR Am J Roentgenol* 1996; 166:1052–1054.
137. Bartz RR, Stern EJ. Airways obstruction in patients with sarcoidosis: expiratory CT scan findings. *J Thorac Imaging* 2000; 15:285–289.
138. Copley SJ, Wells AU, Muller NL, et al. Thin-section CT in obstructive pulmonary disease: discriminatory value. *Radiology* 2002; 223:812–819.
139. Ng CS, Desai SR, Rubens MB, Padley SP, Wells AU, Hansell DM. Visual quantitation and observer variation of signs of small airways disease at inspiratory and expiratory CT. *J Thorac Imaging* 1999; 14:279–285.
140. Chen D, Webb WR, Storto ML, Lee KN. Assessment of air trapping using postexpiratory high resolution computed tomography. *J Thorac Imaging* 1998; 13:135–143.
141. Padley SP, Adler BD, Hansell DM, Muller NL. Bronchiolitis obliterans: high resolution CT findings and correlation with pulmonary function tests. *Clin Radiol* 1993; 47:236–240.
142. Hansell DM, Wells AU, Rubens MB, Cole PJ. Bronchiectasis: functional significance of areas of decreased attenuation at expiratory CT. *Radiology* 1994; 193:369–374.
143. Heremans A, Verschakelen JA, Van Fraeyenhoven L, Demedts M. Measurement of lung density by means of quantitative CT scaning: a study of correlations with pulmonary function tests. *Chest* 1992; 102:805–811.
144. Kauczor HU, Hast J, Heussel CP, Schlegel J, Mildenberger P, Thelen M. CT attenuation of paired HRCT scans obtained at full inspiratory/expiratory position: comparison with pulmonary function tests. *Eur Radiol* 2002; 12:2757–2763.
145. Gefter WB. Functional CT imaging of the lungs: the pulmonary function test of the new millenium? *Acad Radiol* 2002; 9:127–129.
146. Gefter WB. Functional lung imaging: emerging methods to visualize regional pulmonary physiology. *Acad Radiol* 2003; 10:1085–1089.

II | Large Airways

6

Tracheobronchial Stenoses

Phillip M. Boiselle, Jay Catena, Armin Ernst, and David A. Lynch

Summary

Tracheobronchial stenosis is defined as focal or diffuse narrowing of the tracheal lumen. It may arise secondary to a wide variety of benign and malignant causes (Table 1). This chapter describes a general approach to the recognition and characterization of tracheobronchial stenoses and reviews specific clinical and imaging features of various benign causes for this condition. Neoplastic etiologies are reviewed separately in the chapter devoted to tracheobronchial neoplasms. Special emphasis is placed upon post-intubation stenosis, which is by far the most common etiology encountered in daily practice. Other, less common etiologies are subsequently discussed in alphabetical order following this entity.

Key Words: Trachea; bronchi; stenosis; benign; CT.

1. IMAGING TECHNIQUE

Although imaging methods for assessment of tracheobronchial disorders are reviewed in detail in an introductory chapter, it bears repeating that special attention to imaging acquisition and reconstruction parameters will enhance the ability to detect and accurately characterize airway stenoses.

Axial CT images provide exquisite anatomical display of the tracheal wall, tracheal lumen, and adjacent mediastinal and lung structures. Use of narrow collimation (≤3 mm) will enhance the ability to detect and characterize tracheal wall thickening (defined as wall thickness >3 mm) and calcification.

It is important to recognize the limitations of the axial plane for assessing airway stenoses, including a limited ability to detect subtle airway stenoses and underestimation of the craniocaudal extent of disease (1–8). By providing a continuous anatomical display of the airways, multiplanar and 3-D reconstruction images help to overcome these limitations (1–3). Such images also aid procedural planning by surgeons or interventional pulmonologists and assist in determining response to treatment (1,2).

In settings where such reconstructions are not possible, careful review of contiguous thin-section axial images can help to prevent the radiologist from overlooking stenoses. The use of thin-section images is particularly advantageous in the subglottic region, where stenoses are often focal and may be easily overlooked or underestimated on 5-mm sections (Fig. 1).

Intravenous contrast is not generally required for imaging benign stenoses. However, it is recommended in cases such as tuberculosis (TB), in which there is a high likelihood of disease in the adjacent lymph nodes, and for cases in which there is a question of possible primary or secondary airway malignancy.

Airway imaging is routinely performed at end-inspiration during a single breath hold. An additional sequence during dynamic expiration may be helpful to assess for coexisting tracheomalacia (excessive expiratory collapse of the airways), especially among patients with relapsing polychondritis and post-intubation stenoses (9).

From: *Contemporary Medical Imaging: CT of the Airways*
Edited by: P. M. Boiselle and D. A. Lynch © Humana Press, Totowa, NJ

Table 1
Causes of Tracheobronchial Stenosis

Iatrogenic
   Post-intubation
   Lung transplantation
Idiopathic
Infection
   Rhinoscleroma
   Tuberculosis
Laryngotracheal papillomatosis
Neoplasm
   Primary tracheal neoplasm (squamous carcinoma,
   adenoid cystic carcinoma)

   Direct invasion (lung, esophageal, thyroid)
   Secondary neoplasm (breast, renal, melanoma, thyroid)
Saber-sheath deformity
Systemic diseases
   Amyloidosis
   Inflammatory bowel disease
   Relapsing polychondritis
   Sarcoidosis
   Wegener granulomatosis
Tracheobronchopathia osteochondroplastica
Trauma

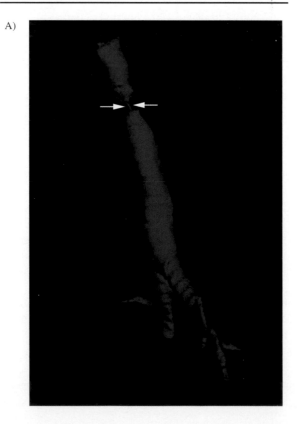

A)

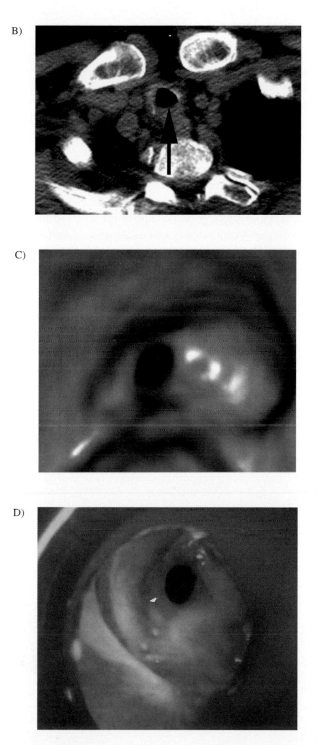

Fig. 1. Focal subglottic stenosis due to traumatic intubation. (**A**) External 3-D rendering of airway in sagittal oblique projection shows high-grade focal subglottic stenosis (arrows). (**B**) Axial 5-mm CT image at the level of stenosis underestimates degree of narrowing (arrow) due to partial volume averaging. (**C**) Virtual endoscopic CT image shows focal high-grade stenosis. (**D**) Conventional bronchoscopic image confirms high-grade stenosis.

2. FRAMEWORK FOR APPROACHING TRACHEOBRONCHIAL STENOSES

When assessing tracheobronchial stenoses, it is important to carefully assess the location, length, and distribution of the stenosis, as well as to characterize the presence, distribution, and type of wall thickening. A consideration of these factors, in combination with ancillary thoracic findings and pertinent clinical and laboratory data, will allow the radiologist to effectively narrow the broad differential diagnosis of tracheobronchial stenosis to two or three likely entities. In certain cases, such as relapsing polychondritis or tracheobronchopathia osteochondroplastica (TBO), a confident diagnosis can be made on the basis of imaging findings alone.

Accurate detection and characterization of tracheal wall thickening requires knowledge of normal tracheal anatomy. As reviewed in the introductory chapter on anatomy, the trachea is supported by a series of C-shaped cartilaginous rings, which comprise the anterior and lateral walls of the trachea (Fig. 2). Notably, the posterior membranous wall is devoid of cartilage. Thus, diseases such as relapsing polychondritis or TBO, which target the cartilage, will characteristically spare the posterior tracheal wall (Fig. 3) *(10)*, whereas most other causes of stenosis will result in circumferential tracheal wall involvement.

Although there is significant overlap in the imaging features of many causes of tracheobronchial stenosis (Table 1), several key imaging features can help to effectively narrow this broad differential diagnosis. As summarized in Table 2, these features include: sparing of the posterior membranous wall, "hourglass" configuration, calcification, coexisting tracheomalacia, and characteristic ancillary thoracic findings.

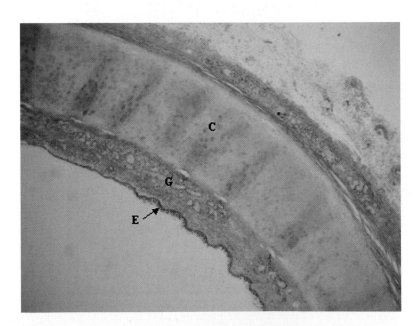

Fig. 2. Histology of anterolateral tracheal wall. Histological specimen of anterolateral tracheal wall shows surface respiratory epithelium (E), tracheal glands (G), and tracheal cartilage (C). (Courtesy of Dr. Olivier Kocher, Department of Pathology, Beth Israel Deaconess Medical Center)

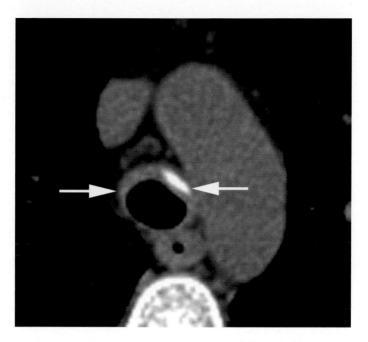

Fig. 3. Relapsing polychondritis. Axial CT image at the level of aortic arch demonstrates partially calcified thickening of anterior and lateral tracheal wall (arrow) with characteristic sparing of posterior, membranous wall.

3. POST-INTUBATION STENOSIS

Definition	Stenosis arising secondary to either endotracheal intubation or tracheostomy tube placement
Etiology	• Cuff-induced pressure necrosis • Direct trauma
Epidemiology	1% following endotracheal intubation, 30% following long-standing tracheostomy tube
Clinical presentation	Dyspnea, stridor, wheezing. Symptoms typically appear several weeks after extubation
Multidetector CT (MDCT) findings	• Eccentric or concentric soft tissue thickening with associated luminal narrowing • Focal subglottic stenosis 1.5–2 cm long • Classic "hourglass" configuration (Fig. 4B) • Thin membrane of granulation tissue projecting into the tracheal lumen less common
Treatment	• Surgical resection with end-to-end anastomosis is preferred primary therapy for surgical candidates • Endoscopic interventions (thermal resection and silicone stenting) for nonsurgical candidates

Table 2
Key Features that Narrow Differential Diagnosis

1. Sparing of posterior membranous wall
   Relapsing polychondritis
   Tracheobronchopathia osteochondroplastica
   Amyloidosis (may also be circumferential)
2. "Hourglass" configuration
   Post-intubation
3. Calcification
   Amyloid
   Relapsing polychondritis
   Tracheobronchopathia osteochondroplastica
   Tuberculosis
4. Tracheomalacia (coexisting with stenosis)
   Post-intubation
   Relapsing polychondritis
   Saber-sheath trachea
5. Ancillary thoracic findings
   Lung nodules
       Amyloid (rare)
       Malignancy
       Papillomatosis
       Tuberculosis
       Wegener granulomatosis
   Lymph node enlargement
       Amyloid (rare)
       Malignancy
       Sarcoid
       Tuberculosis

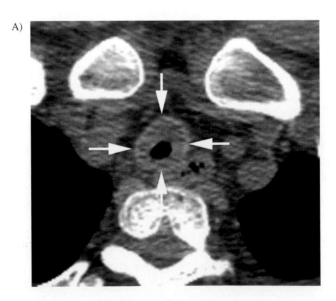

Fig. 4. *(Continued)*

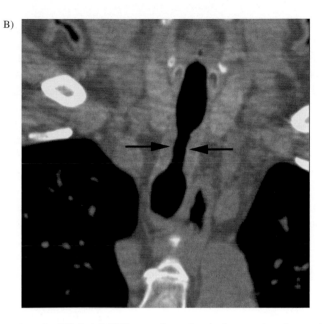

Fig. 4. Post-intubation stenosis. (**A**) Axial CT image shows luminal narrowing due to circumferential tracheal wall thickening. (**B**) Curved oblique multiplanar reformation image of upper trachea shows characteristic "hourglass" configuration of stenosis.

Although post-intubation stenosis is the most common cause of tracheal stenosis, its precise prevalence is unknown. The prevalence of stenosis following endotracheal tube placement has decreased substantially from 20 to 1% following the introduction of low-pressure cuff endotracheal tubes *(11–13)*. By contrast, the prevalence of tracheal stenosis following long-standing tracheostomy tube placement remains high with an estimated rate of approximately 30% *(14)*. Risk factors include difficult or prolonged intubation, infection, mechanical irritation, steroid administration, and use of positive pressure ventilation *(12,15)*.

Affected patients typically present with dyspnea on exertion, stridor, and wheezing *(12)*. It is important to be aware that symptoms of upper airway obstruction are often delayed several weeks following extubation. Moreover, patients with mild stenoses may initially be asymptomatic. However, such patients may eventually develop symptoms when tracheal luminal narrowing is worsened by airway edema and secretions from a coexistent respiratory infection *(16)*.

With regard to the mechanism of development, ischemic necrosis occurs acutely because of compromise of the blood supply to the tracheal mucosa *(11)*. This is followed by a superficial tracheitis with shallow ulcerations. The exposed cartilaginous rings subsequently soften and become fragmented. The softening of the cartilage explains why patients with post-intubation injuries are also at risk of tracheomalacia. This phase is subsequently followed by fibrosis and granulation tissue formation, resulting in concentric or eccentric wall thickening with associated luminal narrowing.

Post-intubation stenosis is thus characterized by eccentric or concentric tracheal wall thickening and associated luminal narrowing. The craniocaudal length usually ranges from 1.5 to 2.5 cm, which is more focal than many other causes of tracheal stenosis *(11,15)*. In patients who have undergone tracheostomy tube placement, the stenosis occurs most commonly at the stoma site and less commonly at the site where the tip of the tube has impinged on the tracheal mucosa *(11,12,17)*. In patients who have undergone endotracheal intubation, stenosis occurs most commonly in the subglottic region at the level of the endotracheal tube balloon *(15)*.

Post-intubation stenoses are often overlooked on conventional radiographs because of their proximal location and because radiologists often fail to carefully review the airway *(12)*. CT is the imaging modality of choice for detecting and characterizing tracheal stenosis. On axial images, CT demonstrates eccentric or concentric soft-tissue thickening with associated luminal narrowing (Fig. 4A) *(15)*. The focal nature and circumferential narrowing may produce a characteristic "hourglass" configuration (Fig. 4B). Less commonly, tracheal stenosis may present as a thin membrane of granulation tissue projecting into the tracheal lumen *(11,12)*. This finding may be difficult to detect on axial CT images. Thus, use of thin-section images and reformation techniques are recommended when imaging a patient with suspected intubation injury.

A variety of interventional bronchoscopic (balloon dilation, laser therapy, stent placement) and surgical (resection and end-to-end anastomosis) techniques may be employed to treat symptomatic tracheal stenoses *(16)*. Specific treatment decisions vary depending upon patient factors, characteristics of the stenosis, and local expertise.

4. AMYLOIDOSIS

Definition	Focal or diffuse extracellular deposition of amyloid fibrils which can be primary, secondary, familial, or senile
Etiology	Primary: clonal expansion of plasma cells in bone marrow. Secondary: response to chronic inflammatory conditions including cystic fibrosis, TB, and bronchiectasis
Epidemiology	Tracheobronchial amyloid is typically not associated with evidence of amyloidosis in other parts of the body
Frequency of airway involvement	Rare
Clinical presentation	Cough, dyspnea, hemoptysis, stridor, and hoarseness
MDCT findings	• Tracheal or bronchial wall thickening secondary to nodular and plaque-like deposition into the submucosa; circumferential or sparing posterior wall • Nodular form may mimic a tracheobronchial neoplasm with or without involvement of the surrounding paratracheal or bronchial tissues • Mural calcification common
Treatment	• Debulking with forceps or laser resection • Silicone stenting • Promising results with external beam radiation therapy and brachytherapy

Amyloidosis may involve the airways because of focal or diffuse submucosal deposits of AL amyloid *(18,19)*. Tracheobronchial amyloid is typically not associated with evidence of amyloidosis in other parts of the body. The mean age of patients with tracheobronchial amyloid in a large review was 53 years, with a range of 16–76 years *(20)*. Twice as many men as women experience the disease *(21)*.

Affected patients are often symptomatic for several years before they finally present *(22,23)*, suggesting that the disease progresses relatively slowly. The major symptoms are cough, dyspnea, hemoptysis, stridor, and hoarseness *(21,22)*. Affected patients may initially be misdiagnosed with asthma *(24,25)*.

Airway amyloid may be focal, multifocal, or diffuse: diffuse involvement seems most common *(19,26)*. It may involve the larynx, trachea, main bronchi, lobar, or proximal segmental bronchi, and often involves contiguous segments of the airway (e.g., larynx and trachea, trachea and main bronchi) *(27)*. Interestingly, tracheal amyloidosis may sometimes be associated with TBO *(27)*. Focal amyloidosis manifests endoscopically as submucosal plaques and nodules, with a cobblestone appearance in 44% of patients, a tumor-like appearance in 28% (Fig. 5), and circumferential wall thickening in

A)

B)

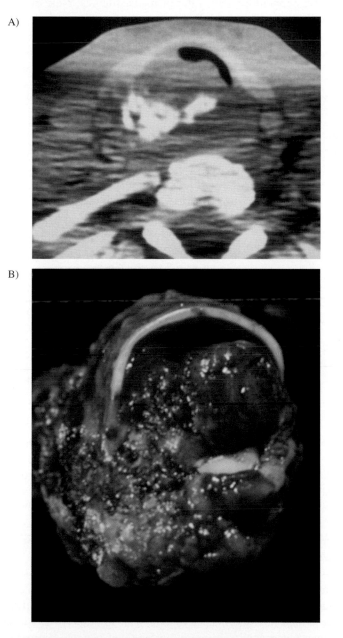

Fig. 5. Amyloidosis. (**A**) Axial CT image demonstrates high-grade proximal tracheal stenosis due to extensive, partly calcified soft tissue surrounding and narrowing the airway lumen. This proved to be due to amyloidosis at biopsy. (**B**) Gross pathological specimen at similar level as (A).

28% of cases *(27)*. There may also be multiple concentric or eccentric strictures. Amyloid tissue is commonly partly calcified, and may be circumferential *(28)*, or may spare the posterior membrane *(29)*. Local lesions give rise to endoluminal masses (amyloidomas) that may be radiologically indistinguishable from neoplasms *(19,30)*. In the trachea, amyloidomas are usually subglottic and may be calcified or ossified *(31)*. On magnetic resonance imaging (MRI), localized airway amyloid shows intermediate signal intensity on T1-weighted images and low signal on T2-weighted images *(31)*. Some patients with amyloidosis have hilar or mediastinal calcified or noncalcified hilar lymph nodes visible on chest radiographs or on CT *(32–34)*.

If treatment is required, the amyloid deposits may be removed by intermittent bronchoscopic resection *(35)* or, more commonly, by laser treatment *(25,27)*. Other treatment options include stenting and radiotherapy *(36,37)*. However, resection is not curative, and lesions often recur 6–12 months after treatment *(21)*.

5. IDIOPATHIC LARYNGOTRACHEAL STENOSIS

Definition	Rare inflammatory disease resulting in cicatricial stenosis of the upper trachea and cricoid
Etiology	Unknown; potential role of gastroesophageal reflux
Epidemiology	Almost exclusively in middle-aged females with no history of infection, trauma, intubation, or systemic disease
Clinical presentation	Progressive shortness of breath, wheezing, stridor, and/or hoarseness
MDCT findings	• Concentric or eccentric stenosis cricoid and proximal trachea • Smooth or lobulated margins
Treatment	• Surgical (preferred therapy)—laryngotracheal resection with laryngotracheoplasty • Endobronchial resection with or without stenting for nonsurgical candidates

Idiopathic laryngotracheal stenosis is a rare inflammatory disease resulting in cicatricial stenosis of the cricoid and upper trachea *(38–40)*. Its precise etiology is unknown, but it occurs almost exclusively in middle-aged females with no history of infection, trauma, intubation, or underlying systemic disease *(38,39)*. Affected patients present clinically with nonspecific signs of airway obstruction, including progressive shortness of breath, wheezing, stridor, and hoarseness *(38,39)*.

Imaging findings are nonspecific and include concentric or eccentric stenosis of the cricoid and proximal trachea with smooth or lobulated wall thickening (Fig. 6) *(38,39)*. Severe lumen compromise may occur in some cases.

Treatment options include surgical and endobronchial approaches *(38–40)*. Surgical treatment is potentially curative and consists of laryngotracheal resection with laryngotracheoplasty. Ashiku et al. *(39)* recently published a large retrospective review of over 70 patients treated surgically for idiopathic laryngotracheal stenosis and reported that laryngotracheal resection was successful in restoring the airway while preserving voice quality in more than 90% of patients. Long-term follow-up showed a stable airway and improvement in voice quality. Palliative endobronchial treatment with repeated dilations should be reserved for patients who are not operative candidates *(38)*.

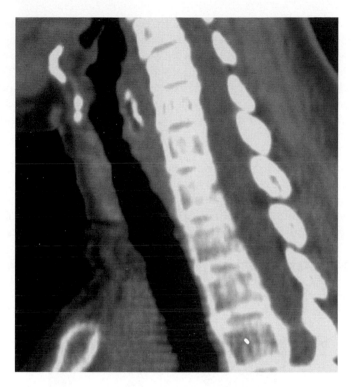

Fig. 6. Idiopathic stenosis. Sagittal reformation CT image demonstrates diffuse subglottic and proximal tracheal narrowing in patient with clinical diagnosis of idiopathic stenosis.

6. INFLAMMATORY BOWEL DISEASE

Definition	Chronic inflammatory diseases of the gastrointestinal (GI) tract of unknown etiology, including ulcerative colitis (UC) and Crohn's disease (CD)
Etiology	Known genetic and environmental risk factors
Epidemiology	More prevalent with UC and among women
Frequency of airway involvement	Rare
Clinical presentation	Tracheal stenosis may produce symptoms of airway obstruction—stridor, dyspnea, and productive cough
MDCT findings	• Edema of the epiglottic and aryepiglottic folds with eventual subglottic inflammation and stenosis
	• Diffuse soft tissue swelling of the hypopharynx
	• Tracheal stenosis and deformity
	• Bronchial wall thickening, with or without impaction
Treatment	• Intravenous or endoscopic injection of steroids
	• Cyclosporine
	• Endoscopic resection (e.g., laser therapy)

Inflammatory bowel diseases, including UC and CD, are chronic inflammatory diseases of the GI tract that demonstrate occasional extraintestinal manifestations, including lung parenchymal and airway disease *(41–43)*. Tracheobronchial complications are rare. They occur more often in association with UC than CD and are observed more frequently in women than in men *(40)*. The diagnosis of inflammatory bowel disease usually, but not always, precedes the presence of airway disease *(40)*.

The most prevalent and distinctive pattern of respiratory involvement is airway mucosal inflammation, which results in luminal narrowing (Fig. 7). Histologically, it is characterized by airway infiltration by inflammatory cells and mucosal ulceration *(40)*. If left untreated, it may progress to potentially irreversible tracheobronchial stenosis *(41)*.

Symptoms may develop directly from submucosal edema or indirectly from inflammation of the cricoarytenoid joint *(12)*. Affected patients typically present with nonspecific symptoms of airway obstruction, including stridor, dyspnea, and cough.

CT findings are nonspecific and include edema of the epiglottis, aryepiglottic folds, and arytenoids; diffuse soft-tissue swelling of the hypopharynx and larynx; tracheal deformity and narrowing; and severe bronchial wall thickening, with or without mucoid impaction *(12)*.

Treatment generally consists of intravenous steroids and cyclosporine. If medical therapy fails to resolve symptoms, interventional bronchoscopic techniques such as dilation and stent placement or endoscopic resection may be considered *(41)*.

A)

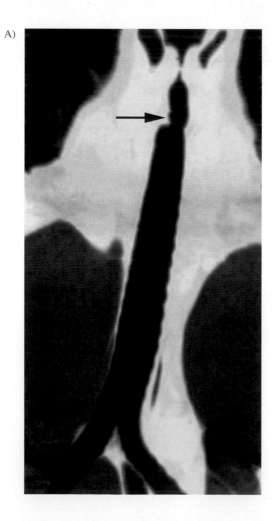

B)

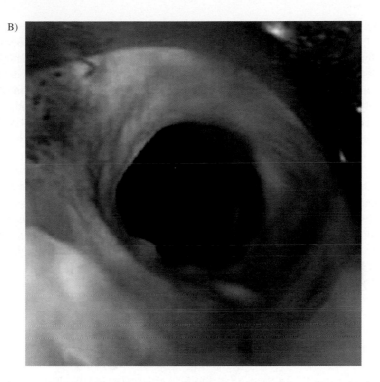

Fig. 7. Subglottic stenosis due to Crohn's disease. (**A**) Coronal minimal intensity projection image demonstrates focal, eccentric subglottic stenosis (arrow). (**B**) Bronchoscopic image shows mucosal erythema and inflammation at stenosis site.

7. RELAPSING POLYCHONDRITIS

Definition	Multisystem disorder characterized by recurrent inflammation of cartilaginous structures (external ear, nose, joints, larynx, trachea, bronchi)
Etiology	Unknown, likely autoimmune
Epidemiology	Rare. Especially Caucasians
Frequency of airway involvement	50%. Respiratory failure leading cause of mortality
Clinical presentation	Hoarseness, aphonia, wheezing, inspiratory stridor, nonproductive cough, dyspnea, and recurrent infections
MDCT findings	• Increased attenuation tracheal wall, subtle to frankly calcified; spares posterior wall • Wall thickening, spares posterior wall • Focal or diffuse stenosis of trachea and/or bronchi • Tracheobronchomalacia
Treatment	• High-dose oral prednisone. Intravenous pulsed steroids for acute airway obstruction • Surgical options: tracheostomy, stenting, external airway splinting, and tracheal reconstruction • Endoscopic interventions (e.g., stenting)

Relapsing polychondritis is a very rare, multisystem disorder that is characterized by recurrent inflammation of the cartilaginous structures of the external ear, nose, peripheral joints, larynx, trachea, and bronchi (44,45). Its etiology is unknown, but it is likely immune-mediated (44). Recent research suggests a genetic susceptibility, an overlap with other disorders associated with immunologic abnormalities, and the potential for multiple inciting events including chemical insults (45).

Relapsing polychondritis is most prevalent among Caucasians (44). Some studies report that men and women are equally affected (44), but a female predominance has also been reported (44). Airway involvement is present in up to 50% of patients and is a major cause of morbidity and mortality (44–46). Women are more likely than men to experience serious respiratory symptoms (45).

The average age of onset is variable, but it most commonly presents in the fifth and sixth decades (45). The diagnosis is established when any three of the following clinical features are present: bilateral auricular chondritis, nonerosive seronegative inflammatory arthritis, nasal chondritis, ocular inflammation, respiratory tract chondritis, and audiovestibular damage (46). Auricular involvement is the most common clinical feature (46). A saddle-nose deformity, which results from collapse of the cartilaginous nasal septum but preservation of the bony nasal septum, is highly characteristic of this condition.

Patients with laryngotracheobronchial involvement may present with various symptoms, including hoarseness, aphonia, wheezing, inspiratory stridor, nonproductive cough, dyspnea, and recurrent infections (46). Notably, airway involvement may be asymptomatic in early stages. Airway involvement may uncommonly occur as an isolated manifestation of relapsing polychondritis, without other perceptible features of this condition (47).

The airway may be involved focally or diffusely. The larynx and upper trachea are most commonly affected, but the disease may also involve the airways more distally to the level of the subsegmental bronchi (2). Glottic, subglottic, laryngeal, and/or tracheobronchial inflammation may result in luminal encroachment. Loss of structural cartilaginous support due to cartilaginous inflammation and destruction may result in tracheomalacia. In the late stages of the disease, there is fibrosis-induced contraction of the airway, with severe luminal narrowing.

There is no biopsy finding that is pathognomonic for relapsing polychondritis, but specimens of inflamed cartilage may show characteristic features of the cartilage including loss of basophilic staining of the matrix and perichondral inflammation (45). Eventually, the cartilage is destroyed and replaced by fibrous tissue.

The most common finding at CT is increased attenuation of the tracheal wall, often accompanied by tracheal wall thickening (Fig. 3) (10,12,15,17). As described earlier in this chapter, because the disease process targets cartilage, the noncartilaginous, posterior membranous wall is characteristically unaffected by this process.

Increased attenuation of the tracheal wall is well demonstrated by CT imaging and may range from subtle to frankly calcified (10). Increased wall thickness is also common and may be calcified or noncalcified (Fig. 3). CT readily identifies wall thickening, but it is unable to distinguish fibrosis from inflammation. A potential advantage of MRI is its ability to distinguish fibrosis from inflammation (48).

When imaging studies depict the presence of characteristic smooth thickening of the anterior and lateral walls of the trachea, a diagnosis of relapsing polychondritis can be made with a high degree of confidence. Although TBO (see Section 11) also spares the posterior membranous wall of the trachea, it is distinguished from relapsing polychondritis by the presence of discrete nodules arising from the submucosa of the tracheal wall and protruding into the airway lumen.

High-dose oral prednisone is usually necessary for treatment of respiratory tract involvement, and intravenous pulse steroids may be useful for treatment of acute airway obstruction (44). Surgical bronchoscopic options include tracheostomy, tracheal stenting, external airway splinting, and tracheal reconstruction (45,49).

8. RHINOSCLEROMA

Definition	Chronic, infectious, granulomatous disease with predilection for the upper respiratory tract with typical origin in the nasal mucosa and subsequent progression to the central airway
Etiology	Infection with *Klebsiella rhinoscleromatis*, a capsulated gram-negative bacterium
Epidemiology	Endemic in tropical and subtropical areas
Frequency of central airway involvement	10%
Clinical presentation	Difficulty breathing, which progresses to stridor
MDCT findings	• Diffuse nodular thickening of the tracheal and proximal bronchi wall with luminal narrowing • Late stage: circumferential fibrosis/strictures of subglottic airway, trachea, and/or bronchi • With or without mediastinal or hilar lymphadenopathy
Treatment	Antibiotics typically result in immediate improvement, but relapse is common

Rhinoscleroma is a chronic infectious granulomatous disease due to *K. rhinoscleromatis*, a capsulated gram-negative bacterium that is endemic in tropical and subtropical areas and has a predilection for the upper respiratory tract *(12)*. The infection typically originates in the nasal mucosa and subsequently progresses to involve the central airway *(12)*.

Laryngeal involvement is reported in 15–80% of cases, but tracheobronchial disease is much less common *(12,50)*. If left untreated, the infection tends to progress slowly over many years with alternating periods of remission and relapse *(12)*.

CT findings include diffuse nodular thickening of the tracheal and proximal bronchi wall with luminal narrowing; nodularity of the tracheal mucosa; and concentric strictures of the subglottic airway, trachea, and/or bronchi (Fig. 8) *(12)*.

Although positive cultures for the organism are diagnostic, they are found in only 60% of cases *(12)*. Antibiotics are standard therapy, but advanced cases with fibrotic stenoses may also benefit from mechanical balloon dilation *(12)*.

9. SABER-SHEATH TRACHEA

Definition	Intrathoracic tracheal deformity defined by narrowing of coronal and elongation of sagittal dimensions (sagittal : coronal diameter >2)
Etiology	Postulated to be a consequence of hyperinflation associated with chronic obstructive pulmonary disease (COPD)
Epidemiology	Strong association with COPD
Clinical presentation	Incidental detection on chest radiograph or CT
MDCT findings	• Abrupt change in configuration from extrathoracic to intrathoracic trachea elevated sagittal:coronal ratio • Often associated with excessive collapsibility of lateral walls resulting in tracheomalacia
Treatment	None

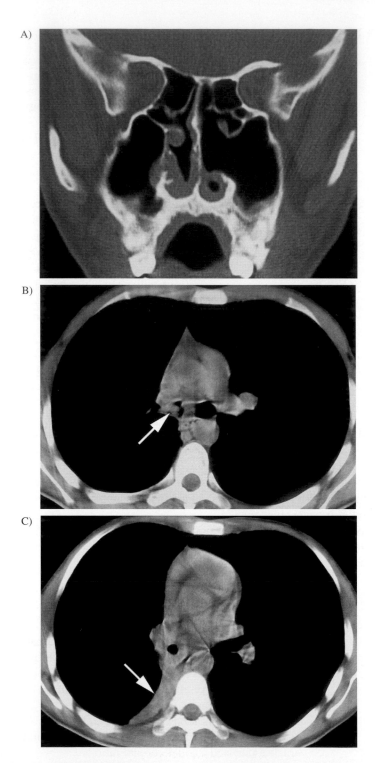

Fig. 8. Rhinoscleroma. (**A**) Coronal CT image of paranasal sinuses shows extensive mucosal thickening. (**B**) Axial CT image at level of proximal main bronchi demonstrates nodular thickening of right main bronchus (arrow). (**C**) Axial CT image at the level of bronchus intermedius shows circumferential thickening around airway lumen and right lower lobe collapse (arrow).

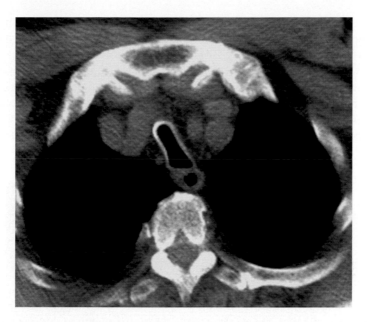

Fig. 9. Saber-sheath trachea in patient with chronic obstructive pulmonary disease (COPD). Axial CT image demonstrates anteroposterior elongation and coronal narrowing of tracheal lumen, consistent with saber-sheath configuration.

A saber-sheath trachea deformity (Fig. 9), defined by a reduction in coronal diameter and elongation of the sagittal diameter (sagittal:coronal diameter >2), may mimic true causes of tracheal stenosis *(17)*. This acquired deformity occurs in the setting of COPD, likely due to a response to mechanical forces related to hyperinflation *(17)*. A helpful distinguishing feature of this condition is that the narrowing is limited to the intrathoracic trachea, with preservation of normal configuration of the extrathoracic trachea *(17)*.

10. SARCOIDOSIS

Definition	Chronic, granulomatous, multisystem disease
Etiology	No clear etiologic mechanism elucidated. Postulated mechanisms include infectious, genetic, and immunological factors
Epidemiology	In US, more common in African Americans and females
Frequency of airway involvement	Tracheal involvement rare; bronchial involvement more common
Clinical presentation	Symptoms of central airway obstruction in advanced cases
MDCT findings	• Smooth, irregular, or nodular thickening of the trachea and bronchi • Focal or diffuse stenoses of bronchi may be complicated by distal collapse • Pulmonary fibrosis usually present
Treatment	• Corticosteroids and immunomodulators • Endoscopic interventions (e.g., stenting)

Tracheal involvement by sarcoidosis is rare *(51)*, and when it occurs it is usually associated with laryngeal involvement. Both the proximal and distal trachea may be affected, and the stenosis can be smooth *(52,53)*, irregular and nodular (Fig. 10) *(54)*, or even mass-like *(55)*.

Bronchial narrowing is much more common than tracheal narrowing as a manifestation of sarcoidosis. Narrowing of both main bronchi due to sarcoidosis may mimic tracheal narrowing *(56)*. Bronchial narrowing in sarcoidosis may be due to endobronchial granulomas, endobronchial fibrosis, bronchial distortion by parahilar conglomerate fibrosis, or some combination of these phenomena *(57)*. Bronchial stenoses are distributed throughout the lung and show no particular lobar or segmental

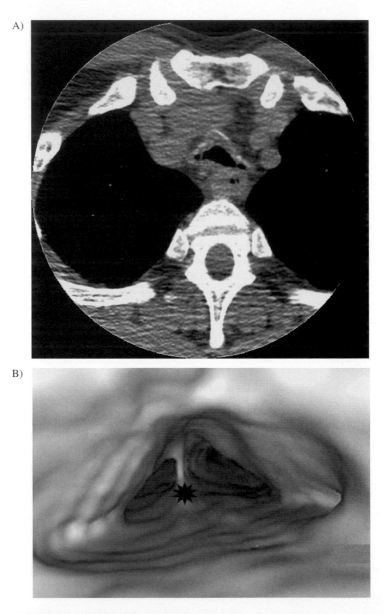

Fig. 10. Sarcoidosis. (**A**) Axial CT image of proximal intrathoracic trachea shows circumferential, nodular wall thickening. (**B**) Virtual bronchoscopic image at the level of carina (asterisk) demonstrates nodularity of airway wall in lower trachea and proximal main bronchi.

predilection. The stenoses may be single *(58,59)* or multiple *(59–61)* and most commonly affect lobar or proximal segmental divisions. At bronchoscopy, depending on the stage of the disease, the mucosa may be granular and hyperemic or even frankly inflamed and edematous. Granulomas may even give rise to a local obstructing endobronchial mass *(62–64)*. Later, when healing by fibrosis occurs, the mucosa may appear normal *(60)*.

Although endobronchial stenoses occur most commonly in well-established sarcoidosis *(58)*, often with pulmonary fibrosis, they have been recorded early in the course of sarcoidosis and with stage 0 radiographic disease *(59,60)*. The frequency of large airway narrowing is about 5% (range 2.5–9%) *(58,59,65)*. Patients present with wheeze, stridor, or airflow limitation *(60,61)* or episodes of lobar or segmental collapse and consolidation. Collapse is a well recognized but uncommon manifestation of sarcoidosis, occurring in about 1% of cases *(66–70)*. Any lobe may be affected, most commonly the middle lobe *(57,68)*. Collapse of an entire lung has been recorded.

In a high-resolution CT (HRCT) study of airways in 60 patients with sarcoidosis, 65% had nodular or smooth thickening of the lobar, segmental, or subsegmental airways *(71)*. Twenty-three percent of patients had smooth or irregular luminal narrowing. Recognition of these abnormalities may be diagnostically important, as endobronchial biopsy of an abnormal site is likely to yield granulomas. Also, patients with endobronchial sarcoidosis have a high prevalence of airway hyperreactivity *(72)*.

The natural history of bronchial stenosis due to sarcoidosis is variable: stenoses may clear spontaneously or with steroid treatment *(73)*. For refractory stenoses, mechanical dilatation or stenting is a therapeutic option *(74–76)*. Because endobronchial stenoses can be very difficult to detect on axial CT images, use of thin-section volumetric acquisition through the central bronchi, with multiplanar reconstructions, is recommended when airway stenosis is suspected, and may be particularly helpful for planning endoscopic interventions *(77)*.

11. TRACHEOBRONCHOPATHIA OSTEOCHONDROPLASTICA

Definition	Benign condition characterized by multiple submucosal osteocartilagenous nodules projecting into the tracheobronchial lumen.
Etiology	Postulated associations include chronic inflammatory processes, chemical irritation, and hereditary factors.
Epidemiology	Prevalence during routine bronchoscopy 0.02% – 0.7%. Especially fifth and sixth decades. 3:1 male predilection.
Clinical Presentation	Most cases asymptomatic but may present with chronic cough and wheezing. Often confused with asthma.
MDCT Findings	• Calcified nodules arising from the anterior and lateral walls of the trachea sparing the posterior membranous wall. • Thickening of the tracheal cartilage. • Saber sheath configuration often present.
Treatment	Asymptomatic cases require no treatment; options for symptomatic cases include: radiation therapy, laser therapy, surgical resection (localized disease) and stent placement.

TBO is a rare, benign disease of unknown etiology *(12,15,17,78,79)*. Several potential causes or associations have been postulated, including chronic inflammatory or degenerative processes, chemical irritation, amyloidosis, infection, and hereditary factors *(78,79)*. Two theories of histogenesis have been proposed: (i) ecchondrosis or exostosis from the tracheal cartilaginous rings; and (ii) cartilaginous and osseous metaplasia of elastic tissue in the internal elastic fibrous membrane of the tracheal wall *(78)*. Its prevalence at routine bronchoscopy is well below 1% *(12)*.

The clinical presentation is variable. The disorder is typically diagnosed during the fifth and sixth decades and has a 3:1 male predilection *(12)*. TBO may be an incidental finding in an asymptomatic patient, or it may present with various respiratory symptoms, including dyspnea on exertion, cough, wheezing, recurrent infections, and hemoptysis *(78)*.

TBO is characterized by multiple submucosal osteocartilaginous nodules that project into the tracheal lumen. At histopathology, the nodules are recognized as submucosal osteocartilaginous growths. The mucosal surface is usually intact, and a connection between the nodule and the perichondrium of the tracheal cartilaginous ring is frequently identified *(12)*.

CT is the imaging modality of choice for this condition *(78)*. It demonstrates a characteristic pattern of calcified nodules arising from the anterior and lateral walls of the trachea and protruding into the lumen, resulting in diffuse luminal narrowing (Fig. 11). The individual nodules typically range in size from 3 to 8 mm *(3)*. Thickening of the tracheal cartilage is also typically visible at CT *(12,15,17,78)*. Similar to relapsing polychondritis, there is sparing of the posterior membranous wall. Interestingly, a saber-sheath configuration of the trachea is frequently observed in patients with TBO *(78)*.

The identification of calcified nodules arising from the anterior and lateral walls of the trachea at CT or bronchoscopy is considered diagnostic of this condition *(12,79)*. The differential diagnosis includes amyloidosis and calcific TB, but these entities do not spare the posterior wall of the trachea. Although relapsing polychondritis has a similar distribution as TBO, it characteristically presents with calcified wall thickening without discrete intraluminal nodules. Moreover, only polychondritis is associated with tracheomalacia.

Treatment is usually supportive and conservative. There is currently no medical therapy to treat this condition or to prevent the growth of new nodules *(12)*. Treatment options for advanced cases

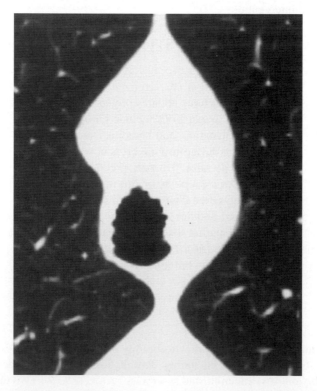

Fig. 11. Tracheobronchopathia osteochondroplastica. Axial CT image at the level of aortic arch demonstrates diffuse nodules arising from the anterior and lateral tracheal walls. (Courtesy of Dr. Michael Gotway)

include laser resection, radiation therapy, surgical resection, or stent placement *(78)*. Interventional therapy is usually tailored for individual cases.

12. TRANSPLANTATION

Definition	Stenosis at bronchial anastomosis site following transplantation
Etiology	Anastomosis site vulnerable because of reliance on low-pressure retrograde perfusion from pulmonary artery collaterals
Epidemiology	• Risk factors: infection, immune suppression
	• 10–15% of lung transplants
Clinical presentation	Failure of anticipated improvement in symptoms in the first months following transplantation; decreased forced expiratory volume in 1s (FEV1)
MDCT findings	Focal bronchial narrowing at the anastomotic site
Treatment	Endoscopic—balloon dilatation with stenting

Bronchial anastomotic stenosis is a relatively common complication following lung transplantation *(12,80)*. Because the bronchial arterial supply of the transplanted lung is not routinely restored during surgery, the transplanted bronchus is vulnerable because of its dependence upon low-pressure retrograde perfusion from pulmonary arterial collateral vessels immediately after surgery *(12)*. Contributing risk factors for stenosis include infection, rejection, and immunosuppression *(12)*. Although initially present in up to 50% of patients following transplantation, its prevalence has decreased to 10–15% following recent improvements in surgical technique and alterations in immunosuppressive regimens *(12,80)*.

Clinically, affected patients typically present with failure of anticipated improvement in symptoms in the first months following transplantation and decline in pulmonary function, especially the FEV1 *(12,80)*. When severe, the stenosis can lead to progressive, often debilitating airflow obstruction that may be difficult to clinically differentiate from other causes of airflow limitation that may occur following transplantation, especially obliterative bronchiolitis *(81)*. Establishing the correct diagnosis is important because treatments for these conditions differ.

At bronchoscopy, the stenosis is characterized by focal, cicatricial narrowing at the anastomotic site *(12)*. Although bronchoscopy is considered the gold standard for diagnosis, it provides only limited information on the length of the stenosis or the patency of the distal airways, which are important factors in planning treatment *(80)*. For this reason, there has been considerable interest in evaluating the ability of CT with virtual bronchoscopic reconstructions in the assessment of this disorder. CT findings are characteristic and consist of focal narrowing at the bronchial anastomotic site (Fig. 12). A study by McAdams et al. *(81)* showed that virtual bronchoscopy depicts over 90% of stenoses found at fiberoptic bronchoscopy. A subsequent study by Shitrit et al. *(80)* that assessed virtual bronchoscopy in 10 patients with stenoses related to lung transplants reported that grading of stenoses by virtual bronchoscopy correlated well with pulmonary function tests. Presently, the role of CT is evolving to include surveillance for stenoses following transplantation and assessment of the patency of the airways distal to high-grade stenoses.

Treatment consists of balloon dilation followed by placement of a silicone stent. The stenosis typically responds well to therapy, and the stent can usually be removed after 1–2 years *(12)*.

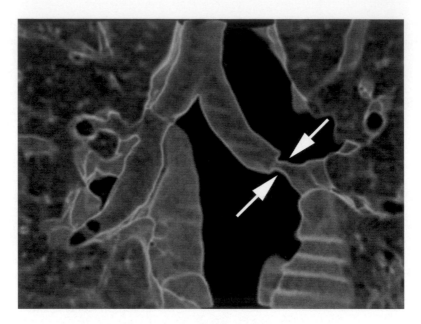

Fig. 12. Post-transplant stenosis. External 3-D rendering of lower trachea and bronchi demonstrates focal stenosis (arrows) of distal left bronchus at site of anastomosis for lung transplantation.

13. TUBERCULOSIS

Definition	Granulomatous infection.
Etiology	Involvement of airway by *Mycobacterium tuberculosis*.
Epidemiology	Tracheobronchial strictures more common in Africans and Asians because of higher prevalence of TB.
Frequency of airway involvement	Endobronchial TB found in 10 – 37% of patients with pulmonary parenchymal tuberculosis. Varying degrees of stenosis in 90% of patients with endobronchial disease.
Clinical Presentation	Barking cough unresponsive to standard treatment. Wheezing and hemoptysis less common.
MDCT Findings	Acute/Subacute: • Thickening and enhancement of the tracheal wall with irregular luminal narrowing. • Lymphadenopathy/mediastinitis. Last Stage: • Concentric stenosis. • Smooth or irregular wall thickening. • Especially distal trachea and left main bronchus.
Treatment	• Standard anti – TB therapy. • Fibrotic strictures: dilation, stent placement.

Tracheobronchial stenosis due to TB may occur in the setting of acute infection or as late as 30 years following infection *(12)*. Endobronchial disease has been reported in up to one-third of patients with pulmonary parenchymal involvement from TB, and a variable degree of airway stenosis has been reported to occur in 90% of cases *(12)*.

TB involvement of the central airways may occur secondary to several mechanisms, including direct implantation of organisms from infected sputum, extension to peribronchial region due to lymphatic drainage from pulmonary parenchymal infection, direct extension from adjacent parenchymal infection, erosion from adjacent lymph nodes, and hematogenous spread *(82,83)*.

Kim et al. *(83)* have described the CT findings of tracheobronchial involvement from TB in 17 patients, comparing and contrasting the imaging features between actively caseating and fibrotic forms of the disease. For example, actively caseating tracheobronchial TB showed circumferential and predominantly irregular luminal narrowing and mediastinitis. The latter findings were present solely in patients with active disease. By contrast, in cases of fibrotic disease, CT showed either smooth or irregular narrowing with a lesser degree of wall thickening compared with patients with active disease.

TB-related airway strictures are typically cicatricial and are often multifocal in distribution (Fig. 13) *(12)*. Interestingly, in the series by Kim et al. *(83)*, tracheal involvement was always accompanied by involvement of the main bronchi and lung parenchyma. Thus, isolated tracheal involvement is likely a rare manifestation.

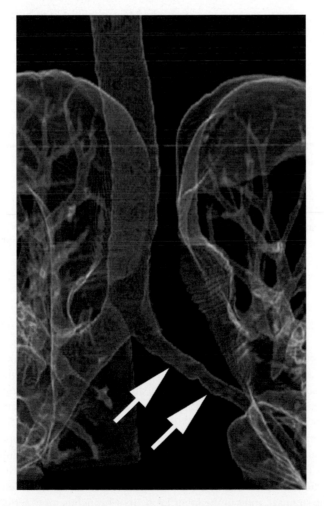

Fig. 13. Tuberculosis stenosis. External 3-D rendering of central airways shows irregular stenosis of left main bronchus (arrows).

Tuberculous stenosis due to active disease is treated with standard antituberculous regimens, sometimes combined with steroids *(12)*. However, once a stenosis has progressed to the fibrotic stage, interventional bronchoscopic procedures such as dilation and stent placement are often required *(12)*. Surgical treatment is generally reserved for cases in which less invasive endoscopic therapy has failed *(12)*.

14. WEGENER GRANULOMATOSIS

Definition	Widespread necrotizing granulomatous vasculitis with a predilection for the respiratory system and kidneys
Etiology	Unknown but likely autoimmune mechanism
Epidemiology	Rare. Especially Caucasians
Frequency of central airway involvement	15–25%
Clinical presentation	Dyspnea, hoarseness, voice change, and stridor
MDCT findings	• Usually subglottic (90%)
	• Smooth or irregular circumferential stenoses, 2–4 cm long, can be smooth or irregular
Treatment	• Corticosteroids—prednisone
	• Immunomodulators—cyclophosphamide, methotrexate, azathioprine

Tracheal narrowing is an important and relatively common manifestation of Wegener granulomatosis, with frequencies of 16 and 23% in two large series *(84,85)*. There is a female predominance and notably all but one of the 17 patients with this complication in a Mayo Clinic series were females *(84)*. Symptoms may occur early in the course of Wegener granulomatosis and may even be a presenting feature in some patients *(84,85)*, whereas in others there is a several year delay *(84)*. Symptoms consist of dyspnea, hoarseness, voice change, and stridor, and these are usually accompanied by nasal involvement *(84)*. However, patients with isolated laryngotracheal disease are recorded *(86,87)*, and in particular subglottic stenosis may be found in Wegener granulomatosis without other evidence of pulmonary involvement *(88)*. In one series, about 50% of tracheal stenoses occurred independently of other features of active Wegener granulomatosis *(85)*. Tracheal stenosis is often unresponsive to systemic therapy and local intervention is favored *(85)*. Endoscopic manifestations of Wegener granulomatosis include inflammatory tracheobronchial stenosis, ulcerating tracheobronchitis, and tracheobronchial stenosis without an inflammatory component *(87)*.

On imaging, tracheal stenoses are most commonly subglottic [90% in one series *(89)*] and usually present as smooth or irregular circumferential stenoses about 2–4 cm long (Fig. 14) *(84,89,90)*. Because of the high prevalence of subglottic stenoses, this area should always be included in the imaging volume in patients with Wegener granulomatosis. CT shows abnormal intratracheal soft tissue, often associated with thickening and calcification of the tracheal rings *(91)*. Cartilaginous erosion may also be seen *(89)*. The mucosal thickening may be irregular or ulcerated, and involvement of adjacent vocal cords may be visible on CT *(89)*. In a study of 18 virtual bronchoscopic examinations performed on 11 patients with Wegener granulomatosis, 32 of 40 bronchoscopically visible stenoses were identified on virtual bronchoscopy by at least one reading radiologist, compared with only 22 on axial CT images *(92)*. The authors emphasized the subtlety of these stenotic lesions and suggested that double reading of virtual bronchoscopic images was important for optimal detection of stenoses. In this series, most of the stenoses were in the lobar bronchi or bronchus intermedius. Bronchial stenoses may result in distal collapse/consolidation of a lobe or lung *(93)*. On MR the abnormal soft tissue

A)

B)

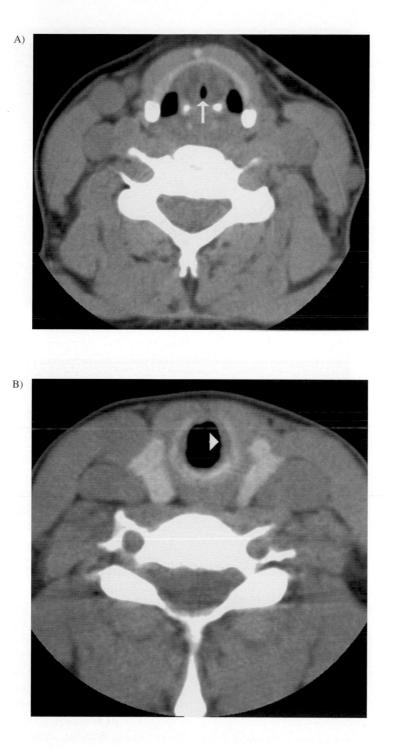

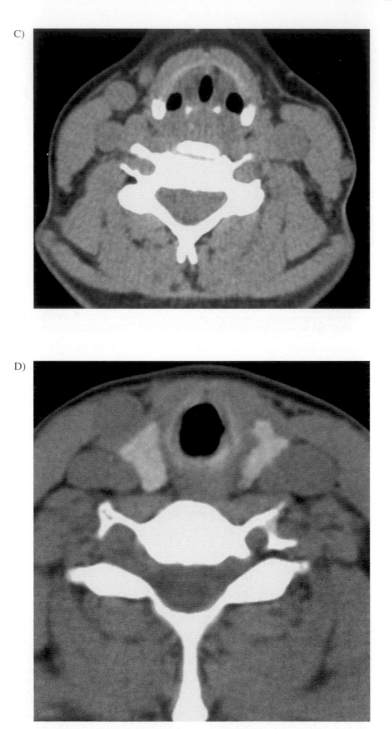

Fig. 14. Wegener granulomatosis. (**A**) Axial CT at the level of the piriform sinuses shows marked thickening of the aryepiglottic folds, with marked narrowing of the supraglottic space (arrow). (**B**) Axial CT through the subglottic region shows moderate soft tissue thickening (arrowhead) and mild narrowing. (**C, D**) Followup CT images at the same levels 6 weeks later, following medical treatment, show decreased supraglottic narrowing and decreased infraglottic soft tissue thickening.

associated with stenoses due to Wegener granulomatosis is of intermediate signal on T1-weighted sequences, high signal on T2-weighted sequences, and enhances with contrast agents *(94)*.

REFERENCES

1. Boiselle PM, Ernst A. Recent advances in central airway imaging. *Chest* 2002;121:1651–1660.
2. Boiselle PM, Reynolds KF, Ernst A. Multiplanar and three-dimensional imaging of the central airways with multidetector CT. *AJR Am J Roentgenol* 2002;179:301–308.
3. Salvolini L, Secchi EB, Costarelli L, De Nicola M. Clinical applications of 2D and 3D CT imaging of the airways—a review. *Eur J Radiol* 2000;34:9–25.
4. Naidich DP, Gruden JF, McGuiness GM, McCauley DI, Bhalla M. Volumetric (helical/spiral) CT (VCT) of the airways. *J Thorac Imaging* 1997;12:11–28.
5. Remy-Jardin M, Remy J, Artaud D, Fribourg M, Naili A. Tracheobronchial tree: assessment with volume rendering-technical aspects. *Radiology* 1998;208:393–398.
6. Remy-Jardin M, Remy J, Artaud D, Fribourg M, Duhamel A. Volume rendering of the tracheobronchial tree: clinical evaluation of bronchographic images. *Radiology* 1998;208:761–770.
7. Remy-Jardin M, Remy J, Deschildre F, Artaud D, Ramon P, Edme JL. Obstructive lesions of the central airways: evaluation by using spiral CT with multiplanar and three-dimensional reformations. *Eur Radiol* 1996;6:807–816.
8. Rubin GD. Data explosion: the challenge of multidetector-row CT. *Eur J Radiol* 2000;36:74–80.
9. Lee KS, Ernst A, Trentham D, Lunn W, Feller-Kopman D, Boiselle, PM. Prevalence of functional airway abnormalities in relapsing polychondritis. *Radiology* 2006;240:565–573.
10. Behar JV, Choi YW, Hartman TA, Allen NB, McAdams HP. Relapsing polychondritis affecting the lower respiratory tract. *AJR Am J Roentgenol* 2002;178:173–177.
11. Fraser RS, Colman N, Müller NL, Pare PD. Upper airway obstruction. In: *Fraser and Pare's Diagnosis of Diseases of the Chest*, 4th Ed. Fraser RS, Colman N, Müller NL, Pare PD, Eds. W.B. Saunders Co, Philadelphia, 1999, pp. 2033–2036.
12. Prince JS, Duhamel DR, Levin DL, et al. Nonneoplastic lesions of the tracheobronchial wall: radiographic findings with bronchoscopic correlation. *Radiographics* 2002;22:S215–S230.
13. Stauffer J, Olson D, Petty T. Complications and consequences of endotracheal intubation and trachostomy. A prospective study of 150 critically ill adult patients. *Am J Med* 1981;70.65–76.
14. Norwood S, Vallina V, Short K, et al. Incidence of tracheal stenosis and other late complications after percutaneous tracheostomy. *Ann Surg* 2000;232:233–241.
15. Webb EM, Elicker BM, Webb WR. Using CT to diagnose nonneoplastic tracheal abnormalities. *AJR Am J Roentgenol* 2000;174:1315–1321.
16. Ernst A, Herth F, Becker H. Overview of the management of central airway obstruction. In: *UpToDate*, Rose, BD, Ed. UpToDate, Waltham, MA, 2006.
17. Marom EM, Goodman PC, McAdams HP. Focal abnormalities of the trachea and bronchi. *AJR Am J Roentgenol* 2001;176:707–711.
18. Toyoda M, Ebihara Y, Kato H, Kita S. Tracheobronchial AL amyloidosis: histologic, immunohistochemical, ultrastructural, and immunoelectron microscopic observations. *Hum Pathol* 1993;24:970–976.
19. Thompson PJ, Citron KM. Amyloid and the lower respiratory tract. *Thorax* 1983;38:84–87.
20. Gottlieb LS, Gold WM. Primary tracheobronchial amyloidosis. *Am Rev Respir Dis* 1972;105:425–429.
21. Rubinow A, Celli BR, Cohen AS, Rigden BG, Brody JS. Localized amyloidosis of the lower respiratory tract. *Am Rev Respir Dis* 1978;118:603–611.
22. Prowse C. Amyloidosis of the lower respiratory tract. *Thorax* 1958;13:308–320.
23. Gross BH, Felson B, Birnberg FA. The respiratory tract in amyloidosis and the plasma cell dyscrasias. *Semin Roentgenol* 1986;21:113–127.
24. Naef AP, Savary M, Gruneck JM, Baumann RP. Amyloid pseudotumor treated by tracheal resection. *Ann Thorac Surg* 1977;23:578–581.
25. Breuer R, Simpson GT, Rubinow A, Skinner M, Cohen AS. Tracheobronchial amyloidosis: treatment by carbon dioxide laser photoresection. *Thorax* 1985;40:87.
26. Hui AN, Koss MN, Hochholzer L, Wehunt WD. Amyloidosis presenting in the lower respiratory tract. Clinicopathologic, radiologic, immunohistochemical, and histochemical studies on 48 cases. *Arch Pathol Lab Med* 1986;110:212–218.
27. Piazza C, Cavaliere S, Foccoli P, Toninelli C, Bolzoni A, Peretti G. Endoscopic management of laryngo-tracheobronchial amyloidosis: a series of 32 patients. *Eur Arch Otorhinolaryngol* 2003;260:349–354.
28. Ozer C, Nass Duce M, Yildiz A, Apaydin FD, Egilmez H, Arpaci T. Primary diffuse tracheobronchial amyloidosis: case report. *Eur J Radiol* 2002;44:37–39.
29. O'Regan A, Fenlon HM, Beamis JF Jr, Steele MP, Skinner M, Berk JL. Tracheobronchial amyloidosis. The Boston University experience from 1984 to 1999. *Medicine (Baltimore)* 2000;79:69–79.

30. Cotton R, Jackson J. Localized amyloid 'tumours' of the lung simulating malignant neoplasms. *Thorax* 1964;19:97–103.
31. Weissman B, Wong M, Smith DN. Image interpretation session: 1996. *Radiographics* 1997;17:244–245.
32. Dalton H, Featherstone T, Athanasou N. Organ limited amyloidosis with lymphadenopathy. *Postgrad Med J* 1992;68: 47–50.
33. Schmidt H, McDonald J, Clagett O. Amyloid tumours of the lower respiratory tract and mediastinum. *Ann Otol Rhinol Laryngol* 1953;62:880–893.
34. Crestani B, Monnier A, Kambouchner M, Battesti JP, Reynaud P, Valeyre D. Tracheobronchial amyloidosis with hilar lymphadenopathy associated with a serum monoclonal immunoglobulin. *Eur Respir J* 1993;6:1569–1571.
35. Flemming AF, Fairfax AJ, Arnold AG, Lane DJ. Treatment of endobronchial amyloidosis by intermittent bronchoscopic resection. *Br J Dis Chest* 1980;74:183–188.
36. Yang S, Chia SY, Chuah KL, Eng P. Tracheobronchial amyloidosis treated with rigid bronchoscopy and stenting. *Surg Endosc* 2003;17:658–659.
37. Kalra S, Utz JP, Edell ES, Foote RL. External-beam radiation therapy in the treatment of diffuse tracheobronchial amyloidosis. *Mayo Clin Proc* 2001;76:853–856.
38. Ashiku SK, Mathieson D. Idiopathic laryngotracheal stenosis. *Chest Surg Clin N Am* 2003;13(2):257–269.
39. Ashiku SK, Kuzucu A, Grillo HC, et al. Idiopathic laryngotracheal stenosis: effective definitive treatment with laryngo-tracheal resection. *J Thorac Cardiovasc Surg* 2004;127(1):99–107.
40. Camus P, Colby TV. The lung in inflammatory bowel disease. *Eur Respir J* 2000;15:5–10.
41. Herrington HC, Weber SM, Andersen PE. Modern management of laryngotracheal stenosis. *Laryngoscope* 2006;116(9):1553–1557.
42. Plataki M, Tzortzaki E, Lambiri I, et al. Severe airway stenosis associated with Crohn's disease: case report. *BMC Pulm Med* 2006;6:7.
43. Ulrich R, Goldberg R, Line WS. Crohn's disease: a rare cause of upper airway obstruction. *J Emerg Med* 2000;19: 331–332.
44. Trentham DE, Le CH. Relapsing polychondritis. *Ann Intern Med* 1998;129:114–122.
45. Herman JH. Relapsing polychondritis. In: *UpToDate*, Rose, BD, Ed. UpToDate, Waltham, MA, 2006.
46. Letko E, Zafirakis P, Baltatzis S, et al. Relapsing polychondritis: a clinical review. *Semin Arthritis Rheum* 2002;31: 384–395.
47. Tsunezuka Y, Sato H, Shimizu H. Tracheobronchial involvement in relapsing polychondritis. *Respiration* 2000;67: 320–322.
48. Heman-Ackhah YD, Remley KB, Goding GS Jr. A new role for magnetic resonance imaging in the diagnosis of laryngeal relapsing polychondritis. *Head Neck* 1999;21:484–489.
49. Gergely P Jr, Poor G. Relapsing polychondritis. *Best Pract Res Clin Rheumatol* 2004;18:723–738.
50. Soni NK. Scleroma of the lower respiratory tract: a bronchoscopic study. *J Laryngol Otol* 1994;108:484–485.
51. Brandstetter RD, Messina MS, Sprince NL, Grillo HC. Tracheal stenosis due to sarcoidosis. *Chest* 1981;80:656.
52. Lefrak S, Di Benedetto R. Systematic sarcoidosis with severe involvement of the upper respiratory tract. *Am Rev Respir Dis* 1970;102:801–807.
53. Henry DA, Cho SR. Tracheal stenosis in sarcoidosis. *South Med J* 1983;76:1323–1324.
54. Kirschner BS, Holinger PH. Laryngeal obstruction in children sarcoidosis. *J Pediatr* 1976;88:263–265.
55. Weisman RA, Canalis RF, Powell WJ. Laryngeal sarcoidosis with airway obstruction. *Ann Otol Rhinol Laryngol* 1980;89:58–61.
56. Miller A, Brown LK, Teirstein AS. Stenosis of main bronchi mimicking fixed upper airway obstruction in sarcoidosis. *Chest* 1985;88:244–248.
57. Rockoff SD, Rohatgi PK. Unusual manifestations of thoracic sarcoidosis. *AJR Am J Roentgenol* 1985;144:513–528.
58. Scadding JG, Mitchell DN. *Sarcoidosis*. London: Chapman and Hall; 1985.
59. Olsson T, Bjornstad-Pettersen H, Stjernberg NL. Bronchostenosis due to sarcoidosis: a cause of atelectasis and airway obstruction simulating pulmonary neoplasm and chronic obstructive pulmonary disease. *Chest* 1979;75:663–666.
60. Hadfield JW, Page RL, Flower CD, Stark JE. Localised airway narrowing in sarcoidosis. *Thorax* 1982;37:443–447.
61. Udwadia ZF, Pilling JR, Jenkins PF, Harrison BD. Bronchoscopic and bronchographic findings in 12 patients with sarcoidosis and severe or progressive airways obstruction. *Thorax* 1990;45:272–275.
62. Conant EF, Glickstein MF, Mahar P, Miller WT. Pulmonary sarcoidosis in the older patient: conventional radiographic features. *Radiology* 1988;169:315–319.
63. Dorman RL Jr, Whitman GJ, Chew FS. Thoracic sarcoidosis. *AJR Am J Roentgenol* 1995;164:1368.
64. Corsello BF, Lohaus GH, Funahashi A. Endobronchial mass lesion due to sarcoidosis: complete resolution with corti-costeroids. *Thorax* 1983;38:157–158.
65. Smellie H, Hoyle C. The natural history of pulmonary sarcoidosis. *Q J Med* 1960;29:539–559.
66. Kirks DR, McCormick VD, Greenspan RH. Pulmonary sarcoidosis. Roentgenologic analysis of 150 patients. *Am J Roentgenol Radium Ther Nucl Med* 1973;117:777–786.

67. Freundlich IM, Libshitz HI, Glassman LM, Israel HL. Sarcoidosis. Typical and atypical thoracic manifestations and complications. *Clin Radiol* 1970;21:376–383.
68. Romer FK. Presentation of sarcoidosis and outcome of pulmonary changes. *Dan Med Bull* 1982;29:27–32.
69. Ellis K, Renthal G. Pulmonary sarcoidosis. Roentgenographic observations on course of disease. *AJR Am J Roentgenol* 1962;88:1070–1083.
70. Rabinowitz JG, Ulreich S, Soriano C. The usual unusual manifestations of sarcoidosis and the "hilar haze"—a new diagnostic aid. *Am J Roentgenol Radium Ther Nucl Med* 1974;120:821–831.
71. Lenique F, Brauner MW, Grenier P, Battesti JP, Loiseau A, Valeyre D. CT assessment of bronchi in sarcoidosis: endoscopic and pathologic correlations. *Radiology* 1995;194:419–423.
72. Shorr AF, Torrington KG, Hnatiuk OW. Endobronchial involvement and airway hyperreactivity in patients with sarcoidosis. *Chest* 2001;120:881–886.
73. Munt PW. Middle lobe atelectasis in sarcoidosis. Report of a case with prompt resolution concomitant with corticosteroid administration. *Am Rev Respir Dis* 1973;108:357–360.
74. Fouty BW, Pomeranz M, Thigpen TP, Martin RJ. Dilatation of bronchial stenoses due to sarcoidosis using a flexible fiberoptic bronchoscope. *Chest* 1994;106:677–680.
75. Iles PB. Multiple bronchial stenoses: treatment by mechanical dilatation. *Thorax* 1981;36:784–786.
76. Mayse ML, Greenheck J, Friedman M, Kovitz KL. Successful bronchoscopic balloon dilation of nonmalignant tracheo-bronchial obstruction without fluoroscopy. *Chest* 2004;126:634–637.
77. Curtin JJ, Innes NJ, Harrison BD. Thin-section spiral volumetric CT for the assessment of lobar and segmental bronchial stenoses. *Clin Radiol* 1998;53:110–115.
78. Restrepo S, Pandit M, Villamil MA, Rojas IC, Perez JM, Gascue A. Tracheobronchopathia osteochondroplastica: helical CT findings in 4 cases. *J Thorac Imaging* 2004;19:112–116.
79. Fraser RS, Colman N, Müller NL, Pare PD. Upper airway obstruction. In: *Fraser and Pare's Diagnosis of Diseases of the Chest*, 4th Ed. Fraser RS, Colman N, Müller NL, Pare PD, Eds. W.B. Saunders Co, Philadelphia, 1999, p. 2042.
80. Shitrit D, Postinikov V, Grubstein A, et al. Accuracy of virtual bronchoscopy for grading tracheobronchial stenosis: correlation with pulmonary function test and fiberoptic bronchoscopy. *Chest* 2005;128:3545–3550.
81. McAdams HP, Palmer SM, Erasmus JJ, et al. Bronchial anastomotic complications in lung transplant recipients: virtual bronchoscopy for noninvasive assessment. *Radiology* 1998;209:689–695.
82. Kim YH, Kim HT, Lee KS, Uh ST, Cung YT, Park CS. Serial fiberoptic bronchoscopic observations of endobronchial tuberculosis before and early after antituberculosis chemotherapy. *Chest* 1993;103:673–677.
83. Kim Y, Lee KS, Yoon JII, et al. Tuberculosis of the trachea and main bronchi: CT findings in 17 patients. *AJR Am J Roentgenol* 1997;168:1051–1056.
84. McDonald TJ, Neel HB 3rd, DeRemee RA. Wegener's granulomatosis of the subglottis and the upper portion of the trachea. *Ann Otol Rhinol Laryngol* 1982;91:588–592.
85. Langford CA, Sneller MC, Hallahan CW, et al. Clinical features and therapeutic management of subglottic stenosis in patients with Wegener's granulomatosis. *Arthritis Rheum* 1996;39:1754–1760.
86. Hellmann D, Laing T, Petri M, Jacobs D, Crumley R, Stulbarg M. Wegener's granulomatosis: isolated involvement of the trachea and larynx. *Ann Rheum Dis* 1987;46:628–631.
87. Daum TE, Specks U, Colby TV, et al. Tracheobronchial involvement in Wegener's granulomatosis. *Am J Respir Crit Care Med* 1995;151:522–526.
88. Utzig MJ, Warzelhan J, Wertzel H, Berwanger I, Hasse J. Role of thoracic surgery and interventional bronchoscopy in Wegener's granulomatosis. *Ann Thorac Surg* 2002;74:1948–1952.
89. Screaton NJ, Sivasothy P, Flower CD, Lockwood CM. Tracheal involvement in Wegener's granulomatosis: evaluation using spiral CT. *Clin Radiol* 1998;53:809–815.
90. Cohen MI, Gore RM, August CZ, Ossoff RH. Tracheal and bronchial stenosis associated with mediastinal adenopathy in Wegener granulomatosis: CT findings. *J Comput Assist Tomogr* 1984;8:327–329.
91. Stein MG, Gamsu G, Webb WR, Stulbarg MS. Computed tomography of diffuse tracheal stenosis in Wegener granulomatosis. *J Comput Assist Tomogr* 1986;10:868–870.
92. Summers RM, Aggarwal NR, Sneller MC, et al. CT virtual bronchoscopy of the central airways in patients with Wegener's granulomatosis. *Chest* 2002;121:242–250.
93. Cordier JF, Valeyre D, Guillevin L, Loire R, Brechot JM. Pulmonary Wegener's granulomatosis. A clinical and imaging study of 77 cases. *Chest* 1990;97:906–912.
94. Park KJ, Bergin CJ, Harrell J. MR findings of tracheal involvement in Wegener's granulomatosis. *AJR Am J Roentgenol* 1998;171:524–525.

7

Tracheal and Bronchial Neoplasms

Karen S. Lee and Phillip M. Boiselle

Summary

Primary central airway neoplasms are rare. These neoplasms present with symptoms of airway obstruction and hemoptysis. Oftentimes, the diagnosis is delayed because of the late presentation of symptoms. Multidetector CT is the imaging modality of choice for diagnosis, staging, and preoperative planning of central airway tumors. The differential diagnosis of central airway neoplasms is broad, but five histologies comprise the majority of lesions. Whereas multidetector CT imaging features can help distinguish benign from malignant entities, only rarely can imaging alone provide a specific diagnosis. Secondary airway malignancies and non-neoplastic processes are mimickers of central airway tumors.

Key Words: Airway; trachea; bronchus; neoplasm; tumor; CT.

1. INTRODUCTION

Primary central airway neoplasms (involving the trachea and main bronchi) are rare, comprising approximately 5% of all primary lung malignancies (1). Primary tracheal tumors are an even rarer subset, as they are estimated to be 100 times less frequent than primary bronchial neoplasms and account for 2% of all respiratory tract tumors (2,3). A neoplasm within the central airways is more likely due to direct airway invasion by an adjacent secondary neoplasm originating from the thyroid, lung, or esophagus, rather than a primary airway neoplasm (4).

Patients with primary central airway neoplasms often remain clinically silent until the airway lumen is narrowed by approximately 75% (5) (Fig. 1). Patients typically present with symptoms of airway obstruction including dyspnea, stridor, cough, and wheezing, as well as hemoptysis and chest pain (1,6). Many of these patients are misdiagnosed as having adult-onset asthma or bronchitis (1,7). Consequently, these airway tumors often escape detection for many months or years and are often large at the time of diagnosis (1,6).

The majority of primary central airway neoplasms in the adult are malignant, unlike in children, where the majority of airway tumors are benign (6,8). The differential diagnosis of central airway neoplasms is broad; however, five histologies comprise the majority of primary tracheobronchial tumors: squamous cell carcinoma, adenoid cystic carcinoma, carcinoid, mucoepidermoid carcinoma, and squamous cell papilloma (9).

2. IMAGING ASSESSMENT

Conventional posteroanterior and lateral chest radiographs have a limited role in the evaluation of central airway neoplasms. Although airway neoplasms are often overlooked initially, they can frequently be identified retrospectively (10). The reported sensitivity of chest radiographs for detecting

From: *Contemporary Medical Imaging: CT of the Airways*
Edited by: P. M. Boiselle and D. A. Lynch © Humana Press, Totowa, NJ

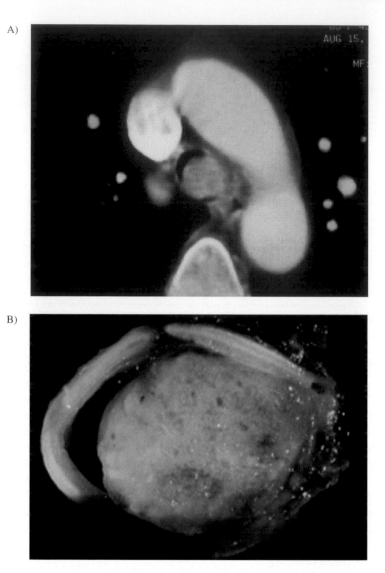

Fig. 1. Mucoepidermoid carcinoma. Axial, contrast-enhanced CT image **(A)** just above the level of the carina demonstrates a large, rounded, endoluminal mass arising from the left posterolateral wall of the trachea with airway wall invasion and significant airway narrowing. Gross pathologic specimen **(B)** confirms extraluminal extension of the tracheal mass.

central airway lesions is poor, ranging from 23 to 66% when compared with computed tomography (CT) *(11,12)*. When visible radiographically, airway neoplasms can appear as intraluminal opacities with irregular, smooth, or lobulated contours *(13)* (Fig. 2). Airway luminal narrowing may also be present. However, determining whether the luminal narrowing is due to an intrinsic airway lesion or to extrinsic compression is difficult with chest radiographs alone. If the extraluminal component of the airway tumor is extensive, the mediastinal contours may appear distorted. Indirect signs of a central, obstructing airway lesion may also be visible including the presence of post-obstructive atelectasis or pneumonia.

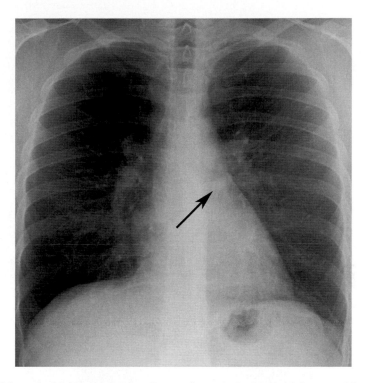

Fig. 2. Bronchial carcinoid. Posteroanterior chest radiograph depicts a subtle, smoothly marginated, round opacity within the left main bronchus (arrow).

Prior to the development of CT, tracheal tomography was utilized as a technique for dedicated evaluation of the trachea. Planar tomography involved the simultaneous motion of the radiograph tube and film cassette, thereby causing intentional blurring of the structures surrounding the trachea *(14)*. Compared with chest radiographs, tracheal tomograms were more sensitive in identifying tracheal neoplasms *(6)* (Fig. 3). Today, these studies are rarely performed and are of historical interest, as they have been supplanted by CT imaging.

Multidetector CT is the imaging modality of choice for detection and staging of central airway neoplasms. The sensitivity of CT for identifying airway abnormalities including neoplasms is 97% *(11)*. Multidetector CT imaging allows for multiplanar reformation and 3-D reconstruction images, which complement conventional axial images by providing a more anatomically meaningful display of the neoplasm and its relationship to adjacent structures, and by accurately determining the craniocaudal extent of disease *(15)*. 3-D external rendering of the airways simulates conventional bronchography whereas virtual bronchographic images provide a unique intraluminal perspective of the tumor and adjacent proximal and distal airways, which may not be accessible with conventional bronchoscopy in cases where there is high-grade luminal narrowing or obstruction (Fig. 4).

Multidetector CT provides crucial information for pre-procedural planning (Fig. 5). If resectable, the optimal therapy for all airway neoplasms, whether benign or malignant, is surgery *(16)*. Multidetector CT can determine amenability of the tumor to complete surgical resection, as well as the approach, type, and extent of surgical resection. Prosthetic reconstruction of the airways and adjuvant therapy can be anticipated based on CT imaging.

Multidetector CT provides critical information for the surgeon (Fig. 6). The 3-D size, including the craniocaudal length, and location of the airway neoplasm can be precisely delineated. Multiplanar

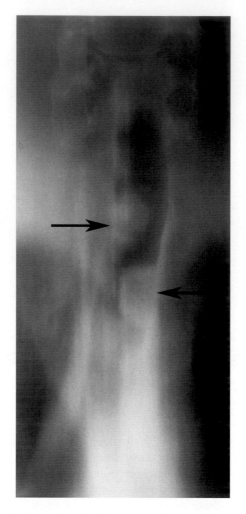

Fig. 3. Tracheal papillomatosis. Coronal tracheal tomogram demonstrating multiple polypoid masses (arrows) protruding into the tracheal lumen.

reformatted images can encapsulate in a single image key anatomic relationships between the neoplasm and surrounding airways and vasculature. Multidetector CT can precisely define intraluminal and extraluminal extension of tumor, as well as demonstrate post-obstructive complications of air trapping, atelectasis, and mucous plugging. Furthermore, multidetector CT can detect the presence of lymphadenopathy and metastases, thereby enhancing tumor staging and guiding biopsy procedures.

For patients who are deemed to be non-surgical candidates, multidetector CT can evaluate patency of the airways distal to the neoplasm, thereby determining suitability of the airways for stent placement.

Magnetic resonance imaging (MRI) plays a limited role in the evaluation of airway neoplasms primarily because of its slower imaging speed and poorer resolution when compared with multidetector CT. Because of its superior soft-tissue contrast, MRI is often reserved as a problem-solving modality for cases in which CT fails to fully characterize an airway lesion. For example, MRI can aid in tissue characterization of lipomatous, fibrous, vascular, and chondroid lesions. Additionally, MRI

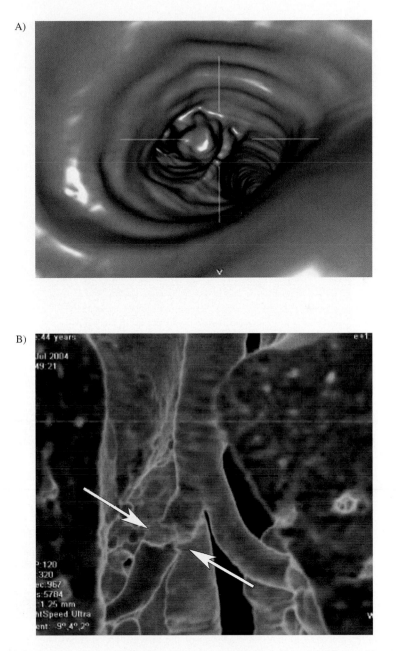

Fig. 4. Bronchial adenoid cystic carcinoma. Virtual bronchoscopic image (**A**) provides an intraluminal perspective of a large, lobulated mass in the right main bronchus which projects superiorly into the carina. 3-D external rendering of the airways (**B**) delineates extent of airway narrowing by the mass (arrows). Patency of the distal airway is depicted.

can provide more accurate assessment of mediastinal invasion and submucosal extension of airway tumors when compared with other imaging modalities *(17,18)*. Although MRI may not serve as the primary imaging modality for central airway neoplasms, it can certainly provide complementary information.

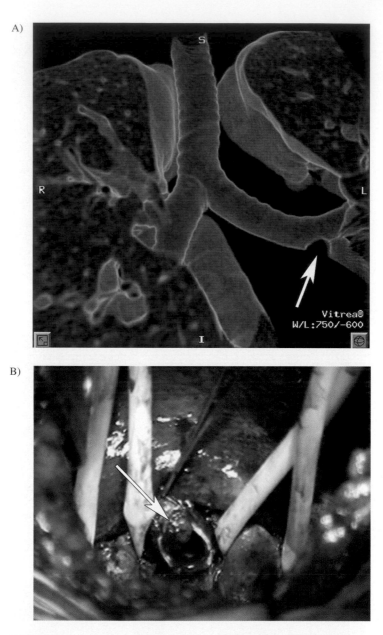

Fig. 5. Bronchial carcinoid. 3-D external rendering of the airways **(A)** demonstrates a smooth, round mass in the distal left mainstem bronchus (arrow). Intraoperative picture **(B)** shows surgical resection of the bronchial mass (arrow).

3. CT CHARACTERIZATION OF AIRWAY NEOPLASMS

Whereas multidetector CT is highly sensitive for identifying central airway neoplasms, CT imaging features only rarely allow for or provide a specific diagnosis. Certain CT imaging characteristics, however, can help predict whether the neoplasm may be of benign or malignant etiology (Table 1).

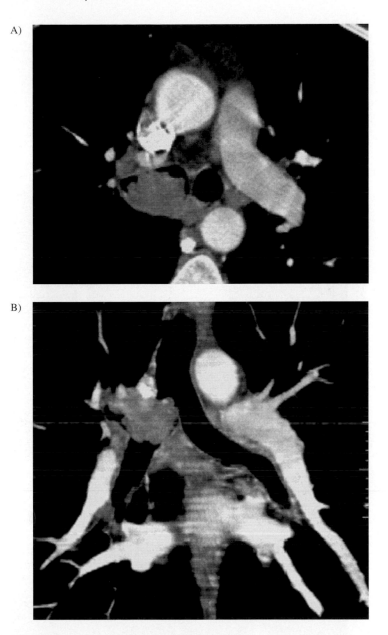

Fig. 6. Bronchial adenoid cystic carcinoma. Axial, enhanced CT image **(A)** demonstrates a lobulated mass within the right main bronchus with posterior extraluminal extension. Coronal reformation image **(B)** depicts both endobronchial and extrabronchial extent of the lesion with direct extraluminal extension into the right hilar region. The position of the mass and the surrounding anatomic relationships are clearly illustrated in a single image. This bronchial adenoid cystic carcinoma is the same neoplasm depicted in Fig. 4.

Benign lesions usually are relatively small in size, measuring less than 2 cm in diameter. Benign neoplasms can appear as round, polypoid, or sessile focal intraluminal masses. These lesions tend to be well circumscribed and smoothly marginated (Fig. 7). Mediastinal invasion and extraluminal extension of the tumor are absent *(6)*.

Table 1
Benign Versus Malignant CT Imaging Characteristics

	Benign	Malignant
Size	<2cm	>2cm
Shape	Round	Lobulated
Margins	Smooth	Irregular
Extraluminal or mediastinal invasion	Absent	Present in some cases

A)

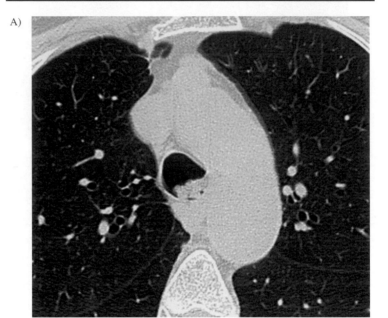

B)

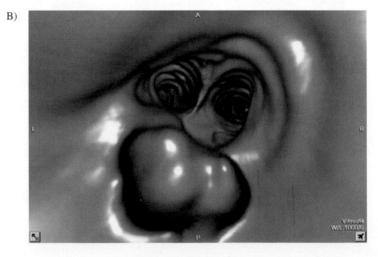

Fig. 7. *(Continued)*

C)

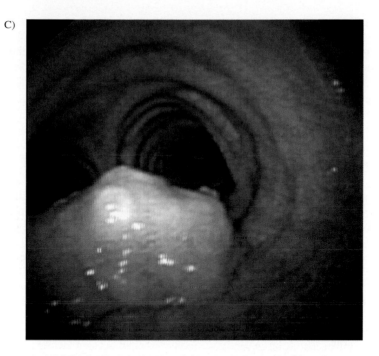

Fig. 7. Fibrolipoma. Axial CT image of the trachea (**A**) along with virtual (**B**) and conventional (**C**) broncho-scopic images demonstrate a well-marginated, polypoid, endoluminal mass within the dependent portion of the trachea without extramural extension, suggestive of a benign etiology. A small amount of fat attenuation was visible within the lesion on soft-tissue windows (not shown).

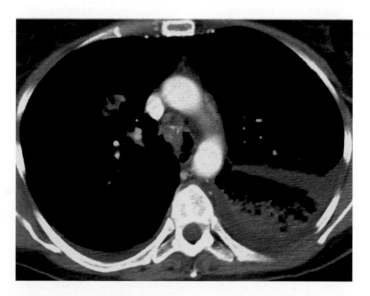

Fig. 8. Carinal adenoid cystic carcinoma. Axial, contrast-enhanced CT image demonstrates an endoluminal carinal mass invading the tracheal wall with an adjacent enlarged precarinal lymph node. Multifocal consolidation and left-sided pleural effusion are also depicted.

On the contrary, malignant airway lesions are frequently larger in size, often measuring 2–4 cm in diameter. Poorly circumscribed, flat or lobulated masses with irregular margins are common malignant features (Fig. 8). Malignant tumors may arise eccentrically from the airway wall and present with contiguous airway wall thickening. 10% of malignant airway tumors demonstrate circumferential airway wall thickening resulting in luminal narrowing, a finding that is virtually diagnostic for malignancy *(19)*, although complex benign stenoses may sometimes demonstrate this appearance. Extramural extension with invasion of the adjacent mediastinal fat can be present in advanced cases of malignancy, a finding that is not encountered in benign lesions *(2,6)*. Mediastinal lymphadenopathy is also more often present in malignancy *(6)*, but reactive benign lymph nodes may be seen in both benign and malignant lesions complicated by post-obstructive pneumonia.

The majority of airway neoplasms on CT are soft tissue in density, a non-specific imaging finding. In a few selected cases, however, the CT density of a lesion can aid neoplastic characterization (Table 2). CT is highly specific and sensitive for the detection of fat, and the presence of fat within a lesion suggests a benign etiology, such as a lipoma or hamartoma *(8)* (Figs 9 and 10). Calcification in an airway lesion may be seen in carcinoids or in cartilaginous tumors such as

Table 2
CT Density and Neoplastic Characterization

Density	Neoplastic Entity
Soft tissue	Non-specific
Fat	Hamartoma, lipoma
Calcification	Chondroma, chondroblastoma, carcinoid
Marked contrast enhancement	Carcinoid

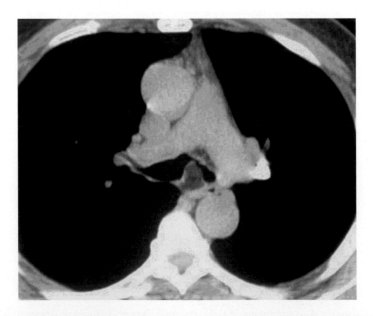

Fig. 9. Endobronchial lipoma. Axial contrast-enhanced CT image through the carina demonstrates a homogeneous, fat-attenuation, endoluminal mass within the proximal left main bronchus resulting in high-grade narrowing of the airway lumen. (Courtesy of Michael Gotway, MD)

chondroma, chondroblastoma, and chondrosarcoma *(2,6)*. The combination of fat and calcification within a lesion is essentially pathognomonic for a hamartoma *(2,6)*. The use of intravenous contrast can also assist in further characterization of a lesion. For example, carcinoid tumors may demonstrate marked, homogenous enhancement post-contrast administration *(20,21)*.

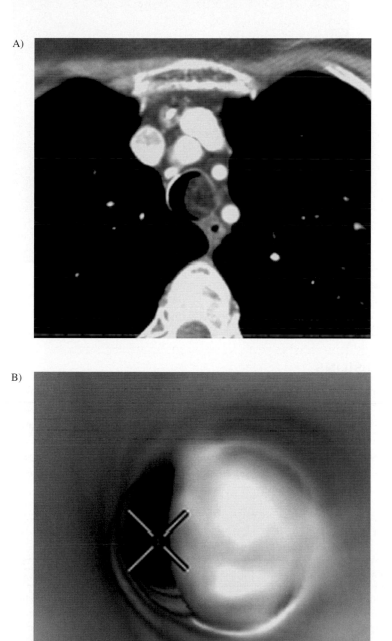

Fig. 10. *(Continued)*

C)

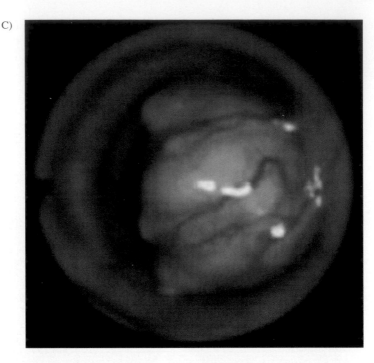

Fig. 10. Tracheal lipomatous hamartoma. Contrast-enhanced axial CT image (**A**) shows a smooth, sharply marginated, round, fat-attenuation, endoluminal mass originating from the left posterolateral wall of the trachea without extra-tracheal involvement. Virtual (**B**) and conventional (**C**) bronchoscopic images demonstrate extent of airway narrowing caused by the tumor.

4. BENIGN LESIONS

Benign airway tumors are much less common than malignant airway neoplasms, comprising approximately 2% of all lung tumors *(8)*. Benign tumors are more common in children than in adults, accounting for >90% of pediatric tracheal neoplasms *(22)*. Many benign neoplasms are clinically and radiographically indistinguishable from malignant lesions. A multitude of histologies are associated with benign airway neoplasms, and these can be classified based on their tissue of origin as either epithelial or mesenchymal (Table 3). Several of the most common benign neoplastic entities are discussed in the following subsections.

Table 3
Benign Central Airway Tumors

Epithelial	Mesenchymal	
Squamous cell papilloma	Hamartoma	Fibrous histiocytoma
Papillomatosis	Neurofibroma	Pseudosarcoma
Pleomorphic adenoma	Schwannoma	Hemangioendothelioma
Glandular papilloma	Fibroma	Leiomyoma
Adenomas of salivary gland-type	Hemangioma	Chondroblastoma
Mucous gland adenoma	Granular cell tumor	Lipoma
Monomorphic adenoma	Chondroma	Glomus tumor
Oncocytoma		Hemangioendothelioma

4.1. Squamous Cell Papilloma

Squamous cell papilloma is the most common benign central airway neoplasm *(6)*. Papillomas result from a proliferation of squamous epithelium around a core of fibrovascular tissue *(23)*. These tumors can arise throughout the airways but have a propensity for the larynx *(23)*. Within the tracheobronchial tree, the majority of papillomas are found within the main and lobar bronchi *(23)*. Males are approximately 4.5 times more frequently affected than females, and patients typically range in age from 50 to 70 years *(23,24)*. Squamous cell papilloma can arise de novo, but smoking is a predisposing risk factor *(6,24)*. On CT imaging, it was found that squamous cell papillomas can appear as a lobulated, polypoid, or sessile intraluminal mass without extraluminal extension or calcification *(6)* (Fig. 11).

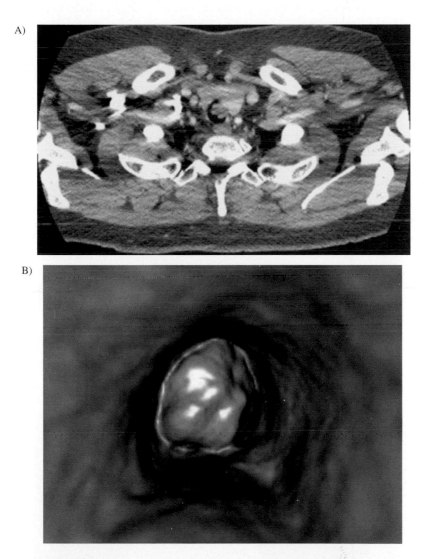

A)

B)

Fig. 11. Tracheal papilloma. Axial CT image **(A)** demonstrates a large polypoid intraluminal mass within the proximal trachea. Virtual bronchoscopic image **(B)** demonstrates extent of airway narrowing caused by this polypoid mass.

4.2. Papillomatosis

Papillomatosis, also known as laryngotracheobronchial papillomatosis and recurrent respiratory papillomatosis, refers to a condition of multiple squamous papillomas throughout the airway. Papillomatosis is histologically similar to solitary squamous cell papilloma but remains a distinct entity *(6,24)*. Papillomatosis is primarily a disease of children with two-thirds of cases diagnosed in patients less than 5 years old *(25,26)*. Approximately one-third of cases present at a later age, in patients from 16 to 50 years *(25)*. Papillomatosis is caused by human papillomavirus (HPV) types 6 and 11, and contraction is believed to primarily occur through the infected maternal genital tract during birth *(27)*. In cases where the disease presents at a later age, HPV is thought to be contracted either at birth followed by a period of dormancy or through sexual activity *(25)*.

In children, papillomatosis is typically confined to the larynx and can spontaneously regress, whereas in adults, papillomatosis more frequently involves the airways distal to the larynx and often recurs *(6)*. Malignant degeneration into squamous cell carcinoma can occur and is more common in adults, occurring in approximately 10% of cases *(26,28)*. Rarely, pulmonary lesions can also develop and gradually progress *(27)*. Although antiviral therapy, interferon, and endoscopic laser ablation have been used, complete excision is the treatment of choice to prevent recurrence and to exclude malignancy *(24)*. When diffuse, complete excision is not usually possible.

On CT imaging, multiple, small, nodular masses may be identified projecting into the airway lumen *(6)* (Fig. 12). When papillomatosis disseminates distally to the lung parenchyma, multiple, small, well-defined nodules may be present which frequently undergo central cavitation *(6,28)*. Cysts of varying size can also be observed *(6)*.

4.3. Lipomas

Lipomas are composed exclusively or nearly exclusively of mature fat and comprise 0.1% of all benign lung tumors *(29)*. Endobronchial lipomas are more common than endotracheal lipomas *(8,30)*. Airway lipomas have a striking male predominance (90%) and usually present in patients in late

A)

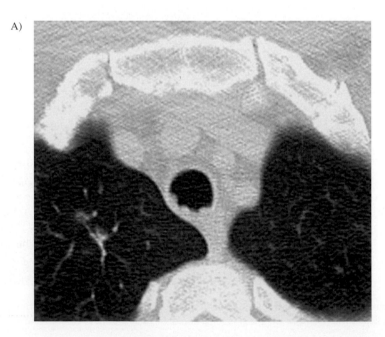

Fig. 12. *(Continued)*

B)

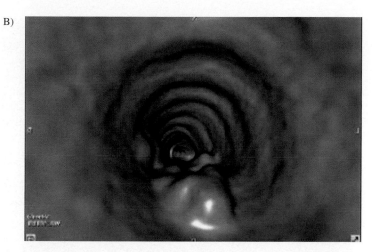

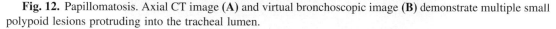

Fig. 12. Papillomatosis. Axial CT image **(A)** and virtual bronchoscopic image **(B)** demonstrate multiple small polypoid lesions protruding into the tracheal lumen.

middle age *(8)*. These neoplasms originate from the submucosal fat of the tracheobronchial tree and commonly appear pedunculated with a narrow stalk *(8)*. Identification of fat on CT within a lesion is suggestive of either a lipoma or hamartoma *(8)* (Fig. 9). Endobronchial removal with laser therapy or surgical resection is the preferred treatment options *(8)*.

4.4. Hamartoma

Hamartomas are slowly growing, benign mesenchymal tumors composed of varying proportions of adipose tissue, loose myxoid fibrous tissue, and hyaline cartilage *(24)*. Although hamartomas are the most commonly encountered benign tumor of the lung, approximately 10% will present within the airways, with a bronchial predominance *(31,32)*. Patients are frequently symptomatic at the time of diagnosis, presenting between the sixth and seventh decades with hemoptysis and post-obstructive pneumonia. Like most other airway tumors, hamartomas have a male predominance *(32)*.

On CT, endobronchial hamartoma may appear as a well-circumscribed, smooth, polypoid, or lobulated intraluminal mass without extramural extension *(24)* (Fig. 10). Punctate or "popcorn"-like calcifications are identified in 25–30% of cases, and the combination of calcification and fat within a lesion is essentially pathognomonic for a hamartoma *(14,33,34)*.

4.5. Peripheral Nerve Sheath Tumors

Benign peripheral nerve sheath tumors, including schwannomas and neurofibromas, are exceedingly rare within the central airways *(6,24)*. These tumors have no gender predilection and the mean age at diagnosis is 36 years *(6)*. Many of these tumors are solitary and not associated with neurofibromatosis *(8)*. CT findings include a round, ovoid, or lobulated, well-defined, intraluminal, homogeneous soft-tissue mass, often without mediastinal invasion *(6,8)* (Fig. 13). When endotracheal in location, neurogenic tumors usually arise within the lower third of the trachea *(6)*. Surgical or endobronchial resection is curative treatment *(8)*.

4.6. Chondroma

Chondromas and their malignant counterparts, chondrosarcomas, are the most common cartilaginous neoplasm of the airway *(6)*. These exceedingly rare endoluminal tumors arise from the cartilaginous rings of the trachea or large bronchi *(6)*. The epicenter of these tumors is on the

A)

B)

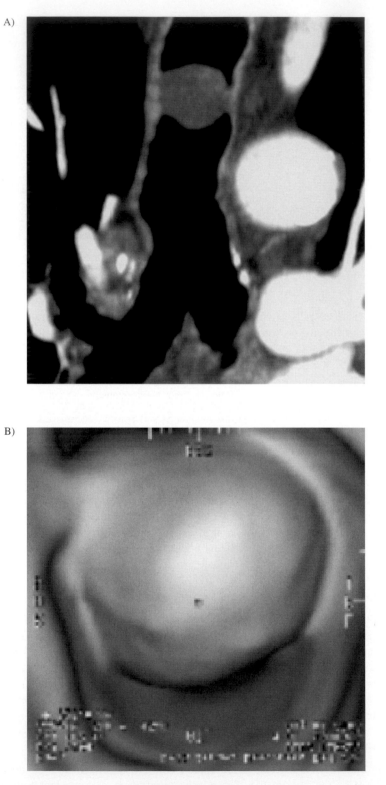

Fig. 13. *(Continued)*

C)

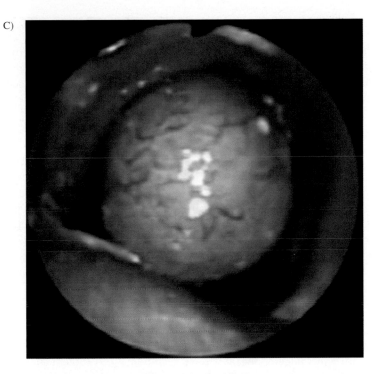

Fig. 13. Tracheal neurofibroma. Coronal reformatted image (**A**) demonstrates a round, smoothly marginated, soft tissue density mass within the trachea without extraluminal extension. These features are suggestive of a benign tracheal neoplasm. Virtual (**B**) and conventional (**C**) bronchoscopic images show near-complete occlusion of the airway by the mass.

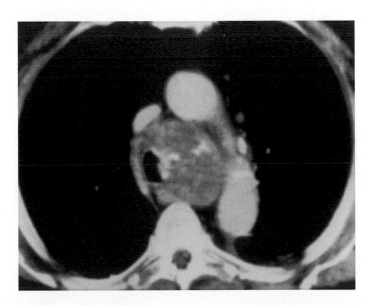

Fig. 14. Tracheal chondrosarcoma. Axial, contrast-enhanced CT image shows an enhancing mass originating from the left lateral tracheal wall containing coarse calcifications. (Courtesy of Jo-Anne Shepard, MD)

cartilaginous ring, and these lesions often demonstrate both intraluminal and extraluminal growth (Fig. 14). These neoplasms range from 1 to 3 cm in size. They are sharply defined and can appear as small, irregular, polypoid endoluminal projections along a broad base *(35,36)*. Notably, 75% of these tumors contain calcifications *(35,37)*. Unfortunately, CT imaging features cannot readily distinguish between chondroma and chondrosarcoma, although invasion of adjacent mediastinal structures strongly favors chondrosarcoma.

5. MALIGNANT LESIONS

The majority of airway neoplasms are malignant in adults. In several case series, 60–88% of all tracheal tumors have been reported as being malignant *(9,38)*. Approximately 75% of primary tracheal neoplasms are accounted for by two histologies, squamous cell carcinoma and adenoid cystic carcinoma *(39)*. As malignant lesions usually behave more aggressively than benign lesions, the duration of symptoms is typically shorter, approximately 6–12 months *(6)*. Like benign lesions, malignant airway neoplasms can be classified based on their tissue of origin as epithelial or mesenchymal (Table 4). The four most common primary central airway malignancies, squamous cell carcinoma, adenoid cystic carcinoma, carcinoid, and mucoepidermoid carcinoma, are discussed in the following sections.

5.1. Squamous Cell Carcinoma

Squamous cell carcinoma is the most common primary central airway malignancy, but at least one series has reported that adenoid cystic is more common *(9)*. Although squamous cell carcinoma is the most frequent primary malignancy within the trachea, this neoplasm occurs more commonly within the main, lobar, and segmental bronchi *(9,36,38,40)*. Multifocal carcinoma is present in approximately 10% of cases *(3,41)*. This neoplasm has a 4:1 male to female predominance and typically presents during the sixth and seventh decades of life *(42)*. Squamous cell carcinoma has a strong association with cigarette smoking *(43)*. These neoplasms are often large at the time of diagnosis, averaging 4 cm *(3)*. They tend to be rapidly progressive and have a poor prognosis *(41)*. Treatment involves surgical resection and oftentimes adjuvant radiation therapy, even when surgical margins are negative *(9,40)*. For unresectable disease, radiation therapy can serve as definitive therapy *(40)*.

Table 4
Malignant Central Airway Tumors

Epithelial	Mesenchymal
Squamous cell carcinoma	Fibrosarcoma
Adenoid cystic carcinoma	Rhabdomyosarcoma
Carcinoid	Angiosarcoma
Mucoepidermoid carcinoma	Kaposi's sarcoma
Adenocarcinoma	Liposarcoma
Small-cell undifferentiated carcinoma	Osteosarcoma
Large-cell carcinoma	Leiomyosarcoma
Acinic cell carcinoma	Chondrosarcoma
Malignant salivary gland type mixed	Paraganglioma
tumors	Spindle cell sarcoma
Carcinomas with pleomorphic,	Lymphoma
sarcomatoid, or sarcomatous elements	Malignant fibrous histiocytoma

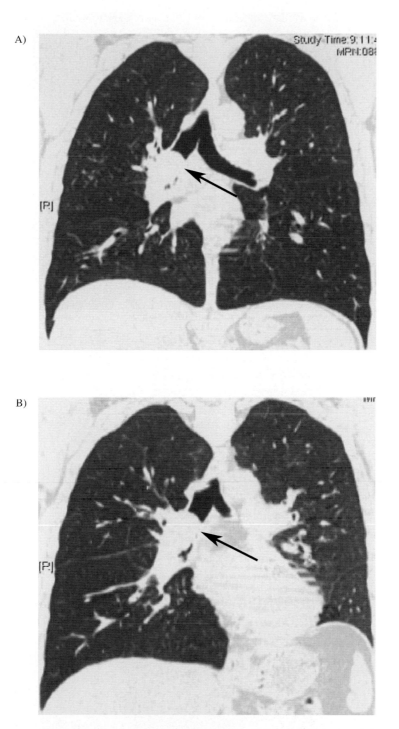

Fig. 15. Squamous cell carcinoma. Coronal reformation CT images during inspiration (**A**) and expiration (**B**) demonstrate an endoluminal mass within the right main bronchus (arrows) with extraluminal extension. Note expiratory air trapping involving the entire right lung.

A)

B)

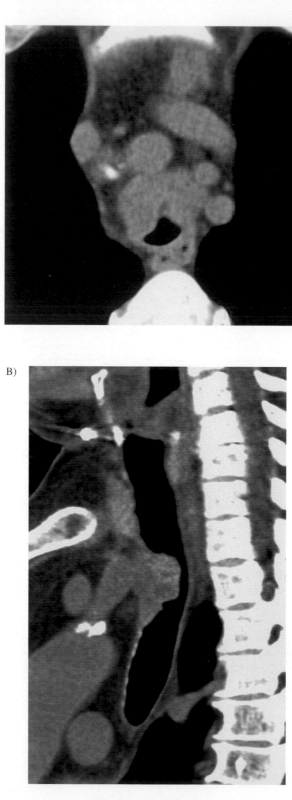

Fig. 16. *(Continued)*

C)

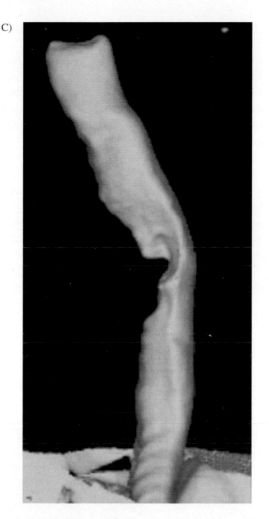

Fig. 16. Tracheal squamous cell carcinoma. Axial non-contrast CT image **(A)** of the trachea demonstrates a polypoid endoluminal mass within the anterior proximal trachea with associated airway wall thickening and luminal narrowing. The neoplasm extends anteriorly into the mediastinal fat, encroaching upon the adjacent great vessels. Sagittal 2-D **(B)** and 3-D **(C)** reformation images define the craniocaudal extent of the airway neoplasm and degree of airway narrowing. (Courtesy of Andetta Hunsaker, MD)

On CT imaging, this airway neoplasm can present in various ways including a large intraluminal, obstructing polypoid mass; a sessile mass with eccentric airway narrowing; or focal lobular airway wall thickening *(6,43,44)* (Figs 15 and 16). A circumferential pattern of growth can be identified in nearly 10% of cases *(19,42)*. The endoluminal component of these tumors may be ulcerative, and exophytic spread is commonly noted *(3,41)*. The neoplasm frequently invades the mediastinal structures and metastasizes to regional lymph nodes *(41)*. Up to 15% of cases may be complicated by the development of a tracheoesophageal fistula *(4,19)*.

5.2. Adenoid Cystic Carcinoma

Adenoid cystic carcinoma, formerly known as "cylindroma" and "adenocystic carcinoma," is a low-grade malignancy arising from the glands in the tracheobronchial mucosa *(6,13)*. These tumors are the most common sialadenoid tumors of the central airways, accounting for 75–80% of cases, and are the second most common primary neoplasm of the trachea and main bronchi *(45–48)*. Unlike squamous cell carcinoma, these tumors do not have a gender predilection and are not associated with smoking *(6)*. The average age of patients at presentation is in their fifth decade. Compared with squamous cell carcinoma, these neoplasms grow more slowly and have a better prognosis, but late recurrence is relatively common after surgical resection *(5,6,9,49)*. Surgical resection is the treatment of choice; however, adjuvant radiation therapy is often required because of the predilection of these tumors to spread perineurally and submucosally *(40,50)*.

Adenoid cystic carcinomas are usually greater than 2 cm at the time of diagnosis and commonly arise from the posterolateral wall of the intrathoracic distal trachea and mainstem bronchi *(6,13, 51,52)* (Fig. 17). Adenoid cystic carcinomas are not encapsulated and have a marked propensity for endophytic spread along submucosal planes *(3,13,51)*. As a result, adenoid cystic carcinomas on CT imaging tend to appear either as an intraluminal soft-tissue density mass with extramural extension or as diffuse or circumferential airway wall thickening *(13)*. These tumors often involve more than 180° of the airway circumference and cause luminal narrowing *(13)*. The longitudinal extent of the tumor is often greater than its transaxial extent *(6)*. The morphology of these lesions is variable, including polypoid, broad-based, annular, and diffusely infiltrating *(6,13,45)* (Fig. 18). The contours of the neoplasm can range from smooth, lobulated, or irregular *(6)*. Calcifications within the tumor are rare *(13)*. Frequently, these neoplasms demonstrate extraluminal spread and invasion of the surrounding tissues *(6,41,53)*. 10% of primary adenoid cystic carcinomas present with regional lymph node metastases at the time of diagnosis *(54)*.

A)

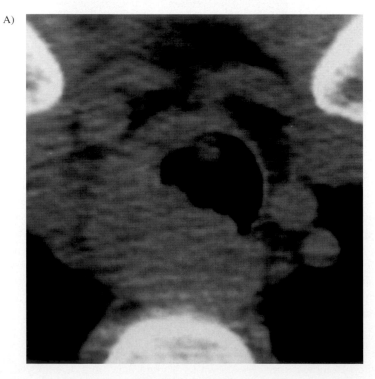

Fig. 17. *(Continued)*

B)

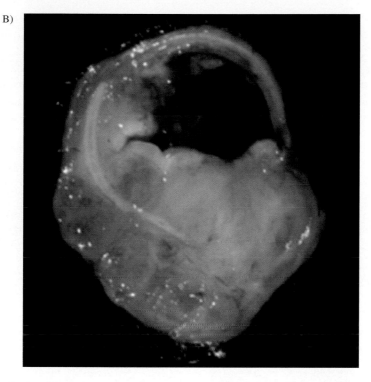

Fig. 17. Tracheal adenoid cystic carcinoma. Axial CT image **(A)** and gross pathologic correlation **(B)** demonstrate a lobulated mass arising from the posterolateral aspect of the trachea with contiguous tracheal wall thickening. (Fig. 17A reprinted with permission from Boiselle PM, McLoud TC. *Case Review: Thoracic Imaging*. St. Louis: Mosby, 2001: 112).

A)

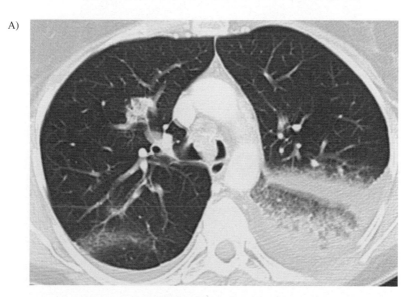

Fig. 18. *(Continued)*

B)

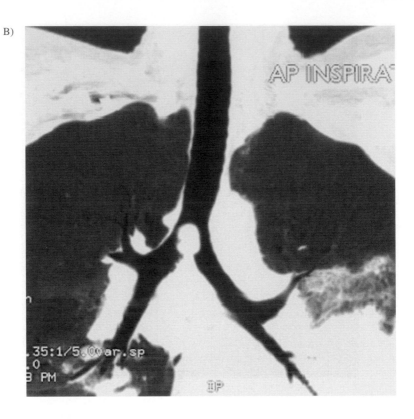

C)

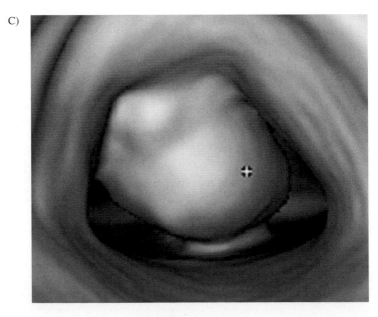

Fig. 18. *(Continued)*

D)

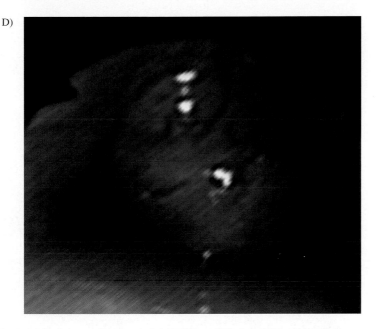

Fig. 18. Carinal adenoid cystic carcinoma. Axial CT image (**A**) shows an endoluminal mass within the carina with multifocal consolidation. Coronal minimal intensity projection image (**B**) delineates the pedunculated nature of this lobulated mass, originating from the carina. Patency of the main and distal bronchi is also depicted. Virtual (**C**) and conventional (**D**) bronchoscopic images demonstrate marked luminal narrowing by the mass.

5.3. Carcinoid

Carcinoid tumors are neuroendocrine neoplasms that typically arise centrally. The majority arise within the mainstem and lobar bronchi, whereas 15% develop within the segmental bronchi or lung periphery (14,55). Carcinoid tumors comprise 1–2% of all lung neoplasms (56). When carcinoids arise in the central airways, affected patients are often symptomatic, presenting with cough, recurrent obstructive pneumonia, and hemoptysis (57,58). Only rarely are systemic hormonal manifestations present with symptoms of carcinoid syndrome seen in less than 5% of patients and Cushing's syndrome in approximately 2% of patients (57). Carcinoids have an equal incidence in males and females and present at an average age of 45 years (24,58).

Carcinoids are classified into two categories: typical and atypical carcinoids. Typical carcinoids are low-grade neoplasms with an excellent prognosis (24). Atypical carcinoids, which comprise 10–20% of all pulmonary carcinoids, are a more aggressive subtype which histologically demonstrate an increased mitotic rate and foci of coagulative necrosis (24). Atypical carcinoids have a greater tendency to invade vascular and lymphatic structures and metastasize to regional lymph nodes and distant sites (24,57,59). Atypical carcinoids usually present a decade later than typical carcinoids, approximately during the sixth decade of life (60,61). Atypical carcinoids have a poorer prognosis with a 5-year survival rate of 40–69% compared with 87–100% for typical carcinoids (57,62–66). Both carcinoid types are treated primarily with surgical resection, and adjuvant chemotherapy is sometimes employed for advanced and atypical carcinoids (16,57).

The CT imaging features of typical and atypical carcinoids are similar. These tumors tend to be large, ranging from 2 to 5 cm in diameter (57). Carcinoids may be well-circumscribed, round or ovoid nodules or masses with a slightly lobulated contour (Fig. 19). Atypical carcinoids may have irregular contours, but this is not a diagnostic feature (20). Whereas the tumor may be completely intraluminal, more commonly, bronchial carcinoids appear as dumbbell-shaped lesions with both endoluminal and parenchymal components *(56,57)*. Some carcinoids contain only a small endobronchial component, which represents the "tip of the iceberg," whereas the bulk of the tumor predominantly extends extraluminally into the adjacent lung parenchyma *(21)*. Carcinoids are highly vascular and can display marked, homogenous enhancement after contrast administration *(21)*. Atypical carcinoids, however,

A)

B)

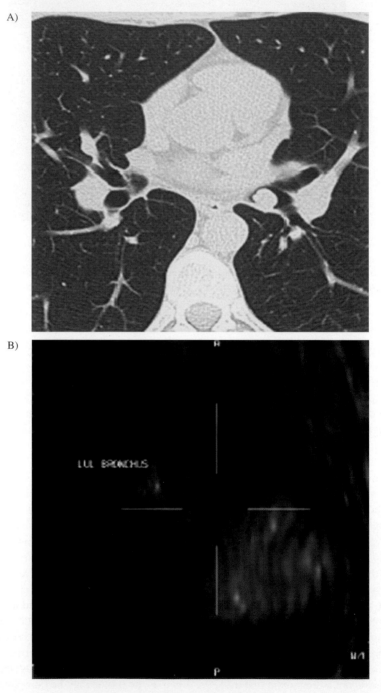

Fig. 19. *(Continued)*

C)

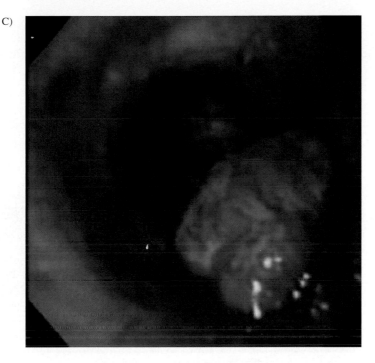

Fig. 19. Bronchial carcinoid. Axial CT image **(A)** and virtual **(B)** and conventional **(C)** bronchoscopic images depict an endobronchial lesion in the distal left mainstem bronchus at the bifurcation of the left upper and lower lobe bronchi, both of which are patent.

may demonstrate heterogeneous enhancement, whereas other carcinoids may not enhance at all *(20,21)*. Approximately 30% of carcinoids exhibit punctate or diffuse calcification and may mimic broncholiths *(67,68)*. Post-obstructive parenchymal changes of atelectasis, consolidation, and mucoid impaction can commonly be seen.

5.4. Mucoepidermoid Carcinoma

Mucoepidermoid carcinomas arise from the minor salivary glands of the tracheobronchial tree and are rare tumors, comprising 0.1–0.2% of all primary lung malignancies *(56,69)*. Affected patients range in age from 4 to 78 years, but almost half are younger than 30 years *(56)*. Mucoepidermoid carcinomas are more commonly located in the segmental bronchi than in the trachea or main bronchi *(46)*.

These tumors can be divided histologically into low-grade and high-grade lesions based on the number of mitoses and the presence of nuclear pleomorphism and necrosis *(56)*. Low-grade tumors are usually confined to the airway wall, whereas nearly 50% of high-grade mucoepidermoid carcinomas tend to exhibit parenchymal invasion *(46,69)*. Because low-grade tumors grow slowly, are non-invasive, and rarely metastasize, this tumor subtype has an excellent prognosis. By contrast, high-grade tumors have a greater risk of transforming into frank bronchogenic carcinoma and are associated with a poorer prognosis *(69)*. Surgical resection is the treatment of choice for both subtypes *(70)*.

CT features may help distinguish between the two classes of mucoepidermoid carcinoma. Low-grade tumors generally appear as well-circumscribed, exophytic endobronchial nodules that are smoothly oval, lobulated, or polypoid in contour *(46,56)* (Fig. 20). High-grade tumors are less likely to be polypoid and more often appear infiltrative, broad-based, and irregular *(52)* (Fig. 1). Regardless of subtype, mucoepidermoid carcinomas are non-spherical in shape, and the long axis of the tumor

A)

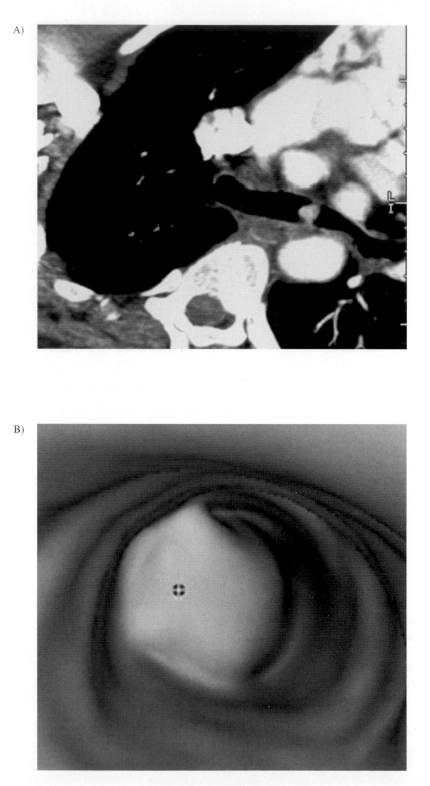

B)

Fig. 20. *(Continued)*

C)

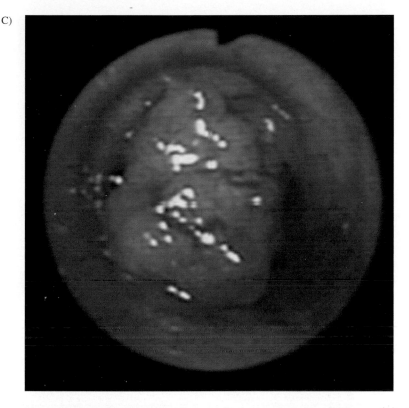

Fig. 20. Mucoepidermoid carcinoma. Curved oblique multiplanar reformation CT image (**A**) along the axis of the left mainstem bronchus shows a well-circumscribed, smoothly lobulated, enhancing endobronchial mass with patency of the distal airway. Virtual (**B**) and bronchoscopic (**C**) images confirm near-complete obstruction of the left mainstem bronchus by this mass.

is oriented parallel to the direction of the airway containing the tumor *(46)*. Punctate calcifications can be seen in up to 50% of tumors *(46)*. Additionally, mild enhancement within the lesion can be noted after contrast administration *(46)*.

6. SECONDARY AIRWAY MALIGNANCIES

The airways can be involved by secondary malignancies, either through direct invasion or through hematogenous metastases to the airway mucosa *(10)*. Neoplasms arising from lung, esophagus, thyroid, and larynx are the most common adjacent malignancies to directly invade the tracheobronchial tree *(6,10)* (Fig. 21). On CT imaging, the primary malignancy and its extension directly into the adjacent airway can be identified. Tracheal invasion by laryngeal carcinoma may appear as a soft-tissue mass extending below the inferior margin of the cricoid cartilage *(6)*. In some cases of invading upper esophageal carcinomas, the tumor may encase the trachea and rarely result in tracheoesophageal fistula formation *(71)* (Fig. 22).

Hematogenous metastases to the airway are exceptionally rare. Reported primary malignancies that metastasize to the tracheobronchial tree include kidney, melanoma, testis, colon, lymphoma, adrenal, uterus, breast, and soft-tissue sarcomas *(10,72)* (Fig. 23). Interestingly, lung carcinomas are not known to metastasize hematogeneously to the airways *(72)*. On CT, solitary or multiple intraluminal polypoid soft-tissue masses may be identified *(6,10)*.

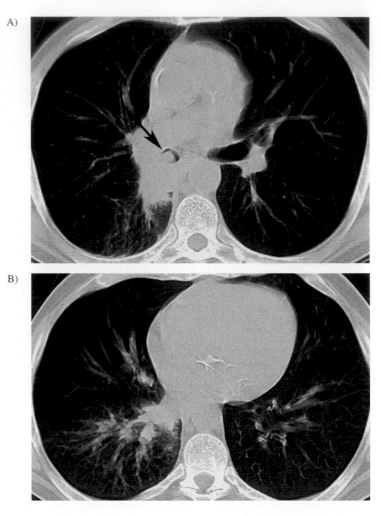

Fig. 21. Bronchogenic adenocarcinoma with direct invasion of the bronchus intermedius. Axial CT image **(A)** demonstrates an occluding endobronchial lesion within the right bronchus intermedius (arrow). A larger, extraluminal component of the mass is seen posteriorly, filling the azygoesophageal recess, which represents the primary lung adenocarcinoma. Axial CT image obtained more inferiorly **(B)** shows mucoid impaction of the right lower lobe airways.

7. NON-NEOPLASTIC MIMICKERS

Several non-neoplastic entities can mimic the appearance of a central airway tumor. These mimickers include tracheobronchopathia osteochondroplastica (TBO), amyloidosis, inflammatory or granulation polyps, and retained airway secretions.

7.1. Tracheobronchopathia Osteochondroplastica

TBO is an idiopathic, rare, benign condition characterized by multiple nodules of cartilage and/or bone arising within the submucosa of the trachea and, to a lesser extent, the major bronchi *(6,10,73)*. The disease may be focal or diffuse, and the nodules typically affect the lower two-thirds of the trachea and proximal main bronchi *(73,74)*. These osteocartilaginous growths are characteristically

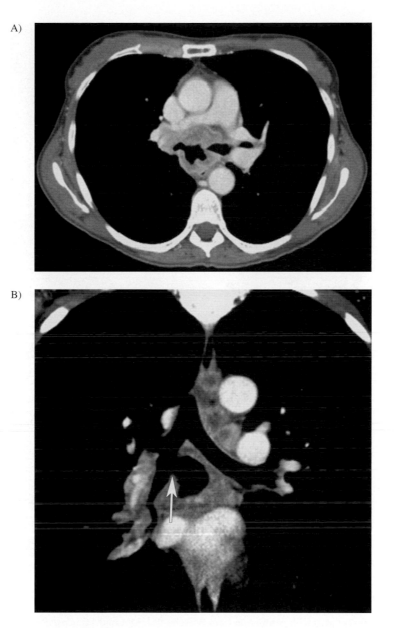

Fig. 22. Esophageal adenocarcinoma with bronchoesophageal fistula. Axial CT image (**A**) demonstrates marked focal dilatation and irregular wall thickening of the esophagus with direct invasion into the adjacent right bronchus intermedius resulting in fistulous communication. Coronal reformatted image (**B**) delineates the extent of the bronchoesophageal fistula (arrow).

located within the anterior and lateral walls of the airway, with sparing of the posterior membranous wall *(6,10,74)*. Patients present in their mid-fifties, and males are affected three times more often than females *(73)*. Usually, though, this disease is an incidental, asymptomatic finding. Currently, no specific treatment is available.

On CT, multiple, small, sessile or polypoid, soft-tissue and calcified nodules can be seen projecting into the lumen of the trachea and main bronchi with pathognomonic sparing of the posterior airway

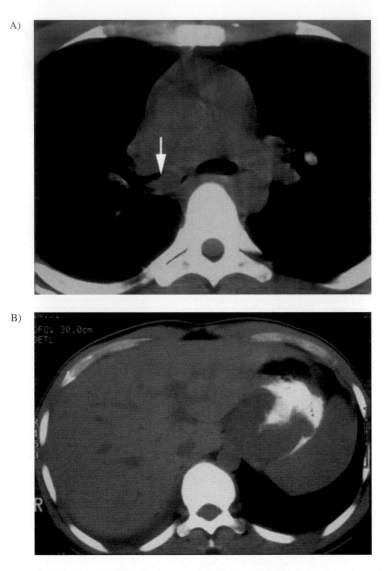

Fig. 23. Endobronchial lymphoma. Non-contrast axial CT image **(A)** demonstrates a large intraluminal mass within the right mainstem bronchus (arrow) causing significant airway narrowing. Axial CT image of the upper abdomen **(B)** in the same patient shows marked wall thickening of the gastric fundus, consistent with gastric lymphoma. (Fig. 23B reprinted with permission from Boiselle PM, McLoud TC. *Case Review: Thoracic Imaging.* St. Louis: Mosby, 2001: 129).

wall *(73)* (Fig. 24). Irregular airway narrowing may result. Additionally, the tracheal cartilage may be thickened and contain irregular calcifications *(10,74)*.

7.2. Amyloidosis

Amyloidosis is a disease that results in the deposition of amyloid, an insoluble fibrillar protein, within the extracellular tissues of various organs *(6,73)*. Amyloidosis can involve the airways either in isolation or as part of a widespread systemic process. Tracheobronchial amyloidosis is usually characterized by diffuse or multifocal amyloid deposits within submucosa and muscle of the airways.

A)

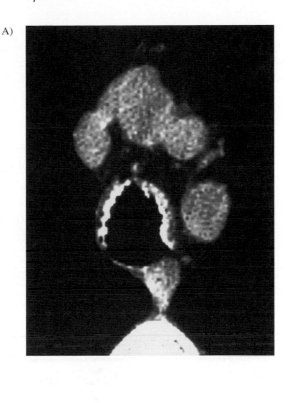

B)

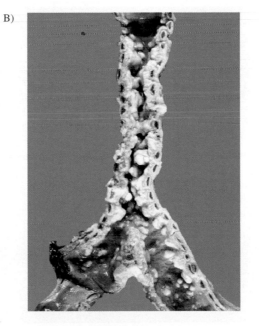

Fig. 24. Tracheobronchopathia osteochondroplastica (TBO). Non-contrast, axial (**A**) CT image of the trachea demonstrates confluent nodular areas of calcification along the anterolateral walls of the trachea with sparing of the posterior membranous wall. Gross airway specimen (**B**) from a different patient with TBO demonstrates innumerable osteocartilaginous growths within the tracheal and proximal main bronchial walls causing irregular, severe airway narrowing. (Courtesy of Michael Gotway, MD)

Less commonly, amyloidosis can present as a single submucosal mass-like lesion *(10)*. The average age at presentation is 53 years, and males are twice as often affected than females *(75)*.

Radiographically, amyloidosis may appear as diffuse mural thickening or solitary or multiple masses within the airway wall, resulting in diffuse or irregular airway narrowing *(6,73,75)* (Fig. 25).

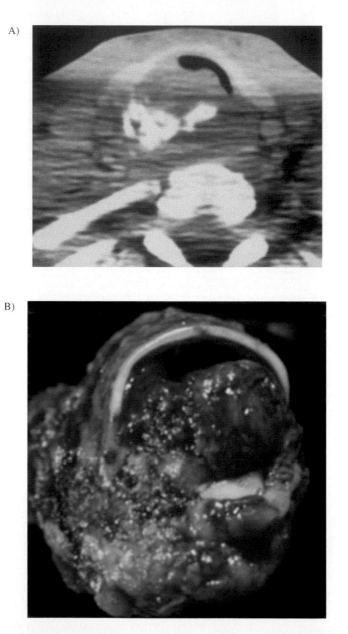

Fig. 25. Tracheal amyloidosis. Axial CT image **(A)** demonstrates a large nodular mass arising from the right posterolateral proximal tracheal wall with coarse calcifications, causing marked airway narrowing. These findings simulate a malignant central airway tumor. Correlative gross pathologic image **(B)** demonstrates the intra- and extra-mural extension of this large nodular tracheal mass.

A)

B)

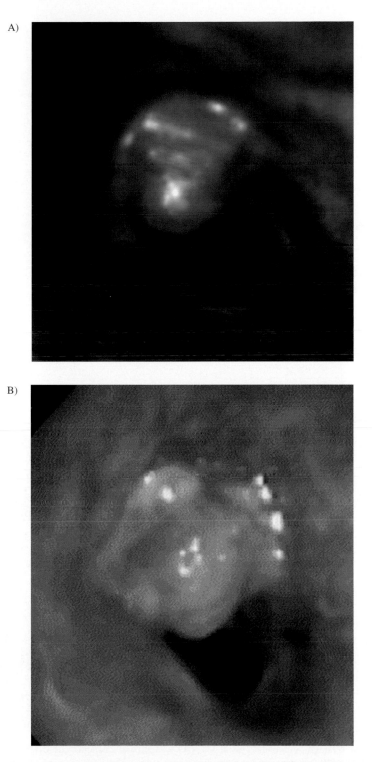

Fig. 26. Granulation polyp. Virtual (**A**) and correlative conventional (**B**) bronchoscopic images show a rounded polypoid intraluminal mass arising from the anterior wall of the trachea causing airway luminal narrowing, findings simulating an airway neoplasm.

A)

B)

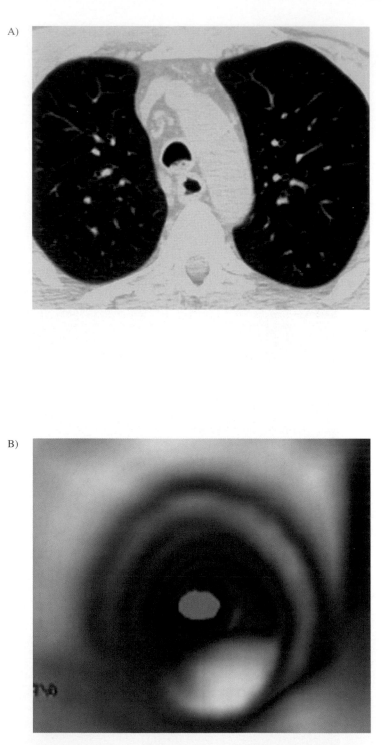

Fig. 27. Tracheal retained secretions. Axial CT **(A)** and virtual bronchoscopic **(B)** images demonstrate a smoothly marginated, well-circumscribed intraluminal opacity within the dependent portion of the trachea with features suggestive of a benign tracheal neoplasm. Air bubbles on axial CT image suggested retained secretions, which were confirmed by repeat imaging following coughing. (Reprinted with permission from ref. *15*)

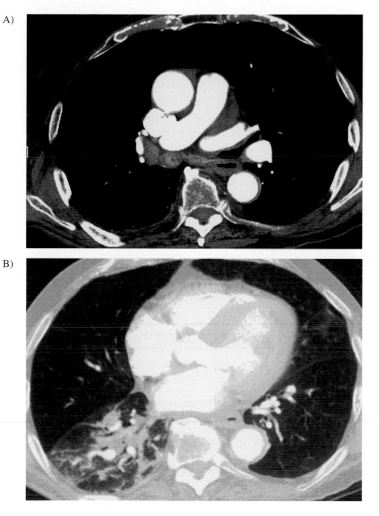

Fig. 28. Aspirated foreign body. Axial, contrast-enhanced CT image (**A**) demonstrates an enhancing endoluminal lesion within the right bronchus intermedius with surrounding thickening of the airway wall. Axial, contrast-enhanced CT image through the lung bases (**B**) shows associated post-obstructive pneumonia and partial atelectasis of the right lower lobe. An aspirated chickpea that incited an intense inflammatory reaction was discovered at bronchoscopy.

Mural or nodular calcification may be identified, thereby simulating TBO; however, the posterior membranous airway wall is not spared in amyloidosis, allowing for differentiation of these two entities *(6,19,73)*.

7.3. Miscellaneous

Other mimickers of central airway tumors on imaging include endoluminal granulation or inflammatory polyps, retained airway secretions, and aspirated foreign bodies. Endoluminal polyps may arise secondary to chronic underlying inflammation or irritation. On CT, polyps often appear as smooth, well-defined, round soft-tissue endoluminal projections, similar to other central airway neoplasms *(8)* (Fig. 26). Airway narrowing and obstruction may also result.

Retained airway secretions can also simulate the appearance of a central airway tumor. Secretions usually appear as focal, smoothly marginated, well-defined intraluminal "masses" along the dependent portions of the airways. Oftentimes, tiny bubbles of gas can be identified within these secretions, allowing them to be differentiated from a solid lesion (Fig. 27). Repeat imaging in the prone position or following coughing can confirm the diagnosis and exclude a fixed lesion.

Aspirated foreign bodies can also mimic endoluminal neoplasms. Foreign body aspiration occurs more frequently in children than in adults. Aspirated objects tend to be lodged within proximal airways, with a predilection for the right bronchial tree due to the more vertical orientation of the right main bronchus when compared with the left *(76)*. Aspirated organic substances are rapidly broken down by enzymes within tracheobronchial secretions, leading to exuberant exudative and inflammatory responses within the airway, findings that can resemble a central airway malignancy (Fig. 28) *(77)*.

REFERENCES

1. Sternam DH, Sztejman E, Rodriquez E, Friedberg J. Diagnosis and staging of "other bronchial tumors." *Chest Surg Clin N Am* 2003;13:79–94.
2. Shepard JO. The trachea. In: McLoud TC, ed. *Thoracic Radiology: The Requisites*. St. Louis: Mosby, 1998:347–371.
3. Hajdu SI, Huvos AG, Goodner JT, Foote FW, Beattie EJ. Carcinoma of the trachea: clinicopathologic study of 41 cases. *Cancer* 1970;25:1448–1456.
4. Dennie CJ, Coblentz CL. The trachea: pathologic conditions and trauma. *Can Assoc Radiol J* 1993;44:157–167.
5. Weber AL, Grillo HC. Tracheal tumors: a radiological, clinical, and pathological evaluation of 84 cases. *Radiol Clin North Am* 1978;16:227–246.
6. McCarthy MJ, Rosado-de-Christenson ML. Tumors of the trachea. *J Thorac Imaging* 1995;10:180–198.
7. Heitmiller RF, Mathisen DJ, Ferry JA, Mark EJ, Grillo HC. Mucoepidermoid lung tumors. *Ann Thorac Surg* 1989;47: 394–399.
8. Ko JM, Jung JI, Park SH, et al. Benign tumors of the tracheobronchial tree: CT-pathologic correlation. *AJR Am J Roentgenol* 2006;186:1304–1313.
9. Grillo HC, Mathisen DJ. Primary tracheal tumors: treatment and results. *Ann Thorac Surg* 1990;49:69–77.
10. Kwong JS, Müller NL, Miller RR. Diseases of the trachea and main-stem bronchi: correlation of CT with pathologic findings. *Radiographics* 1992;12:647–657.
11. Kwong JS, Adler BD, Padley SPG, et al. Diagnosis of diseases of the trachea and main bronchi: chest radiography vs CT. *AJR Am J Roentgenol* 1993;161:519–522.
12. Manninen MP, Paakkala TA, Pukander JS, et al. Diagnosis of tracheal carcinoma at chest radiography. *Acta Radiol* 1992;33:546–547.
13. Kwak SH, Lee KS, Chung MJ, Jeong YJ, Kim GY, Kwon OJ. Adenoid cystic carcinoma of the airways: helical CT and histopathologic correlation. *AJR Am J Roentgenol* 2004;183:277–281.
14. Parsons RB, Milestone BN, Adler LP. Radiographic assessment of airway tumors. *Chest Surg Clin N Am* 2003;13:63–77.
15. Boiselle PM, Reynolds KF, Ernst A. Multiplanar and three-dimensional imaging of the central airways with multidetector CT. *AJR Am J Roentgenol* 2002;179:301–308.
16. Kaminski JM, Langer CJ, Movsas B. The role of radiation therapy and chemotherapy in the management of airway tumors other than small-cell carcinoma and non-small-cell carcinoma. *Chest Surg Clin N Am* 2003;13:149–167.
17. Shanley DJ, Daum-Kowalski R, Embry RL. Adenoid cystic carcinoma of the airway: MR findings. Letters. *AJR Am J Roentgenol* 1991;156:1321–1322.
18. Akata S, Ohkubo Y, Park J, et al. Multiplanar reconstruction MR image of primary adenoid cystic carcinoma of the central airway: MPR of central airway adenoid cystic carcinoma. *Clin Imaging* 2001;25:332–336.
19. Gamsu G, Webb WR. Computed tomography of the trachea and mainstem bronchi. *Semin Roentgenol* 1983;18:51–59.
20. Naidich DP. CT/MR correlation in the evaluation of tracheobronchial neoplasia. *Radiol Clin North Am* 1990;28:555–571.
21. Aronchick JM, Wexler JA, Christen B, Miller W, Epstein D, Gefter WB. Computed tomography of bronchial carcinoid. *J Comput Assist Tomogr* 1986;10:71–74.
22. Gilbert JG Jr, Mazzarella LA, Feit LJ. Primary tracheal tumors in the infant and adult. *Arch Otolaryngol* 1953;58:1–9.
23. Naka Y, Nakao K, Hamajii Y, Nakahara M, Tsujimoto M, Nakahara K. Solitary squamous cell papilloma of the trachea. *Ann Thorac Surg* 1993;55:189–193.
24. Litzky L. Epithelial and soft tissue tumors of the tracheobronchial tree. *Chest Surg Clin N Am* 2003;13:1–40.
25. Strong MS, Vaughn CW, Healy GB, Cooperband SR, Clemente MACP. Recurrent respiratory papillomatosis. Management with the CO_2 laser. *Ann Otol Rhinol Laryngol* 1976;85:508–516.

26. Takasugi JE, Godwin JD. The airway. *Semin Roentgenol* 1991;26:175–190.
27. Byrne JC, Tsao MS, Fraser RS, Howley PM. Human papillomavirus-11 DNA in a patient with chronic laryngotracheo-bronchial papillomatosis and metastatic squamous-cell carcinoma of the lung. *N Engl J Med* 1987;317:873–878.
28. Gruden JF, Webb WR, Sides DM. Adult-onset disseminated tracheobronchial papillomatosis: CT features. *J Comput Assist Tomogr* 1994;18:640–642.
29. Wilson RW, Kirejezyk W. Pathological and radiological correlation of endobronchial neoplasm. Part I. Benign tumors. *Ann Diagn Pathol* 1997;1:31–46.
30. Politis J, Funahashi A, Gehlsen JA, DeCock D, Stengel BF, Choi H. Intrathoracic lipomas: report of three cases and review of the literature with emphasis on endobronchial lipoma. *J Thorac Cardiovasc Surg* 1979;77:550–556.
31. Van den Bosch JM, Wagenaar SS, Corrin B, Elbers JR, Knaepen PJ, Westermann CJ. Mesenchymoma of the lung (so called hamartoma): a review of 154 parenchymal and endobronchial cases. *Thorax* 1987;42:790–793.
32. Cosío BG, Villena V, Echave-Sustaeta J, et al. Endobronchial Hamartoma. *Chest* 2002;122:202–205.
33. Ahn JM, Im JG, Seo JW, et al. Endobronchial hamartoma: CT findings in three patients. *AJR Am J Roentgenol* 1994;163:49–50.
34. Bennett LL, Lesar MS, Tellis CJ. Multiple calcified chondrohamartomas of the lung: CT appearance. *J Comput Assist Tomogr* 1985;9:180–182.
35. Weber AL, Shortsleeve M, Goodman M, Montgomery W, Grillo HC. Cartilaginous tumors of the larynx and trachea. *Radiol Clin North Am* 1978;16:261–271.
36. Carter D, Patchefsky AS. *Tumors and Tumor-Like Lesions of the Lung.* 1st ed., vol. 36. Philadelphia, PA: WB Saunders, 1998.
37. Frank JL, Schwartz BR, Price LM, Neifeld JP. Benign cartilaginous tumors of the upper airway. *J Surg Oncol* 1991;48:69–74.
38. Regnard JF, Fourquier P, Levasseur P. Results and prognostic factors in resections of primary tracheal tumors: a multi-center retrospective study—The French Society of Cardiovascular Surgery. *J Thorac Cardiovasc Surg* 1996;111:808–813.
39. Grillo HC. Development of tracheal surgery: a historical review. Part 2: treatment of tracheal diseases. *Ann Thorac Surg* 2003;75:1039–1047.
40. Webb BD, Walsh GL, Roberts DB, Sturgis EM. Primary tracheal malignant neoplasms: the University of Texas MD Anderson Cancer Center experience. *J Am Coll Surg* 2006;202:237–246.
41. Mathisen DJ. Surgical management of tracheobronchial disease. *Clin Chest Med* 1992;13:151–171.
42. Houston HE, Payne WS, Harrison ED Jr, Olsen AM. Primary cancers of the trachea. *Arch Surg* 1969;99:132–140.
43. Rosado-de-Christenson M, Templeton PA, Moran CA. Bronchogenic carcinoma: radiologic pathologic correlation. *Radiographics* 1994;14:429–446.
44. Foster WL Jr, Roberts L Jr, McLendon RE, Hill RC. Localized peribronchial thickening: a CT sign of occult bronchogenic carcinoma. *AJR Am J Roentgenol* 1985;144:906–908.
45. Kim TS, Lee KS, Han J, Kim EA, Yang PS, Im J. Sialadenoid tumors of the respiratory tract: radiologic-pathologic correlation. *AJR Am J Roentgenol* 2001;177:1145–1150.
46. Kim TS, Lee KS, Han J, et al. Mucoepidermoid carcinoma of the tracheobronchial tree: radiographic and CT findings in 12 patients. *Radiology* 1999;212:643–648.
47. Fraser RS, Paré JAP, Fraser RG, Paré PD. Neoplastic disease of the lungs. In: Fraser RS, Paré JAP, Fraser RG, Paré PD, eds. *Synopsis of Diseases of the Chest,* 2nd ed. Philadelphia: Saunders, 1994:445–539.
48. Li W, Ellerbroek NA, Libshitz HI. Primary malignant tumors of the trachea: a radiologic and clinical study. *Cancer* 1990;66:894–899.
49. Pearson FG, Todd TRJ, Cooper JD. Experience with primary neoplasms of the trachea and carina. *J Thorac Cardiovasc Surg* 1984;88:511–518.
50. Clough A, Clarke P. Adenoid cystic carcinoma of the trachea: a long-term problem. *Aust N Z J Surg* 2006;76:751–753.
51. Zunker HO, Moore RL, Baker DC, Lattes R. Adenoid cystic carcinoma (cylindroma) of the trachea. Case report with 9-year follow-up. *Cancer* 1969;23:699–707.
52. Conlan AA, Payne WS, Woolner LB, Sanderson DR. Adenoid cystic carcinoma (cylindroma) and mucoepidermoid carcinoma of the bronchus. Factors affecting survival. *J Thorac Cardiovasc Surg* 1978;76:369–377.
53. Spizarny DL, Shepard JO, McLoud TC, Grillo HC, Dedrick CG. CT of adenoid cystic carcinoma of the trachea. *AJR Am J Roentgenol* 1986;146:1129–1132.
54. Xu LT, Sun ZF, Li ZJ, Wu LH, Zhang ZY, Yu XQ. Clinical and pathologic characteristics in patients with tracheo-bronchial tumor: report of 50 patients. *Ann Thorac Surg* 1987;43:276–278.
55. Okike N, Bernatz PE, Woolner LB. Carcinoid tumors of the lung. *Ann Thorac Surg* 1976;22:270–277.
56. Colby TV, Koss MN, Travis WD. Carcinoid and other neuroendocrine tumors. In: Colby TV, Koss MN, Travis WD, eds. *Atlas of Tumor Pathology: Tumors of the Lower Respiratory Tract,* fasc 13, ser 3. Washington, DC: Armed Forces Institute of Pathology, 1995;287–317.
57. Rosado-de-Christenson ML, Abbott GF, Kirejczyk WM, Galvin JR, Travis WD. Thoracic carcinoids: radiologic-pathologic correlations. *Radiographics* 1999;19:707–736.

58. Dusmet ME, McKneally MF. Pulmonary and thymic carcinoid tumors. *World J Surg* 1996;20:189–195.
59. Fink G, Krelbaum T, Yellin A, et al. Pulmonary carcinoid: presentation, diagnosis, and outcome in 142 cases in Israel and review of 640 cases from the literature. *Chest* 2001;119:1647–1651.
60. Schreurs AJM, Westermann CJJ, van den Bosch JMM, Vanderschueren RGJRA, de la Riviere AB, Knaepen PJ. A twenty-five year follow-up of ninety-three resected typical carcinoid tumors of the lung. *J Thorac Cardiovasc Surg* 1992;104:1470–1475.
61. Grote TH, Macon WR, Davis B, Greco FA, Johnson DH. Atypical carcinoid of the lung: a distinct clinicopathologic entity. *Chest* 1988;93;370–375.
62. Marty-Ané CH, Costes V, Pujol JL, Alauzen M, Baldet P, Mary H. Carcinoid tumors of the lung: do atypical features require aggressive management? *Ann Thorac Surg* 1995; 59:78–83.
63. Ducrocq X, Thomas P, Massard G, et al. Operative risk and prognostic factors of typical bronchial carcinoid tumors. *Ann Thorac Surg* 1998;65:1410–1414.
64. Soga J, Yakuwa Y. Bronchopulmonary carcinoids: an analysis of 1875 reported cases with special reference to a comparison between typical carcinoids and atypical varieties. *Ann Thorac Cardiovasc Surg* 1999;5:211–219.
65. McCaughan BD, Martini N, Bains MS. Bronchial carcinoids. *J Thorac Cardiovasc Surg* 1985;89:8–17.
66. Attar S, Miller JE, Hankins J, et al. Bronchial adenoma: a review of 51 patients. *Ann Thorac Surg* 1985;40:126–132.
67. Magid D, Siegelman SS, Eggleston JC, Fishman EK, Zerhouni EA. Pulmonary carcinoid tumors: CT assessment. *J Comput Assist Tomogr* 1989;13:244–247.
68. Shin MS, Berland LL, Myers JL, Clary G, Zorn GL. CT demonstration of an ossifying bronchial carcinoid simulating broncholithiasis. *AJR Am J Roentgenol* 1989; 153:51–52.
69. Yousem SA, Hochholzer L. Mucoepidermoid tumors of the lung. *Cancer* 1987;60:1346–1352.
70. Scott WJ. Surgical treatment of other bronchial tumors. *Chest Surg Clin N Am* 2003;13:111–128.
71. Martini N, Goodner JT, D'Angio GJ, Beattie EJ Jr. Tracheoesophageal fistula due to cancer. *J Thorac Cardiovasc Surg* 1970;59:319–324.
72. Morency G, Chalaoui J, Samson L, Sylvestre J. Malignant neoplasms of the trachea. *Can Assoc Radiol J* 1989;40:198–200.
73. Prince JS, Duhamel DR, Levin DL, Harrell JH, Friedman PJ. Nonneoplastic lesions of the tracheobronchial wall: radiologic findings with bronchoscopic correlation. *Radiographics* 2002;22:S215–S230.
74. Braman SS, Grillo HC, Mark EJ. A 44-year-old man with tracheal narrowing and respiratory stridor. Massachusetts General Hospital Case Records, case 32–1999. *N Engl J Med* 1999;341:1292–1299.
75. Choplin RH, Wehunt WD, Theros EG. Diffuse lesions of the trachea. *Semin Roentgenol* 1983;18:38–50.
76. Karakoc F, Karadag B, Akbenlioglu C, et al. Foreign body aspiration: what is the outcome? *Pediatr Pulmonol* 2002;34:30–36.
77. Oguz F, Citak A, Unuvar E, Sidal M. Airway foreign bodies in childhood. *Int J Pediatr Otorhinolaryngol* 2000:52:11–16.

8

Tracheobronchomalacia

Ronaldo Hueb Baroni, Rodrigo Caruso Chate,
Daniel Nobrega da Costa, and Phillip M. Boiselle

Summary

Tracheomalacia is a condition characterized by weakness of the airway walls and/or supporting cartilage, resulting in excessive expiratory collapse. It may be either congenital or acquired. Although the earliest reports of this condition date to the 1930s and 1940s, it has only recently been recognized as a relatively common and potentially treatable cause of chronic cough, dyspnea, and recurrent infections. The diagnosis relies upon identification of excessive collapsibility of the airway during expiration or other functional maneuvers. Although bronchoscopy has been widely considered as the reference gold standard for diagnosis, recent advances in CT imaging provide the opportunity to non-invasively diagnose this condition with similar accuracy to bronchoscopy. This chapter provides a comprehensive review of the current knowledge of this condition, including its epidemiology, histopathology, clinical features, natural history, diagnosis, and treatment. A special emphasis is placed upon the evolving role of multidetector-row CT for diagnosing this condition.

Key Words: Tracheomalacia; bronchomalacia; tracheobronchomalacia; trachea; bronchi; CT; bronchoscopy.

1. INTRODUCTION

The general term airway malacia refers to a weakness of the airway walls and/or supporting cartilage, resulting in a softer airway that is more susceptible to collapse during expiration (1–3). The intrathoracic trachea normally dilates during inspiration and narrows with expiration in response to changes between intrathoracic and intraluminal pressures during the phases of respiration (Fig. 1) (3,5,6). However, in airway malacia, there is exacerbation of this process leading to excessive expiratory collapse of the trachea and/or bronchi (Fig. 2) (1–3, 5–7).

This condition may involve the central airways focally or diffusely (6,8). Tracheomalacia (TM) refers to involvement of all or part of the trachea with sparing of the bronchi. The term tracheobronchomalacia (TBM) is employed when both the trachea and the mainstem bronchi are involved. Isolated involvement of one or both main bronchi without tracheal involvement is referred to as bronchomalacia (BM), which is much less common than TM and TBM (3).

TBM occurs in both children and adults. Although the earliest reports of this condition date to the 1930s and 1940s, TBM has only recently been recognized as a relatively common and potentially treatable cause of chronic cough, dyspnea, and recurrent infections (3). Despite recent advances in diagnosis and treatment, there are still many unanswered questions about this relatively elusive condition in terms of its prevalence, natural history, and treatment. In this chapter, we provide a comprehensive review of the current knowledge about this condition, with an emphasis on recent advances in non-invasive imaging diagnosis using multidetector-row CT (MDCT) scanners.

From: *Contemporary Medical Imaging: CT of the Airways*
Edited by: P. M. Boiselle and D. A. Lynch © Humana Press, Totowa, NJ

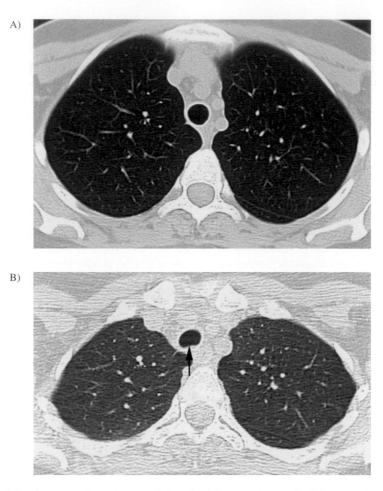

Fig. 1. Normal inspiratory and expiratory CT tracheal lumen changes in 36-year-old woman. (**A**) End-inspiratory CT scan demonstrates a round shape of the tracheal lumen. (**B**) Dynamic-expiratory CT scan demonstrates normal degree of expiratory tracheal luminal narrowing with slight anterior bowing of posterior membranous wall. [Reprinted with permission from ref. *4.*]

2. CLASSIFICATION

Although different classification schemes for TBM have been proposed *(9)*, the most accepted system classifies this condition into congenital and acquired forms *(3)*.

2.1. Congenital or Primary Form

TBM is the most common congenital anomaly of the trachea *(10)*. Although it can be an isolated finding in normal infants, it is more commonly encountered among premature infants *(11)*. TBM may be associated with congenital disorders related to abnormalities of cartilage such as polychondritis *(12)* and chondromalacia *(13)*. TBM is also associated with the mucopolysaccharidoses, including Hunter's and Hurler's syndromes *(8,14,15)*, as well as other genetic syndromes.

Idiopathic giant trachea, or congenital tracheomegaly (also known as Mounier-Kuhn disease), is a rare congenital condition that most commonly presents in adulthood *(3)*. It is characterized by severe atrophy of the longitudinal elastic fibers and thinning of the muscularis mucosa, which allows both

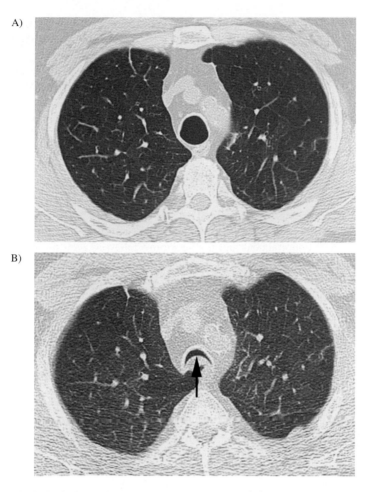

Fig. 2. Tracheomalacia in 51-year-old man with chronic cough. (**A**) End-inspiratory CT scan demonstrates a normal oval shape of the tracheal lumen. (**B**) Dynamic expiratory CT scan demonstrates excessive expiratory collapse, consistent with tracheomalacia. Note frown-like, crescenteric configuration of tracheal lumen (arrow). [Reprinted with permission from ref. *4.*]

the cartilaginous and the membranous portions of the trachea and main bronchi to dilate. This results in increased luminal diameter and increased expiratory compliance of the airway.

Several other conditions have been associated with TBM, most commonly tracheoesophageal fistula *(16,17).* TBM has also been associated with cardiovascular abnormalities, bronchopulmonary dysplasia, and gastroesophageal reflux disease *(3).*

In the majority of infants, primary TBM is a self-limiting disease *(3).* Indeed, most infants outgrow the condition by the age of 2 years. However, in patients with connective tissue disorders and congenital syndromes, TBM usually persists and may even be fatal *(3).*

2.2. *Acquired or Secondary Form*

Acquired or secondary TBM is more common than the congenital form and is associated with various risk factors and comorbidities, most notably chronic obstructive pulmonary disease *(3).*

A sentinel review by Feist et al. in 1975 reported that intubation with endotracheal or tracheostomy tubes was the most common cause of acquired TM *(6)*. Prolonged endotracheal intubation is associated with tracheal damage due to pressure necrosis, impairment of blood supply, inflammation due to friction of the tube upon the tracheal mucosa, and recurrent infections *(8)*. Premature infants with respiratory distress syndrome are the group most predisposed to developing TM from intubation, but this complication occurs in all age groups *(3)*. Tracheostomy also predisposes patients to acquired TM. Areas at the highest risk include the stoma site, cuff site, and impingement point at the distal aspect of the tube *(3)*. Other etiologies of TBM include various causes of cartilage loss or damage, including external trauma, surgery, and radiation therapy.

Recently, there has been a growing emphasis on the role of chronic inflammation and irritants, such as cigarette smoke, as the most important contributors to the development of acquired TBM *(3)*. For example, a recent study of adult patients with acquired TBM by Lee et al. *(18)* found that COPD was by far the most common risk factor for this condition. The greater proportion of patients with COPD compared with prior intubation in this recent study is likely related to technological advances in the design of endotracheal and tracheostomy tubes, as well as increased recognition of TBM among patients with COPD compared with the time of Feist's study.

Additional causes of secondary TBM include various causes of extrinsic compression of the trachea, including thyroid goiter *(11,19)*, paratracheal malignancies *(16,20,21)*, skeletal disorders (scoliosis and pectus excavatum) *(22,23)*, congenital paratracheal cysts *(8,16,24,25)*, and paratracheal vascular anomalies *(8, 26–39)*.

It is important to be aware that TM is relatively common among patients with extrinsic tracheal compression because of paratracheal vascular anomalies, especially among patients with innominate artery compression. Although surgical correction of vascular anomalies is potentially curative, up to 30% of patients will experience residual postoperative symptoms from malacia because of airway wall weakening as a result of long-standing extrinsic airway compression *(40)*. Chan et al. *(40)* recommend that MDCT dynamic airway imaging be performed routinely in the preoperative assessment of patients with vascular rings. In this way, both the extrinsic compression and the intrinsic malacia can be addressed at the time of surgery, avoiding the need for future interventions.

3. EPIDEMIOLOGY

The true incidence of TBM is uncertain because reports are based on bronchoscopic assessment of selected patients rather than the general population *(3)*. The incidence of congenital TBM has been estimated at 1 per 1445 infants and 1 per 2100 children *(41,42)*. The most recent incidence data in adults are from Japan, where airway malacia was detected in 542 (12.7%) of 4283 patients suffering from pulmonary disease who underwent bronchoscopy *(7)*.

Although some investigators report no gender predominance in the primary form of the disease *(43)*, others suggest a definite male predominance *(8,21,32)*. In patients with the acquired form of TBM, a male predominance has been demonstrated, but the reasons for this gender predominance are unknown *(2,3,7,18)*.

4. HISTOPATHOLOGY

Because the diagnosis of TBM is made by visualization of excessive airway collapsibility rather than by pathological analysis, relatively little is known about the histopathology of this condition in children or adults.

Pioneering work in the pediatric form of this disease has been reported by Wailoo and Emery, who performed 1000 sequential autopsies of children of all ages *(44)*. They found an increased tracheal internal perimeter and increased cartilage length as compared with the mean values of a "normal" population *(44)*. Membranous tracheal measurements were also larger than the mean, but the ratio of the cartilage to muscle was reduced, implying easier collapsibility of the trachea. These investigators later studied the membranous trachea of 560 children and found that the transverse muscle was consistently uniformly arranged, but there was considerable variability in the longitudinal muscle fibers, which are considered important for preventing collapse of the intrathoracic trachea (45). The lowest incidence of longitudinal muscle was found in preterm infants, and the highest incidence was found in children over 1 year of age. These results suggest that lack of muscular development may play a role in primary TBM associated with prematurity in addition to lack of cartilage development.

Autopsy studies of adults with TBM have revealed that the pars membranacea is typically dilated and flaccid, with anteroposterior narrowing of the bronchial lumen (45,46). Atrophy of the longitudinal elastic fibers of the pars membranacea (47,48) and "fragmentation" of the tracheal cartilage (49) have also been described.

5. CLINICAL PRESENTATION

In pediatric patients, the onset of signs and symptoms may occur at birth or may be delayed to the first weeks and months or life (3). Expiratory stridor and cough are the most commonly reported symptoms (3,36). Other symptoms and signs include recurrent respiratory infections, wheezing, cyanosis, spontaneous hyperextension of the neck, and breath-holding spells (3). With increasing respiratory distress, sternal, substernal, and intercostal retractions can be seen. Feeding difficulties have also been reported, particularly in children with TM because of vascular compression.

The most common symptoms in adults are dyspnea, cough, sputum production, recurrent infections, and hemoptysis (3,7,18). Although non-specific, a history of intractable cough is particularly common. In patients with TBM, cough is thought to occur secondary to the close juxtaposition of the walls of the airway during expiration, resulting in recurrent vibrations and irritation of the airway (3). The mechanical failure of the weakened airway walls causes central airway obstruction, resulting in progressive dyspnea. Excessive expiratory collapse also impairs clearance of respiratory secretions, which may lead to recurrent infections. In patients with both TM and COPD, large pressure swings in the thorax may occur because of bronchospasm, exacerbating the degree of expiratory airway collapse; the associated increase in airway resistance and work of breathing may lead to respiratory failure (3). If left untreated, TBM can cause significant respiratory dysfunction, and it may rarely prove fatal (3). Thus, a prompt diagnosis of TM is particularly important in patients with underlying COPD.

6. NATURAL HISTORY

Although the natural history of this disorder is not yet fully understood, limited data from longitudinal bronchoscopic studies suggest that this condition is frequently progressive. Jokinen et al. (2) performed follow-up bronchoscopies in 17 patients with malacia and found progression of disease in 13. In a larger study, Nuutinen (50) reported the serial bronchoscopic findings in 94 patients with malacia with an average follow-up of 5.2 years. In this series, the majority of patients with mild-to-moderate disease worsened, and no patients showed improvement over time. Thus, in the absence of intervention, most cases progress, but the factors that influence disease stability or progression are unknown.

Because the available longitudinal data are from bronchoscopic studies, they are biased toward symptomatic cases. Thus, the natural history of this disorder among asymptomatic and mildly symptomatic patients is unknown.

7. TRADITIONAL DIAGNOSTIC APPROACH

Because of the non-specific nature of its symptoms, TBM often goes unrecognized or misdiagnosed, thereby contributing to the morbidity of the disease. TBM is often difficult to distinguish clinically from other respiratory conditions, including asthma, emphysema, chronic bronchitis, and intraluminal obstruction (e.g., airway neoplasms and foreign body aspiration). A contributing difficulty is the fact that airway malacia may coexist with other respiratory disorders such as chronic bronchitis and emphysema *(3)*.

The challenge of diagnosing this condition on clinical grounds has been illustrated by a recent retrospective review of bronchoscopies performed in a series of children age 0–17 years by Boogaard et al. *(42)*. In this series, airway malacia was diagnosed in 160 of 512 children. Notably, airway malacia was unsuspected clinically in roughly half of all cases. Most of these cases were misdiagnosed clinically as asthma. On the basis of their findings, these investigators recommend an assessment for TBM for all pediatric patients with otherwise unexplained impaired exercise tolerance, recurrent lower airway infections, and therapy-resistant, irreversible, or atypical asthma.

Traditional diagnostic methods for diagnosing TBM include pulmonary function tests and bronchoscopy. Although pulmonary function studies (PFTs) may be useful in evaluating a patient with suspected TBM, they are not diagnostic *(3)*. PFTs commonly reveal obstruction in proportion to the severity of malacia. The pattern is usually that of a decreased forced expiratory volume in 1 s and low peak flow rate with a rapid decrease in flow. On forced expiratory spirograms, patients with TBM frequently show a characteristic "break" or notch in the expiratory phase of the flow-volume loop *(3)*. However, this pattern may also be seen in patients with emphysema without coexisting TBM.

As bronchoscopy is the only method that allows direct visualization of the airways during real-time maneuvers, it is widely considered the reference gold-standard for diagnosing TBM (Fig. 3) *(3)*. However, it is interesting to note that the role of bronchoscopy as the "gold-standard" for diagnosing this condition has recently been called into question *(51)*. Although bronchoscopy is a sensitive method for detecting TBM when specific maneuvers such as forced expiration and coughing are employed to elicit airway collapse, these maneuvers are not routinely performed during a standard bronchoscopic study. Thus, TBM can be overlooked at routine bronchoscopy. Furthermore, the use of sedation for bronchoscopy has the potential to impair the ability of the patient to cooperate with the desired maneuvers, and the introduction of the endoscope prevents the depiction of the trachea in a physiologic setting *(52)*. There are also problems in assessing tracheal dimension quantitatively at bronchoscopy. First, because of the wide angle design of the endoscopic lens, the images seen are spatially distorted and presented in a circular ("fisheye") form; this means that central parts of the image appear enlarged, whereas peripheral parts appear reduced in size. Second, quantitative area measurements are not usually performed, because they require not only knowledge of the distance

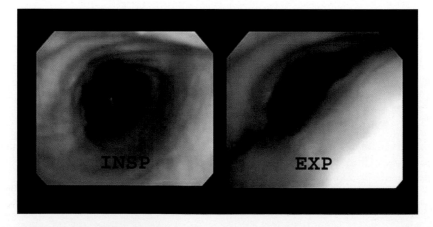

Fig. 3. Bronchoscopic diagnosis of tracheomalacia (TM). Paired inspiratory (INSP) and expiratory (EXP) bronchoscopic images of trachea demonstrate excessive expiratory narrowing of the airway lumen, consistent with TM. Note anterior bulging of posterior wall of trachea on expiratory image.

between the bronchoscopic lens and the area of interest *(53)* but also using a specific cross-sectional area measurement device that is not available in most centers *(54)*.

Finally, because bronchoscopy is an invasive procedure with small but inherent risks, it is not clinically feasible or desirable to perform this invasive test in all patients who present with chronic cough and other non-specific respiratory symptoms *(18)*. Fortunately, recent advances in MDCT imaging afford the opportunity to non-invasively diagnose TM with similar sensitivity to conventional bronchoscopy *(18,55,56)*. In the following section, we describe non-invasive imaging methods for diagnosing this condition, beginning with a historical perspective and ending with the latest generation of MDCT scanners.

8. HISTORICAL REVIEW OF NON-INVASIVE IMAGING METHODS

During the past few decades, various non-invasive imaging methods have been applied to the diagnosis of TM. Historically, cine-fluoroscopy was employed, with a degree of collapse equal to or greater than 50% in the anterior and left anterior oblique positions considered positive for the diagnosis *(1)*. However, this method was limited by several factors, including a relatively poor display of anatomic detail, the subjective and operator-dependent nature of this technique, an inability to simultaneously display the antero-posterior and lateral walls of the trachea, and a tendency to underestimate the degree of collapse compared with bronchoscopy.

With the advent of CT imaging, it became possible to obtain a more objective and reproducible display of the airways and to quantitatively measure the degree of collapse. The introduction of helical CT technology further improved imaged quality, but early single-detector helical scanners were limited by a relatively long acquisition time, a significant rate-limiting factor for functional imaging. The advent of electron beam CT, which acquired images with a temporal resolution of 50–100 ms per slice, made it possible to obtain "real-time" cross-sectional images of the airways during dynamic breathing and coughing *(54,57,58)*. However, this technique was limited by its relatively low spatial resolution, limited *z*-axis coverage, and restricted availability.

Recently, the advent of MDCT has overcome the limitations of previous CT technologies by providing a successful combination of fast speed, high spatial resolution, and large anatomic coverage. These factors have facilitated the ability to acquire a helical data set of the entire airways during a single expiratory maneuver (dynamic expiratory CT) *(18,55,56)*.

Magnetic resonance imaging (MRI) may also be employed for the evaluation of TBM *(59)*. Fast techniques such as T1-weighted turbo-FLASH (fast-low-angle-shot) provide good contrast resolution with a temporal resolution as low as 150 ms per slice. A potential advantage of this technique is the lack of ionizing radiation, which allows for repeated assessments during respiratory maneuvers without concern for radiation exposure. Although preliminary results have been promising *(59)*, there has been relatively little work in this area to date. Larger studies are necessary to determine the relative sensitivity and specificity of this method in comparison with bronchoscopy.

The following section describes the various provocative maneuvers that may be used for functional imaging of TBM, with an emphasis on physiological correlations.

9. PROVOCATIVE MANEUVERS FOR NON-INVASIVE FUNCTIONAL AIRWAY IMAGING

Unlike traditional anatomical imaging, in which the airways are evaluated at maximal end-inspiration, functional imaging requires acquiring imaging data during or after provocative maneuvers such as expiration and coughing.

When considering these provocative maneuvers, it is important to review the relationship of tracheal collapse to intrathoracic pressures. Changes in size of malacic trachea and bronchi depend on the difference between the intraluminal pressure inside the airways and the pleural (intrathoracic)

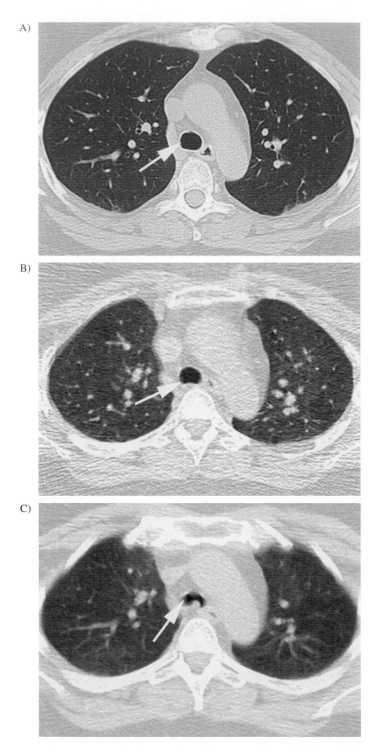

Fig. 4. Comparison of airway collapse during different expiratory maneuvers. These images show normal tracheal appearance at the level of aortic arch at end-inspiration (**A**), with small degree of collapse at end-expiration (**B**) and significant (>50%) collapse during dynamic-expiration (**C**). Arrows denote tracheal lumen. [Reprinted with permission from ref. *51*.]

pressure outside *(3,51)*. Pleural pressure depends mostly on respiratory muscles and is high during expiratory efforts. In contrast, intraluminal pressures are highly variable and depend on airflow. When airflow is zero, intraluminal pressure equals alveolar pressure and differs from pleural pressure only by the elastic recoil pressure of the lung, which depends on lung volume. At maximal lung volume with no flow (end-inspiration), the intraluminal pressure is 20–30 cm H_2O greater than pleural pressure, and the pressure difference expands the trachea. At low lung volumes with no flow (end-expiration), the intraluminal pressure is nearly equal to pleural pressure, and the trachea is unstressed. The trachea is most compressed during cough and dynamic expiration at low lung volume, when pleural pressure is high ($\sim$100 cm H_2O), and expiratory flow limitation in the small airways prevents transmission of the high alveolar pressures to the central airways. Under these conditions, intraluminal pressure is nearly atmospheric, and the large transmural pressure causes tracheal collapse *(60)*.

Baroni et al. *(51)* directly compared the ability of end-expiratory and dynamic expiratory CT imaging methods to elicit TM. Consistent with the principles of respiratory physiology, this study showed that dynamic expiratory CT elicited a significantly greater degree of tracheal collapse than end-expiratory CT (Fig. 4). In this study, the mean percentages of airway collapse measured with the two techniques at three levels were: (i) aortic arch: dynamic-expiration = 53.9% versus end-expiration = 35.7% ($p = 0.0046$); (ii) carina: dynamic-expiration = 53.6% versus end-expiration = 30.9% ($p < 0.001$); and (iii) bronchus intermedius: dynamic-expiration = 57.5% versus end-expiration = 28.6% ($p = 0.0022$).

It is known that cough elicits an even higher level of intrathoracic–extratracheal pressure than forced exhalation. Thus, imaging during coughing should theoretically be the most sensitive method for eliciting tracheal collapse in patients with malacia. Using dynamic MRI, Suto and Tanabe *(59)* have shown that coughing elicits a greater degree of collapse than forced end-expiration. In an early study of eight adult patients with suspected TM evaluated with electron-beam CT, Hein et al. *(53)* also elicited a much higher average percentage of collapse during coughing (71%) than at end-expiration (36%). However, this CT method was limited to imaging a single slice of the trachea during each cine sequence. This resulted in a "sampling" of the trachea, with the need for repeated acquisitions, resulting in a relatively high radiation exposure and long exam time.

More recently, the advent of 64-slice MDCT has helped to overcome the limitations of electron-beam CT because of its high spatial and temporal resolution, combined with its large anatomic coverage capability. During a single cine acquisition, 64-slice MDCT provides anatomic coverage of 3–4 cm in the *z*-axis, allowing simultaneous assessment of portions of the trachea and proximal main bronchi. Preliminary clinical experience with this method shows that it is both technically feasible and highly sensitive for detecting malacia *(61)*.

At present, cine 64-MDCT is still somewhat limited in its *z*-axis coverage, resulting in either a single "sampling" of the trachea or the need for several acquisitions to provide complete anatomical coverage. Fortunately, future advances in CT imaging will soon provide greater coverage, allowing simultaneous cine evaluation of the entire intrathoracic airways during a single imaging acquisition *(61)*.

10. DIAGNOSTIC CRITERION FOR TBM

The vast majority of studies reported in the literature support the use of a threshold of greater than or equal to 50% collapse as diagnostic of TBM when using either bronchoscopy or CT. However, it is important to note that several studies have advocated the adoption of different threshold values. For example, Stern et al. *(62)* obtained a degree of tracheal collapse greater than 50% at end-expiration in 4 of 10 healthy young adult male volunteers scanned with an electron-beam CT. On the basis of their findings, these authors recommended a more conservative threshold of 70% of collapse as indicative of TM. Similarly, Heussel et al. *(58)* have reported that healthy volunteers can sometimes exceed the standard diagnostic criterion. On the contrary, Aquino et al. *(63)* studied 23 normal subjects and 10 patients with bronchoscopically proven acquired TM using end-expiratory CT scans and obtained a positive-predictive value of 89–100% using a threshold of >18% collapse for the upper trachea and >28% for the mid-trachea. Although the use of a lower threshold when imaging at end-expiration fits well with physiological principles, the low threshold values of 18 and 28% likely overlap substantially with those of normal subjects and will require further validation. In contrast, based on preliminary experience with 64-MDCT "cine" imaging during coughing, a higher threshold value of 70% should be considered when using this robust provocative maneuver to elicit tracheal collapse *(61)*.

On the basis of these studies, it seems reasonable that the recommended threshold criterion of collapse for diagnosing TBM will vary depending on which provocative maneuver has been employed. However, the precise values for accurate diagnosis have yet to be validated in large studies. Thus, there is a need to obtain normative data regarding the range of tracheal collapse using different provocative maneuvers among patients of varying ages, ethnicities, and both genders, both with and without coexistent pulmonary disease. Until these data have been published, it seems reasonable to employ a diagnostic threshold of >50% reduction for dynamic expiration and >70% reduction during coughing. However, one should keep in mind that there is likely overlap with normal at the lower range of positive.

11. HOW TO PERFORM A FUNCTIONAL MDCT STUDY

To ensure a high-quality study, technologists should be trained to coach and monitor patients as they perform the respiratory techniques (end-inspiration, dynamic expiration, coughing) that are included in the functional imaging protocol that is being employed. Technologists should also be trained to recognize the characteristic appearance of inspiratory and expiratory CT scans to ensure that the imaging sequences have been successfully performed during the appropriate respiratory maneuvers. For centers that are just beginning to use this technique, it is recommended that the radiologists observe and monitor cases until the technologists have become comfortable coaching patients with these maneuvers.

In the following paragraphs, functional airway imaging protocols are reviewed, including paired inspiratory-dynamic expiratory CT and cine CT during coughing. The end-expiratory imaging technique is not reviewed because it has been supplanted by the more effective dynamic expiratory imaging method.

Paired inspiratory-dynamic expiratory CT includes imaging during two different phases of respiration: end inspiratory (imaging during suspended end inspiration) and continuous dynamic expiratory (imaging *during* forceful exhalation). This protocol can be successfully performed with any type of MDCT scanner. However, in the author's experience, the best results are produced with scanner configurations of eight or more detector rows. Before helical scanning, initial scout topographic images are obtained to determine the area of coverage, which extends from the proximal trachea through the main bronchi, corresponding to a length of approximately 10–12 cm. Helical scanning is performed in the craniocaudal dimension for both end inspiratory and dynamic expiratory scans. The end inspiratory scan is performed first (170 mAs, 120 kVp, 2.5 mm collimation, pitch equivalent of 1.5). Following the end inspiratory scan, patients are subsequently coached with instructions for the dynamic expiratory component of the scan (40 mAs, 120 kVp, 2.5 mm collimation, high-speed mode, with pitch equivalent of 1.5). For this sequence, patients are instructed to take a deep breath in and to blow it out *during* the CT acquisition, which is coordinated to begin with the onset of the patient's forced expiratory effort. Patients should not purse their lips during exhalation.

Cine CT during coughing requires use of a 64-MDCT scanner. At the author's institution, this protocol is performed with detector collimation 0.5 × 64 mm; mA = 80; kVp = 120; gantry rotation = 0.4 s.

An initial scout topographic image is obtained to determine the area of coverage, which extends 3.2 cm in craniocaudad length. To "sample" the trachea and proximal main bronchi within a single acquisition, the inferior aspect of the acquisition is set at the level of the carina, and the superior aspect of the acquisition is set 3.2 cm above this level, which corresponds to approximately the level of the aortic arch. A 5-s acquisition is acquired in cine mode beginning at end-inspiration and followed by repeated coughing maneuvers. Images are reconstructed at 8-mm collimation in a standard algorithm, creating four contiguous cine data sets from a single acquisition.

This protocol can also be modified for use with 64-MDCT scanners from other vendors. Depending on the scanner configuration, there is a potential to increase the z-axis coverage (e.g., $0.625 \times 64 = 4.0$ cm z-axis coverage).

12. DOSE-REDUCTION FOR MDCT

Because paired inspiratory-dynamic expiratory CT requires imaging during two phases of respiration, it has the potential to result in a "double dose" compared with a traditional single-phase CT scan unless methods for dose reduction are employed. Similarly, there is a potential for high radiation exposure using cine techniques unless dose-reduction methods are used.

Fortunately, the high inherent contrast between the air-filled trachea and soft-tissue structures allows for significant reductions in dose without negatively influencing image quality for assessing luminal dimensions of the airway (56). For example, a clinical study by Zhang et al. (56) showed no difference between standard (240–260 mA) and low-dose (40–80 mA) images for assessing the tracheal lumen during dynamic expiration in the evaluation of suspected malacia.

As reviewed in the previous section on protocols, a low-dose (30–40 mAs) technique is recommended when imaging during coughing or expiration. In contrast, a standard-dose technique should be employed for the end-inspiratory scan, which is also used for comprehensive anatomical assessment of the airways and lungs. The estimated radiation dose (expressed as dose-length product) for a dual-phase study (standard dose end-inspiratory sequence + low-dose dynamic expiratory sequence) for a 70-kg patient is approximately 500 mGy.cm, which is comparable to a routine chest CT (reference value 600 mGy.cm) (64). By comparison, the estimated dose for a low-dose cine CT is approximately 200–220 mGy.cm. However, unlike the dual-phase scan, which covers the entirety of the central airways, a single cine acquisition only covers 3.2–4.0 cm in the z-axis (depending on the scanner configuration). If repeated at multiple levels to provide similar coverage to the dual-phase CT, the total dose for serial cine acquisitions would be greater than the dual-phase technique.

13. MULTIPLANAR REFORMATIONS AND 3-D CT RECONSTRUCTIONS

Volumetric data acquisition using MDCT allows for the creation of three-dimensional (3-D) reconstructions and multiplanar reformations (MPR), which have the potential to aid diagnosis and preoperative planning (65,66). Virtual bronchoscopic images, which provide an intraluminal perspective similar to conventional bronchoscopy, are particularly helpful for assessing dynamic changes in the lumen of the main bronchi, which course obliquely to the axial plane and are not optimally evaluated by traditional axial CT images (Fig. 5). Paired end-inspiratory and dynamic-expiratory sagittal reformation images along the axis of the trachea are helpful for displaying the craniocaudad extent of excessive tracheal collapse during expiration and may aid planning for stent placement or corrective tracheoplasty procedures (Fig. 6) (65,66). Similar information can also be obtained using 3-D external renderings (Fig. 7).

14. DIAGNOSTIC INTERPRETATION OF FUNCTIONAL MDCT STUDIES

Interpretation of CT images for the diagnosis of TM requires careful review and comparison of both end-inspiratory and dynamic-expiratory images. End-inspiratory images provide important anatomical information about the tracheal size and shape, the thickness of the tracheal wall, and the

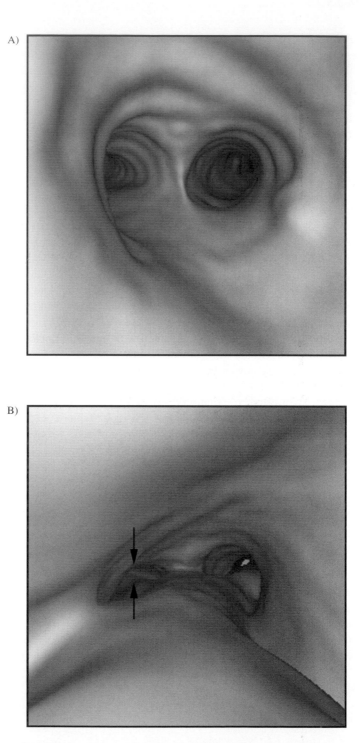

Fig. 5. Virtual bronchoscopic assessment of tracheobronchomalacia. Virtual-bronchoscopy images at carinal level obtained at end-inspiration (**A**) and dynamic-expiration (**B**) show excessive anterior protrusion of the posterior wall of the distal trachea, carina and main bronchi at expiration, significantly reducing the airway caliber. Left main bronchus (paired arrows, b) shows more marked narrowing than the right main bronchus.

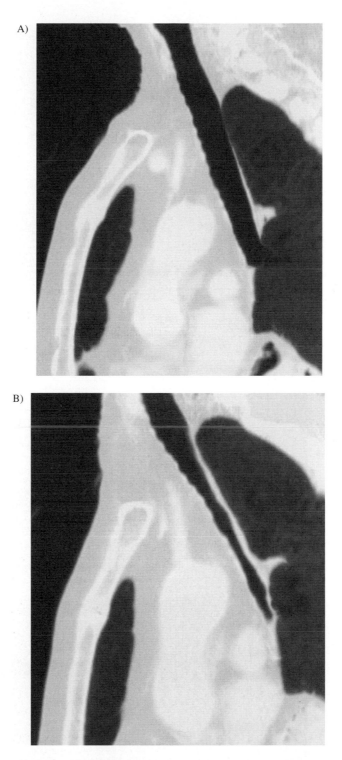

Fig. 6. Multiplanar reformation images. Sagittal multiplanar reformations at end-inspiration (**A**) and dynamic expiration (**B**) demonstrate longitudinal length of tracheomalacia, involving entire intrathoracic trachea with extrathoracic sparing.

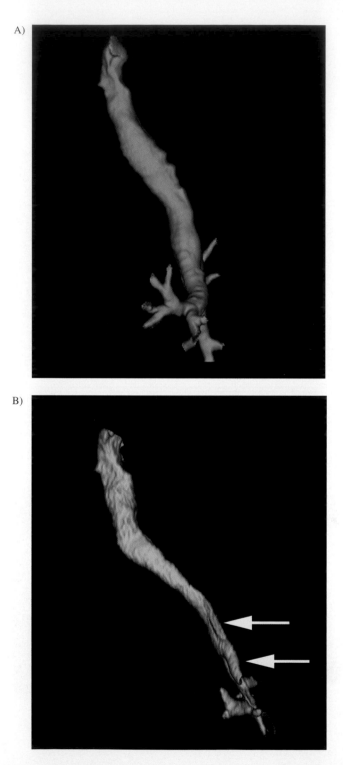

Fig. 7. Three-dimensional segmentation of tracheal lumen in patient with diffuse tracheomalacia (TM). End-inspiratory (**A**) 3-D segmentation of trachea in lateral projection shows normal caliber. Note marked narrowing (arrows) of anteroposterior dimension of intra-thoracic trachea during dynamic expiration (**B**), consistent with TM.

presence or absence of extrinsic masses compressing the trachea. It is important to be aware that the tracheal lumen is almost always normal in appearance on end-inspiration CT *(4)*. Notable exceptions include (a) patients with relapsing polychondritis (Fig. 8), who may demonstrate characteristic wall thickening and calcification that spares the posterior membranous wall of the trachea; (b) patients with lunate tracheal shape (coronal > sagittal dimension), which is frequently associated with TM (Fig. 9); and (c) patients with extrinsic tracheal compression from adjacent vascular anomalies or thyroid masses, in whom long-standing compression has been complicated by TM.

The most accurate means for diagnosing malacia on CT is to use an electronic tracing tool to calculate the cross-sectional area of the airway lumen on images at the same anatomic level obtained at inspiration and dynamic expiration (Fig. 10) *(67)*. Such tools can be found on commercially available PACS stations as well as with 3-D workstations. As described in the previous section, >50% expiratory reduction in cross-sectional area is considered diagnostic. Care should be taken to ensure that the same anatomical level is compared between the two sequences by comparing vascular structures and other anatomical landmarks.

Obviously, in the setting of severe malacia, in which there is near complete collapse of the airway lumen during expiration, the diagnosis can be confidently made based on visual analysis of the images. Interestingly, about half of patients with acquired TM will demonstrate an expiratory "frown-like" configuration, in which the posterior membranous wall is excessively bowed forward and parallels the convex contour of the anterior wall with <6 mm distance between the anterior and posterior walls (Fig. 2B) *(4)*. This appearance, which has been coined the "frown sign," is highly suggestive of TM and has the potential to aid the detection of TM when patients inadvertently breathe during routine CT scans *(4)*. Ideally, however, the diagnosis of TM should be confirmed and quantified by a dedicated study.

With regard to interpreting cine coughing CT studies, they are ideally viewed in "cine" fashion at either a PACS workstation or a 3-D workstation. Quantitative measurements are obtained on individual static images in a similar fashion to the technique described for paired inspiratory-dynamic expiratory CT. As described earlier, >70% reduction in cross-sectional area during coughing is considered diagnostic. A commercial software program (Analyze 6.0, AnalyzeDirect, Inc., Lenexa

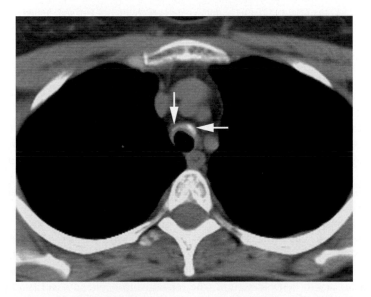

Fig. 8. Relapsing polychondritis. Axial CT image demonstrates calcified thickening of the anterior and lateral tracheal walls (arrows) with sparing of posterior membranous wall.

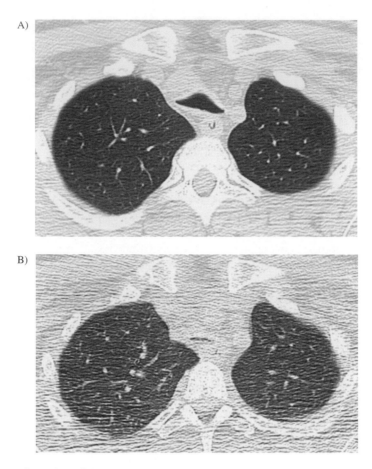

Fig. 9. Lunate configuration of the trachea in a 39-year-old man with chronic cough, dyspnea, and recurrent respiratory infections. (**A**) Inspiratory CT image demonstrates widening of coronal diameter of trachea consistent with a lunate configuration. (**B**) Expiratory CT image demonstrates complete collapse of airway lumen, consistent with tracheomalacia. Excessive image noise, most prominent posteriorly, relates to use of low-dose technique and large body habitus of the patient. [Reprinted with permission from ref. *4.*]

KS) can also be used to provide automated measurement of changes in tracheal lumen cross-sectional area values during the cine sequence *(61)*.

When interpreting functional CT scans of patients with TM, it is important to report the severity, distribution, and morphology. These factors have an important impact on treatment decisions, which are based on a combination of symptoms, severity and distribution of disease, and underlying cause of TM *(68)*.

Because there is not a single widely accepted scale for reporting the severity of TM, it is important to report the quantitative degree of collapsibility rather than simply using a qualitative descriptor. A severity scale that has been employed by other investigators includes three grades of severity based on the degree of airway collapse: (a) mild: 50–74%; (b) moderate: 74–99%; and (c) severe: 100% collapse *(55,68)*. It is the authors' opinion that 100% collapsibility is too limited a definition for severe disease and that a range of 91–100% expiratory collapse is more appropriate. However, further work is necessary to better determine the relationship between severity of collapse at CT or bronchoscopy and severity of symptoms and functional limitations.

Regarding assessment of distribution of disease, Murgu and Colt *(68)* have recently proposed a multifaceted classification system for TM that combines various factors, including functional class

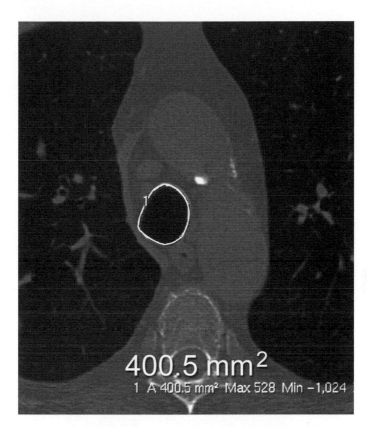

Fig. 10. Example of electronic tracing method for measuring cross-sectional area of tracheal lumen at the level of the aortic arch. The tracing line has been electronically thickened to enhance visibility for photographic reproduction. [Reprinted with permission from ref. *51*.]

of symptoms, extent of disease, morphology, origin, severity, and distribution. In their proposed classification system, distribution is considered focal if present in one tracheal region (upper, middle, or lower) or in one main or lobar bronchus; multifocal if present in two contiguous or at least two non-contiguous regions; and diffuse if present in more than two contiguous regions. From a practical perspective, accurate determination of the distribution of malacia has implications for treatment. For example, focal areas of malacia may benefit from stenting, whereas diffuse disease is more amenable to tracheoplasty surgery.

Regarding morphology, one should describe whether the collapse occurs circumferentially, or if it occurs primarily because of either excessive bulging of the posterior membranous wall or collapse of the anterolateral cartilaginous structures. For example, patients with collapse primarily because of bulging and flaccidity of the posterior membranous wall are potential candidates for tracheoplasty surgery, a novel surgical technique described in the following section.

15. TREATMENT

Various therapies have been employed for the treatment of TBM, including conservative/supportive measures, continuous positive airway pressure (CPAP), airway stent placement, and surgical intervention *(3)*. Preliminary data suggest that surgery is the most effective means of long-term therapy for patients with severely symptomatic TBM in whom excessive flaccidity of the posterior membranous wall is the major factor contributing to malacia *(3)*. With regard to stent placement, a recent evaluation

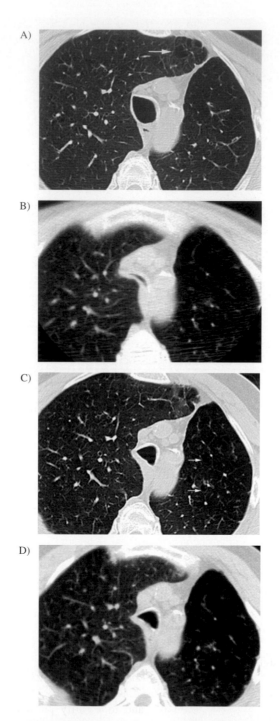

Fig. 11. A 62-year-old man with tracheobronchomalacia treated by tracheoplasty: comparison of preoperative and postoperative dynamic CT scans. Before surgery, the trachea has a biconvex ("fishmouth") shape at end-inspiration (**A**), and it shows a marked collapse at dynamic-expiration (**B**), acquiring a "lunate" shape. After tracheoplasty, the trachea has a normal, horseshoe-shape at end-inspiration (**C**), which persists at dynamic-expiration despite a mild degree of collapse (**D**). [Reprinted with permission from ref. *69.*]

of over 50 patients with severe TBM who were treated at Beth Israel Deaconess Medical Center with silicone stents demonstrated that most patients experienced improvement in respiratory symptoms, quality of life, and functional status [personal communication, Armin Ernst, MD]. However, stenting was associated with a high number of short- and long-term complications, which were mostly reversible. Thus, the role of long-term stenting for TBM is unclear. At present, stenting should probably be considered as a temporary measure for airway stabilization to determine whether eventual surgical airway stabilization is likely to be effective in improving airway symptoms, especially among patients with coexisting COPD and TBM, in whom airway symptoms may be due to either or both conditions.

For some patients, intervention is unnecessary. For example, in the pediatric population, as the child grows, the tracheal cartilage strengthens and stiffens. Symptoms often resolve in mild to moderate cases by age 1–2 *(3)*.

For both pediatric and adult patients with only mild symptoms, a conservative approach is often employed, including treatment of respiratory infections, humidified oxygen therapy, and pulmonary physiotherapy *(3)*. For patients with more severe and progressive symptoms, more aggressive treatment options include CPAP, stent placement, or surgical intervention *(3)*. The latter is reserved for patients with severe or life-threatening TM that is unresponsive to medical management.

Tracheoplasty has recently emerged as a potentially curative therapy for severely symptomatic adult patients with acquired TBM. This novel surgical approach involves reinforcement of the posterior membranous wall of the trachea and/or main bronchi by a Marlex graft *(69)*. Surgical reinforcement of the posterior membranous wall enhances the rigidity of this structure and makes it less susceptible to bowing during expiration (Fig. 11). CT plays several potentially important roles in evaluating patients who are undergoing evaluation for curative tracheoplasty surgery *(69)*. Preoperative roles include (a) precise characterization of airway shape and determination of which parts of the airway wall contribute to excessive airway collapsibility; (b) evaluation for airway wall thickening and calcification (in combination with airway malacia, these findings suggest polychondritis, a disorder that is not treated surgically); (c) evaluation for extrinsic paratracheal masses, which may preclude surgery; and (d) baseline measure of airway collapsibility by which to compare postoperative scans for evaluating response to surgery. In the postoperative setting, CT provides a non-invasive method for assessing for postoperative complications and non-invasively quantifying the degree of improvement in airway collapsibility. Finally, CT has the unique ability to visualize the characteristic thickening of the posterior wall of the airways after surgery, which may serve as a clue to the radiologist that tracheoplasty has been performed.

16. CONCLUSIONS

TBM, a condition characterized by excessive collapsibility of the airway, has recently been increasingly recognized as a relatively common and potentially treatable cause of chronic respiratory symptoms. Recent advances in MDCT imaging afford the opportunity to non-invasively diagnose TM with similar sensitivity to conventional bronchoscopy by using either paired inspiratory-dynamic expiratory CT or cine coughing techniques.

Future studies are necessary to determine the range of normal tracheal compliance among people of varying ages and both sexes; to better define threshold values for diagnosing TBM; to further elucidate the natural history of this condition; and to identify predictors of response to specific interventions.

REFERENCES

1. Johnson TH, Mikita JJ, Wilson RJ, Feist JH. Acquired tracheomalacia. *Radiology* 1973;109:576–580.
2. Jokinen K, Palva T, Sutinen S, Nuutinen J. Acquired tracheobronchomalacia. *Ann Clin Res* 1977;9:52–57.

3. Carden K, Boiselle PM, Waltz D, Ernst A. Tracheomalacia and tracheobronchomalacia in children and adults: an in-depth review of a common disorder. *Chest* 2005;127:984–1005.
4. Boiselle PM, Ernst A. Tracheal morphology in patients with tracheomalacia: prevalence of inspiratory "lunate" and expiratory "frown" shapes. *J Thor Imaging* 2006;21:190–196.
5. Heinbecker P. A method for the demonstration of calibre changes in the bronchi in normal respiration. *J Clin Invest* 1927;4:459–469.
6. Feist JH, Johnson TH, Wilson RJ. Acquired tracheomalacia: etiology and differential diagnosis. *Chest* 1975;68:340–345.
7. Nuutinen J. Acquired tracheobronchomalacia. *Eur J Respir Dis* 1982;63:380–387.
8. Mair EA, Parsons DS. Pediatric tracheobronchomalacia and major airway collapse. *Ann Otol Rhinol Laryngol* 1992;101:300–309.
9. Masaoka A, Yamakawa Y, Niwa H, et al. Pediatric and adult tracheobronchomalacia. *Eur J Cardiothorac Surg* 1996;10:87–92.
10. Holinger LD. Etiology of stridor in the neonate, infant, and child. *Ann Otol Rhinol Laryngol* 1980;89:397–400.
11. Jacobs IN, Wetmore RF, Tom LW, Handler SD, Potsic WP. Tracheobronchomalacia in children. *Arch Otolaryngol Head Neck Surg* 1994;120:154–158.
12. Johner CH, Szanto PA. Polychondritis in a newborn presenting as tracheomalacia. *Ann Otol Rhinol Laryngol* 1970;79:1114–1116.
13. Cox WL, Shaw RR. Congenital chondromalacia of the trachea. *J Thorac Cardiovasc Surg* 1965;49:1033–1039.
14. Morehead JM, Parsons DS. Tracheobronchomalacia in Hunter's syndrome. *Int J of Pediatr Otorhinolaryngol* 1993;26:255–261.
15. Shapiro J, Strome M, Crocker AC. Airway obstruction and sleep apnea in Hurler and Hunter syndromes. *Ann Otol Rhinol Laryngol* 1985;94:458–461.
16. Benjamin B. Tracheomalacia in infants and children. *Ann Otol Rhinol Laryngol* 1984;93:438–442.
17. Paston F, Bye M. Tracheomalacia. *Pediatr Rev* 1996;17:328.
18. Lee KS, Sun ME, Ernst A, Feller Kopman D, Boiselle PM. Comparison of dynamic expiratory CT with bronchoscopy in diagnosing airway malacia. *Chest* 2007;131:758–764.
19. Shaha AR, Alfonso AE, Jaffe BM. Operative treatment of substernal goiters. *Head Neck Surg* 1989;11:325–330.
20. Geelhoed GW. Tracheomalacia from compressing goiter: management after thyroidectomy. *Surgery* 1988;104: 1100–1108.
21. Krivchenia DI, Slepov AK, Chumakova LF. [Intrathoracic compression of the respiratory airways by mediastinal teratomas in children] Russian. *Lik Sprava* 2001;4:92–95.
22. Blair GK, Cohen R, Filler RM. Treatment of tracheomalacia: eight years' experience. *J Pediatr Surg* 1986;21:781–785.
23. Andrews TM, Myers CMI, Gray SP. Abnormalities of the bony thorax causing tracheobronchial compression. *Int J Pediatr Otorhinolaryngol* 1990;19:139–144.
24. Godfrey S. Association between pectus excavatum and segmental bronchomalacia. *J Pediatr* 1980;96:649–652.
25. Krivchenia DI, Slepov AK, Chumakova LF. [Intrathoracic compression of the respiratory tracts caused by broncho- and enterogenic mediastinal cysts in children] Russian. *Lik Sprava* 1999;7(8):87–90.
26. Krivchenia DI, Slepov AK, Zavodii VG, Chumakova LF, Golopara GV. [Surgical treatment of bronchogenic and enterogenic mediastinal cysts complicated by intrathoracic compression of respiratory tracts in children] Russian. *Klin Khir* 2001;1:26–28.
27. Dailey ME, O'Laughlin MP, Smith RJ. Airway compression secondary to left atrial enlargment with increased pulmonary artery pressure. *Int J Pediatr Otorhinolaryngol* 1990;19:33–44.
28. Krivchenia DI, Slepov AK, Zavodii VG, Chumakova LF, Golopara GV. [Surgical correction of intrathoracic compression of respiratory airways due to double aortic arch in children] Russian. *Klin Khir* 2000;6:27–30.
29. Sebening C, Jakob H, Tochtermann U, et al. Vascular tracheobronchial compression syndromes – experience in surgical treatment and literature review. *Thorac Cardiovasc Surg* 2000;48:164–174.
30. Snelling CE, Erb IH. Double aortic arch. *Arch Dis Child* 1933;8:401–408.
31. Heck HAJ, Moore HV, Lutin WA, et al. Esophageal-aortic erosion associated with double aortic arch and tracheomalacia. Experience with 2 infants. *Tex Heart Inst J* 1993;20:126–129.
32. Vasko JS, Ahn C. Surgical management of secondary tracheomalacia. *Ann Thorac Surg* 1968;6:269–272.
33. Adler SC, Isaacson G, Balsara RK. Innominate artery compression of the trachea: diagnosis and treatment by anterior suspension. A 25-year experience. *Ann Otol Rhinol Laryngol* 1995;104:924–927.
34. Ardito JM, Ossoff RH, Tucker GFJ, DeLeon SY. Innominate artery compression of the trachea in infants with reflex apnea. *Ann Otol Rhinol Laryngol* 1980;89:401–405.
35. Fearon B, Shortreed R. Tracheobronchial compression by congenital cardiovascular anomalies in children: syndrome of apnea. *Ann Otol Rhinol Laryngol* 1963;72:949–969.
36. Holinger PH. Clinical aspects of congenital anomalies of the larynx, trachea, bronchi, and oesophagus. The Semon lecture. *J Laryngol Otol* 1961;75:1–44.

37. Koopot R, Nikaidoh H, Idriss FS. Surgical management of anomalous left pulmonary artery causing tracheobronchial obstruction. Pulmonary artery sling. *J Thorac Cardiovasc Surg* 1975;69:239–246.

38. Potts WJ, Holinger PH, Rosenblum AH. Anomalous left pulmonary artery causing obstruction to right main bronchus: report of a case. *J Am Med Assoc* 1954;155:1409–1411.

39. Rivilla F, Utrilla JG, Alvarez F. Surgical management and follow-up of vascular rings. *Z Kinderchir* 1989;44:199–202.

40. Chan MS, Chan M, Chu WCW, et al. Angiography and dynamic airway evaluation with MDCT in the diagnosis of double aortic arch associated with tracheomalacia. *Am J Roentgenol* 2005;185:1248–1251.

41. Callahan CW. Primary tracheomalacia and gastroesophageal reflux in infants with cough. *Clin Pediatr* 1998;37:725–731.

42. Boogaard R, Huijsmans SH, Pijnenburg MWH, et al. Tracheomalacia and bronchomalacia in children: Incidence and patients characteristics. *Chest* 2005;128:3391–3397.

43. Baxter JD, Dunbar JS. Tracheomalacia. *Ann Otol Rhinol Laryngol* 1963;72:1013–1023.

44. Wailoo M, Emery JL. The trachea in children with respiratory diseases including children presenting as cot deaths. *Arch Dis Child* 1980;55:199–203.

45. Pohl R. Universal conditions of malacia at the level of the tracheobronchial system (universelle erweichungszustande am tracheobroncialsystem (tracheo-bronchopthia malacica). *Futaschr Geb Rontgens* 1951;74:40–43.

46. Campbell AH, Faulks LW. Expiratory air-flow pattern in tracheobronchial collapse. *Am Rev Respir Dis* 1965;92:781–791.

47. Kiener M, Koblet H, Wyss F. [Pathology of stenosed bronchial collapse with pulmonary emphysema]. Schweiz Med Wochenschr 1957;87:660–663.

48. Herzog H. [Expiratory stenosis of the trachea and great bronchi by loosenig of the membraneous portion; plastic chip repair]. *Thoraxchururgie* 1958;5:281–319.

49. Ikeda S, Hanawa T, Konishi T, et al. [Diagnosis, incidence, clinicopathology and surgical treatment of acquired tracheobronchomalacia] Japanese. *Nihon Kyobu Shikkan Gakkai Zasshi* 1992;30:1028–1035.

50. Nuutinen J. Acquired tracheobronchomalacia: a bronchological follow-up study. *Ann Clin Res* 1977;9:359–364.

51. Baroni R, Feller-Kopman D, Nishino M, Hatabu H, Loring S, Ernst A, Boiselle PM. Tracheobronchomalacia: comparison between end-expiratory and dynamic-expiratory CT methods for evaluation of central airway collapse. *Radiology* 2005;2:635–641.

52. Kao SC, Smith WL, Sato Y, Franken EA, Jr., Kimura K, Soper RT. Ultrafast CT of laryngeal and tracheobronchial obstruction in symptomatic postoperative infants with esophageal atresia and tracheoesophageal fistula. *Am J Roentgenol* 1990;154:345–350.

53. Hein E, Rogalla P, Hentschel C, Taupitz M, Hamm B. Dynamic and quantitative assessment of tracheomalacia by electron beam tomography: correlation with clinical symptoms and bronchoscopy. *J Comput Assist Tomogr* 2000;24: 247–252.

54. Rozycki HJ, Van Houten ML, Elliott GR. Quantitative assessment of intrathoracic airway collapse in infants and children with tracheobronchomalacia. *Pediatr Pulmonol* 1996; 21(4):241–245.

55. Gilkeson RC, Ciancibello LM, Hejal RB, Montenegro HD, Lange P. Tracheobronchomalacia: dynamic airway evaluation with multidetector CT. *Am J Roentgenol* 2001;176:205–210.

56. Zhang J, Hasegawa I, Feller-Kopman D, Boiselle PM. 2003 AUR Memorial Award. Dynamic expiratory volumetric CT imaging of the central airways: comparison of standard-dose and low-dose techniques. *Acad Radiol* 2003;10: 719–724.

57. Brasch RC, Gould RG, Gooding CA, Ringertz HG, Lipton MJ. Upper airway obstruction in infants and children: evaluation with ultrafast CT. *Radiology* 1987;165:459–466.

58. Heussel CP, Hafner B, Lill J, Schreiber W, Thelen M, Kauczor H-U. Paired inspiratory/expiratory spiral CT and continuous respiration cine CT in the diagnosis of tracheal instability. *Eur Radiol* 2001;11:982–989.

59. Suto Y, Tanabe Y. Evaluation of tracheal collapsibility in patients with tracheomalacia using dynamic MR imaging during coughing. *Am J Roentgenol* 1998;171:393–394.

60. Wilson TA, Rodarte JR, Butler JP. Wave speed and viscous flow limitation. In: Macklem PT, Mead J, eds. *Handbook of Physiology, The Respiratory System*. Vol 3, *Mechanics of Breathing*, Part 1. Bethesda, MD: The American Physiological Society, 1986;55–61.

61. Boiselle PM, Lee KS, Lin S, Raptopoulous V. Cine CT during coughing for assessment of tracheomalacia: preliminary experience with 64-multidetector-row CT. *Am J Roentgenol* 2006;187:438.

62. Stern EJ, Graham CM, Webb WR, Gamsu G. Normal trachea during forced expiration: dynamic CT measurements. *Radiology* 1993;187(1):27–31.

63. Aquino SL, Shepard JA, Ginns LC, et al. Acquired tracheomalacia: detection by expiratory CT scan. *J Comput Assist Tomogr* 2001;25(3):394–399.

64. Mayo JR, Aldrich J, Müller NL. Radiation exposure at chest CT: a statement of the Fleischner Society. *Radiology* 2005;228:15–21.

65. Boiselle PM, Ernst A. State-of-the-art imaging of the central airways. *Respiration* 2004;70(4):383–394.

66. Boiselle PM. Multislice helical CT of the central airways. *Radiol Clin North Am* 2003;41:561–574.

67. Boiselle PM, Feller-Kopman D, Ashiku S, Weeks D, Ernst A. Tracheobronchomalacia: evolving role of dynamic multislice helical CT. *Radiol Clin North Am* 2003;41:627–636.
68. Murgu SD, Colt HG. Recognizing tracheobronchomalacia. *J Respir Dis* 2006;27:327–335.
69. Baroni RH, Ashiku S, Boiselle PM. Dynamic-CT evaluation of the central airways in patients undergoing tracheoplasty for tracheobronchomalacia. *Am J Roentgenol* 2005;184:1444–1449.

John D. Newell, Jr.

Summary

Bronchiectasis is defined as the permanent dilatation of bronchi. The Reid classification includes three grades of progressively more severe bronchial injury: cylindrical, varicose, and cystic. Clinically, bronchiectasis is usually classified into either cystic fibrosis (CF)-related bronchiectasis or non-CF-related bronchiectasis. Physiologically, bronchiectasis is characterized by airflow obstruction. Significant complications that occur in bronchiectasis include hemoptysis, recurrent pneumonia, empyema, pneumothorax, and abscesses. Multidetector-row CT scanning is used in the assessment of obstructive airway disease where bronchiectasis is one component of lung injury that needs to be assessed on every study. Disease entities with a high association with bronchiectasis include CF, non-tuberculous mycobacterial infection, allergic bronchopulmonary aspergillosis (ABPA), alpha-1 antitrypsin deficiency, immunodeficiencies, and primary ciliary dyskinesia.

Key Words: Bronchiectasis; multidetector-row computed tomography; cystic fibrosis; non-tuberculous mycobacterial disease; allergic bronchopulmonary aspergillosis; alpha-1 antitrypsin deficiency; immunodeficiencies; primary ciliary dyskinesia.

1. INTRODUCTION

The purpose of this chapter is to provide a concise review of how to diagnose the presence of bronchiectasis by using multidetector-row CT (MDCT). The chapter will begin with the definition of bronchiectasis. This is followed by a description of the clinical importance and presentation of bronchiectasis. The etiologies of focal, diffuse, and traction bronchiectasis will be described next. Subsequently, the techniques that are necessary to diagnose bronchiectasis using MDCT will be discussed. This is followed by a description of what relevant findings can be detected on MDCT to reliably diagnose bronchiectasis. Finally, a discussion of a number of disease entities that are associated with bronchiectasis will be discussed in more detail along with some of the MDCT features that are seen with bronchiectasis when it is associated with these diseases.

2. DEFINITION OF BRONCHIECTASIS

The morphologic definition of bronchiectasis as described by Lynn Reid in 1950 has proved to be the best working definition of bronchiectasis to this point *(1–3)*. This is fortunate, because it readily aids in the application of MDCT techniques to identify bronchiectatic airways. Reid described bronchiectasis as the permanent dilatation of bronchi. She described three grades of progressively more severe bronchial injury, cylindrical, varicose, and cystic.

Cylindrical bronchiectasis occurs as the mildest form of bronchiectasis where there is loss of tapering of the bronchus, thickening of the bronchial wall, and dilatation of the bronchial lumen (Fig. 1). As the bronchiectasis progresses, varicoid bronchiectasis develops next with irregularities developing in the bronchial wall producing a varicoid appearance with further dilatation of the

From: *Contemporary Medical Imaging: CT of the Airways*
Edited by: P. M. Boiselle and D. A. Lynch © Humana Press, Totowa, NJ

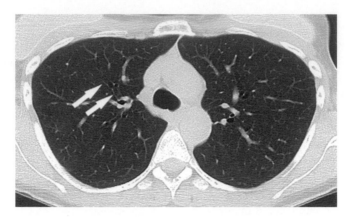

Fig. 1. This multichannel spiral CT image using 5-mm collimation demonstrates mild cylindrical bronchiectasis, arrows, in the right upper lobe.

bronchial lumen and significant foreshortening of the number of identifiable airway branches (Fig. 2). The most severe grade of bronchiectasis is cystic bronchiectasis with progressive dilatation of the bronchial lumen terminating in a large cystic structure, which often has air-fluid levels from accumulated secretions within the bronchial lumen (Fig. 3). There is also further loss of airway divisions with foreshortening of the airway tree in cystic bronchiectasis.

She also pointed out, as alluded to above, that starting from the trachea, there were a normal number of divisions in the microscopic sections of the lung involving cylindrical bronchiectasis, 16 on average, but only eight divisions on average in varicose bronchiectasis and only four on average in cystic bronchiectasis *(1)*. This loss of distal bronchial divisions in more severe bronchiectasis is an important hallmark of progressive more severe bronchiectasis and emphasizes the severity of the chronic inflammatory process in its ability to remodel the lung.

Several factors make a more complete definition of bronchiectasis difficult *(2)*. Bronchiectasis blends into the more general airway disease entity of chronic bronchitis, which smoking is the most common cause *(2)*. This is illustrated by the recent report that showed most patients with

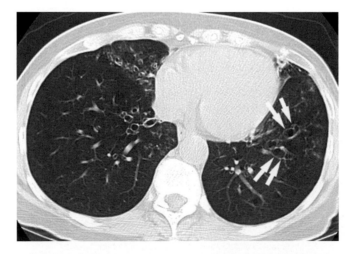

Fig. 2. This multichannel spiral CT image using 5-mm collimation demonstrates varicoid bronchiectasis, arrows, in the left lower lobe.

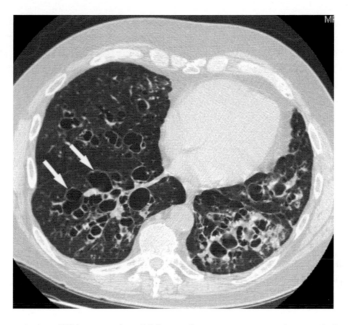

Fig. 3. This high-resolution CT image using 1.25 mm demonstrates extensive cystic bronchiectasis, arrows, in the right lower lobe as well as in the right middle lobe, lingula, and left lower lobe.

bronchiectasis have had symptoms of chronic bronchitis for more than 20 years before a diagnosis of bronchiectasis was made *(4)*. It should be remembered that bronchiectasis is the result of a variety of different mechanisms with the dominant feature being recurrent airway infection from bacteria with associated airway obstruction *(2)*. Bronchiectasis is a heterogenous condition defined best as a syndrome rather than a specific disease entity *(2)*. The infected and obstructed airway will incur airway wall damage by direct effects of microorganisms and secondary effects of the host response *(2)*. Bronchiectasis can be characterized as a disease of both the bronchi and the bronchioles that involves a vicious cycle of transmural infection and inflammation with mediator release *(3)*. The illness is related to retained inflammatory secretions and microbes that cause recurrent infection, airway obstruction, and damage to the airway wall *(3)*. Enhanced cellular and mediator response in patients with bronchiectasis are supported by reports on patients with known bronchiectasis that had bronchial mucosal biopsies that show infiltration by neutrophils and T lymphocytes with increased levels of elastase, interleukin-8, tumor necrosis factor alpha and prostanoids *(3)*.

3. CLINICAL SIGNIFICANCE AND PRESENTATION OF BRONCHIECTASIS

Bronchiectasis is usually classified into either cystic fibrosis (CF)-related bronchiectasis or non-CF-related bronchiectasis *(2)*, see further discussion regarding this issue in the next section. The following discussion is directed toward non-CF bronchiectasis in adults.

It is estimated that there are at least 110,000 adult patients with bronchiectasis in the USA, *(2)*. The principle disease in the differential of bronchiectasis is chronic obstructive pulmonary disease (COPD). It has been recently reported that 29–50% of COPD patients have associated bronchiectasis identified by CT scanning and those patients with COPD who also have bronchiectasis have a higher rate of exacerbation *(2)*.

Bronchiectasis is more common in women (65%) than in men (35%) *(2)*. Bronchiectasis most commonly presents in the sixth decade of life, mean age 56 years *(2)*. The predominant symptom is chronic productive cough, 94%, with associated increased daily sputum production, 73% *(2)*. The cough is typically worse in the early morning because of accumulation of secretions in dependent portions of the bronchiectatic lung *(5)*. Bronchiectasis occurring mainly or exclusively in the upper lobes may present with little or no productive cough because the upper lobes would drain effectively and the pooling of secretions would be unlikely. This is typically the case in secondary tuberculosis *(5)*.

Rhinosinusitus and fatigue are two very common symptoms in bronchiectasis patients. Rhinosinusitus is seen in up to 60–70% of patients *(2)*, and fatigue is seen in up to 70% of patients *(2)*. Fatigue may be the dominant symptom in many patients *(2)*. CT scans of the sinuses will be abnormal in most patients with bronchiectasis *(2)*. Hemoptysis (31%), dyspnea (73%) are also commonly associated with bronchiectasis *(2)*. Rarely, patients with bronchiectasis present with large volume hemoptysis (greater than 200 mL/h) *(2)*. This may necessitate emergency evaluation and possible surgery or transcatheter bronchial artery embolization. Chest pain is reported in up to 50% of patients *(3)*. Weight loss, anemia, and fever are also associated with bronchiectasis *(5)*.

The principle finding on physical examination are crackles, 60%, over the affected lobes. The crackles are commonly bilateral and lower lobe *(2)*. Rhonchi can be heard in 44% of patients *(3)*. Wheezing is heard in 20% of patients *(2)*. Localized wheezing may suggest focal bronchial obstruction by tumor, mucus, or foreign body *(5)*. Diffuse wheezing is associated with asthma and allergic bronchopulmonary aspergillosis (ABPA) *(5)*. Clubbing is seen in only 2% of patients and is usually present only in long-standing and more severe bronchiectasis *(2)*.

Physiologically, bronchiectasis is characterized by airflow obstruction *(2)*. Spirometrically determined measures of airflow obstruction in a number of reports on patients with bronchiectasis have been tabulated and reported to be FEV1% predicted mean 64%, FVC % predicted mean 78%, FEV1/FVC ratio mean 66, 15% increase in FEV1% predicted following bronchodilator mean 32% *(2)*. The bronchodilator response or airway hyperresponsiveness is thought to be related to chronic bronchial inflammation rather than asthma *(2)*. Some patients may develop a rapid decline in respiratory function of unknown etiology, but may be related to specific lung pathogens *(2)*. For this reason, spirometric testing should be performed every 2–5 years in patients with bronchiectasis.

Significant complications that occur in bronchiectasis include hemoptysis, see discussion above, recurrent pneumonia, empyema, pneumothorax, abscesses *(2)*.

4. ETIOLOGIES OF BRONCHIECTASIS

Bronchiectasis is usually classified into CF-type bronchiectasis and non-CF-type bronchiectasis *(2)*. Published reports on bronchiectasis in adult patients refer to the non-CF type of bronchiectasis unless otherwise indicated *(2)*. There continues to be some controversy regarding this distinction largely do to the large number of mutations that have been identified in the CF transmembrane conductance regulator *(CFTR)* gene or *CF* gene, which now number over 1000 *(2)*. The prevalence of CFTR mutations in adults with bronchiectasis is not known, and recently, it has been recognized that CF can present atypically in adults. Recent research reports support the notion that the prevalence of undiagnosed CF in adults with bronchiectasis is low *(2,6,7)* and that retaining the distinction between CF- and non-CF-type bronchiectasis is still useful.

It is helpful to distinguish three distinct morphologic forms of bronchiectasis for the purpose of discussing etiologies of bronchiectasis. These three forms include focal inflammatory bronchiectasis, diffuse inflammatory bronchiectasis, and traction bronchiectasis, which is not directly related to chronic infection and airway obstruction.

Traction bronchiectasis is associated with decreased lung compliance in the setting of focal or diffuse lung fibrosis where the stiff lung pulls the airways open and is not related to recurrent airway infection and obstruction as discussed above (Fig. 4). The focal form of traction bronchiectasis may be seen in chronic mycobacterium tuberculosis infection and in radiation-induced lung fibrosis. Diffuse traction bronchiectasis occurs commonly in the case of interstitial pneumonitis, and the extent of traction bronchiectasis may be useful in the differential diagnosis of diffuse infiltrating lung disease *(8)*.

A recent study has shown that the most proximal extent of traction bronchiectasis is increased in UIP compared with cellular NSIP and is useful in trying to distinguish between these two entities *(8)*. The most proximal extent of traction bronchiectasis and the number of lung segments affected by traction bronchiectasis helps distinguish UIP from RB-ILD, DIP, and LIP where the most proximal extent of traction bronchiectasis and the number of segments with traction bronchiectasis are both increased in UIP compared with RB-ILD, DIP, and LIP *(8)*.

Focal inflammatory bronchiectasis can occur from intrinsic luminal airway obstruction, extrinsic airway compression, and obstruction from postsurgical distortion of the airway *(3)*. The first two forms of focal bronchiectasis present with persistent or recurrent lobar pneumonia and recognition is important because palliation and occasionally cure may result form interventional bronchoscopic techniques or surgery *(3)*.

Intrinsic luminal airway obstruction can occur from obstruction by a foreign body, broncholith, and slowing growing tumor. Extrinsic airway compression and obstruction can occur from enlarged peribronchial lymph nodes compressing the airways. This is particularly a problem for the right middle lobe that has a small angulated lobar bronchial orifice that is surrounded by a ring of lymph nodes. Table 1 summarizes these causes of focal inflammatory bronchiectasis.

Diffuse inflammatory causes of bronchiectasis can be sub-divided into a number of subcategories. The manner in which this is done is not uniform in published reports *(2,3,5,9,10)*. I have chosen to subdivide the broad categories of diffuse inflammatory bronchiectiasis into the following broad categories, idiopathic, postinfection, COPD, inhalational injury, inherited molecular and cellular defects, immune disorders, immunodeficiencies, primary ciliary dyskinesia, inherited structural abnormalities, and other. These subcategories along with a number of entries in each subcategory are summarized in Table 1. A few select subcategory entries will be discussed in more detail below.

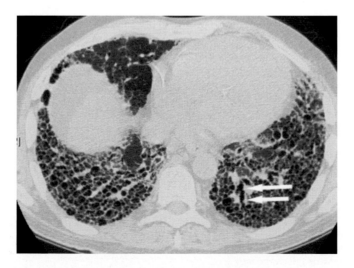

Fig. 4. This high-resolution CT image using 1.25-mm collimation demonstrates traction bronchiectasis in the left lower lobe, arrows, in a patient with IPF. Note the extensive honeycomb cyst formation in both lungs.

Table 1
Causes Of Bronchiectasis

Focal airway obstruction
Intrinsic airway narrowing
      Tumor
      Foreign body
      Broncholith
Extrinsic airway narrowing
      Enlarged lymph nodes
      Post-surgical distortion of bronchial anatomy
Idiopathic
Post-infectious conditions
      Bacteria
            Pseudomonas aeruginosa
            Haemophilus influenza
            Staphylococcus aureus
            Streptococcus pneumoniae
            Mycobacterium tuberculosis (MTB)
            Mycobacterium avian complex (MAC) and other non-tuberculosis
            mycobacterium species
            Bordetella pertussis (whooping cough)
      Viruses
            Measles
            Adenovirus
            Influenzavirus
      Fungi
            Histoplasma capsulatum
            Pneumocystis carinii
Chronic obstructive pulmonary disease (COPD)
Inhalational injury
      Aspiration
      Toxic gases
            Ammonia
            Chlorine
Inherited molecular and cellular defects
      Cystic fibrosis
      Alpha-1 antitrypsin deficiency
Immune disorders
      Allergic bronchopulmonary aspergillosis
      Rheumatoid arthritis
      Sjogren's syndrome
      Inflammatory bowel disease
      Relapsing polychondritis
      Lung allograft rejection
      Graft versus disease in post bone marrow transplant
Immunodeficiencies
      HIV infection
      X-linked agammaglobulinemia
      Selective IgG deficiency
      Selective IgA, IgM or IgE deficiency
      Common variable immunodeficiency
      Chronic granulomatous disease of childhood

Primary ciliary dyskinesia
    Kartagener's syndrome
Inherited bronchial structural abnormalities
    Bronchopulmonary sequestration
    Bronchial atresia
    Tracheobronchomegaly (Mounier-Kuhn syndrome)
    Congenital cartilage deficiency (Williams–Campbell syndrome)
Other
    Yellow nail syndrome
    Young's syndrome
Traction bronchiectasis
    Interstitial pneumonitis (UIP, NSIP, LIP, DIP)
    Chronic granulomatous disease infection-induced fibrosis (I.E. tuberculosis)

5. CT TECHNIQUE FOR THE DIAGNOSIS OF BRONCHIECTASIS

Multichannel CT scanning is used in the assessment of obstructive airway disease where bronchiectasis is one component of lung injury that needs to be assessed on every study. The elements of the examination that need to be done routinely to assess bronchiectasis is a multi-channel acquisition using 1.25-mm detector collimation or less. Reconstructions of this 3-D data set can be done in a number of ways, but the minimum would be to reconstruct 5 mm contiguous axial images using a reconstruction kernal appropriate for the lung, that is, GE "Lung" kernal, and 1.25 mm reconstructions at 10-mm intervals using a reconstruction kernal that is appropriate for high-resolution CT (HRCT), that is, GE "Bone". For additional problem solving on individual cases, additional reconstructions can be done. Typically, this will involve an isotropic reconstruction, that is, the reconstructed image slice thickness, image thickness in the z-axis, equals the x-y plane voxel dimension, so that the resultant voxels are cubes, that is, the voxel would measure $0.625 \times 0.625 \times 0.625$ mm. Near isotropic reconstructions may be sufficient, that is 1.25 (z-axis) $\times$ 0.625 $\times$ 0.625 mm. Multi-planar reconstructions (MPRs) can be obtained from the isotropic data sets in the coronal and sagital planes or along the long axis of the particular airway of interest. The isotropic data sets can also be viewed on special software that can render the data in 3-D as a shaded surface display of the anatomy or can be rendered in a virtual bronchoscopic fashion as well.

A recent study described the superior ability of MDCT using 1-mm reconstructed collimation over HRCT images done at 10-mm intervals in the assessment of the presence and extent of bronchiectasis *(11)*.

6. CT CRITERIA FOR THE DIAGNOSES OF BRONCHIECTASIS

The severity of bronchiectasis on CT has two components. One, the individual bronchus that is affected is graded as to the severity of the morphologic disease injury using the pathology scheme described above, cylindrical, varicoid, and cystic. This CT scheme was first introduced by David Naidich in 1982 *(12)*, and it directly follows the pathologic approach of Lynn Reid's 1950 report, described above. Two, the number of individual pulmonary lobes that have bronchiectasis are described, that is, proximal, varicoid bronchiectasis is noted involving the right upper lobe, right middle lobe, and the left upper lobe. Semi-quantitative and quantitative schema have been developed to more accurately assess total lung involvement by bronchiectasis in CF populations *(13,14)*.

The visual analyses of a bronchus for the detection of cylindrical bronchiectasis (Fig. 1) should include looking for loss of bronchial tapering over a distance of 2 cm, bronchial dilatation with the bronchus exceeding the size of the adjacent pulmonary artery at sea level or exceeding 1.5 times the size of the adjacent artery at altitude, that is, 1600 m *(10)*. More recently, it has been shown that visualization of a bronchus within 1 cm of the costal pleura or abutting the mediastinal pleura indicates bronchiectasis *(10)*. Bronchial wall thickening is often present in all grades of bronchiectasis but is not diagnostic of bronchiectasis. The absence of bronchial wall thickening does not exclude bronchiectasis, for example, thin-walled bronchiectasis seen in both congenital bronchiectasis (Williams–Campbell syndrome) and tracheobroncomegaly (Mounier-Kuhn syndrome) *(5)*.

Varicoid bronchiectasis (Fig. 2) is a more severe form of bronchial injury than cylindrical bronchiectasis and has more severe lack of tapering, irregular beading of the bronchial wall, and alternating segments of bronchial dilatation and constriction giving a "varicoid" appearance to the airway *(5)*.

Cystic bronchiectasis (Fig. 3) represents the most severe form of bronchiectasis affecting an individual airway and shows more severe dilatation of the bronchial lumen than cylindrical or varicoid bronchiectasis, progressive dilatation of the bronchial lumen as the airway progresses distally, termination of the airway in a large cystic structure with no identifiable bronchus beyond the cystic structure. A string of cyst appearance, cluster of cyst appearance, and atelectasis are often seen in cystic bronchiectasis *(5)*. The criteria for diagnosing cylindrical, varicoid, and cystic bronchiectasis are summarized in Table 2.

Recently, the presence of interlobular septal thickening has been associated with idopathic bronchiectasis *(15)*. Significant interlobular septal thickening was seen in 56 of 94 patients, 60%,

Table 2
CT Criteria For Bronchiectasis

Cylindrical bronchiectasis	Varicoid bronchiectasis	Cystic bronchiectasis
Lack of bronchial tapering over a distance of 2 cm	More severe lack of tapering than cylindrical bronchiectasis	Progressive dilatation of the bronchial lumen distally
Bronchial to arterial ratio greater than 1. (greater than 1.5 at 1600 m or higher)	More severe luminal dilatation than cylindrical bronchiectasis	More severe luminal dilatation than in varicoid bronchiectasis
Thickening of the airway wall	Irregular or beaded thickening of the bronchial wall	Termination of the bronchus in a large cystic structure
Visualization of the bronchus within 1 cm of the costal pleura	Alternating bronchial segments of luminal dilatation and constriction	No identifiable bronchus beyond the terminating cystic structure
Visualization of the bronchus abutting the mediastinal pleura	Mucus plugs	Linear collection of cysts ("string of cysts")
Presence of interlobular septal thickening		Several cysts closely grouped together ("cluster of cysts")
		Atelectasis in the affected lung segment or lobe
		Air fluid levels

with idiopathic bronchiectasis. About 514 of 748 lobes, 69%, with bronchiectasis had interlobular septal thickening. There was a strong correlation between the extent of interlobular septal thickening and the extent and severity of bronchiectasis. Interlobular septal thickening was not associated with measures of airflow obstruction or measures of restrictive lung disease.

7. CT OF BRONCHIECTASIS IN SPECIFIC DISEASE STATES

As outlined above, there are many diseases that are associated with both focal and diffuse bronchiectasis. In 40% of patients with bronchiectasis, a cause of the bronchiectasis may not be discovered *(16)*. It should also be noted that even though there are characteristic features of the bronchiectasis associated with idopathic bronchiectasis, CF, ABPA, immunodeficiencies, and primary ciliary dyskinesia, in an individual patient, there is considerable overlap of findings between these disease entities *(17)*. In this section, we will discuss in more detail the disease entities and the specific CT features of bronchiectasis in several important disorders with a high association with bronchiectasis including CF, non-tuberculous mycobacterial (NTM) infection, ABPA, alpha-1 antitrypsin deficiency (A1AD), immunodeficiencies, and primary ciliary dyskinesia.

8. CYSTIC FIBROSIS

CF is the most common lethal genetically transmitted disease in Caucasians *(18)*. It affects 1:3400 Caucasians born in the United States *(19)*. CF is transmitted as an autosomal recessive trait *(18)*. The gene that is responsible for CF was identified in 1989 and is located on the long arm of chromosome 7 and is referred to as *CFTR* gene *(18)*. The *CFTR* gene product is a 1480 amino acid protein that functions as a cyclic adenosine monophosphate-regulated chloride channel in the apical membrane of airway epithelial cells, tracheobronchial gland cells, and in fetus type II pneumocytes *(18)*. This protein is important in the transport of chloride and water from the cell interior to the lumen of the airway. CF is secondary to genetic mutations in this chloride ion channel protein. These mutations are divided up into five categories or classes. The mutation of the *CFTR* gene that produces a three base pair deletion that results in the loss of the amino acid phenylalanine at position 508 of the protein, referred to as deltaF508, accounts for about 70% of the mutant alleles on the *CFTR* gene *(18)*. There are over 1000 *CFTR* gene mutations recognized to date *(2)*. The more severe mutations present earlier in life and typically have more advanced bronchiectasis then the less severe mutations.

The decrease in normal transport of water and chloride, secondary to the defective epithelial cell chloride ion channel protein, into the airway lumen in CF patients is believed to be the origin of the thick tenacious secretions in the airways that leads to early and chronic progressive airway wall inflammation and recurrent airway infections. It is also associated with the pathogenesis of pancreatic insufficiency and other bowel complications. The median survival for CF patients has increased from 10 years in the 1960s to 32 years in 2004 secondary to CF specialty care treatment centers, improved nutrition through liberal fat diets, improved airway clearance therapies, and improved antibiotic therapies *(19)*.

The initial insults produce bronchitis, bronchiolitis, and mucus plugging in both large and small airways. The earliest HRCT signs of CF are believed to be mosaic air trapping on expiratory HRCT scans and branching centrilobular nodules *(5,9)*. Subsequently, the typical CT appearance of CF develops with panlobar involvement but often with more central and upper lobe evidence of bronchiectasis and bronchioloectasis (Fig. 5). Extensive upper lobe cystic bronchiectasis with extensive mucus plugging is not unusual in the patients with more severe *CFTR* gene mutations such as deltaF508. There is usually involvement of all five lobes of the lung particularly as the disease progresses. There is also associated hyperinflation, hilar lymphadenopathy, and superimposed consolidative pneumonias. Pneumothorax is also a known complication of CF. Respiratory failure is a common cause of death for CF patients secondary to advanced lung disease. Cor pulmonale is a complication that is seen later in advanced cases of CF-related lung disease *(18)*.

A)

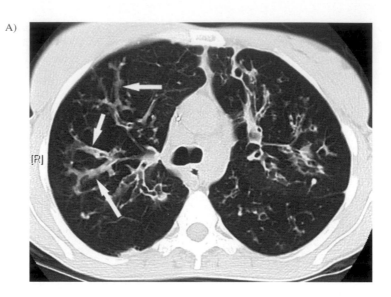

B)

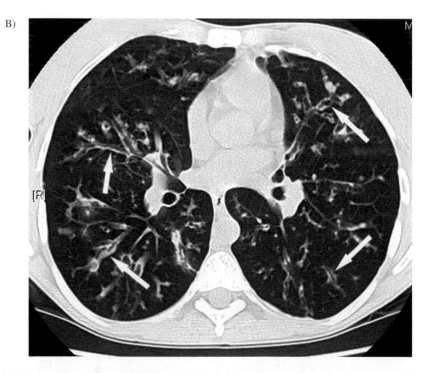

Fig. 5. (**A**) This multidetector-row CT (MDCT) scan using 5-mm collimation demonstrates extensive upper lobe bronchiectasis and mucus plugging, arrows, in a young woman with cystic fibrosis and delta f508 homozygous mutation in the *CFTR* gene. (**B**) This is the same patient as shown in Figure 5A showing bronchiectasis in the right middle lobe, lingula, and lower lobes, arrows, on an MDCT axial image using 5-mm collimation. (**C**) This again is the same patient as shown in Figures 5A and 5B with evidence of lower lobe bronchiectasis and mucus plugging, arrows, on this MDCT axial image using 5-mm collimation.

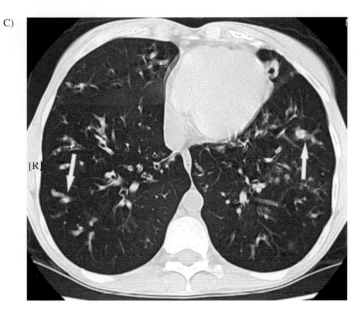

Fig. 5. *(Continued)*

The most common pulmonary infections in CF are *Pseudomonas aeruginosa*, *Staphylococcus aureus*, *Haemophilus influenzae*, and *Burkholderia cepacia (18)*. These bacteria play a major role in the pathogenesis of CF *(18)*. There is increasing recognition of ABPA and NTM infections in CF patients as well (Fig. 6). Chronic infection with severe bronchiectasis puts CF patients at risk for hemoptysis because of the angiogenesis that is stimulated in the chronically inflamed airway. The hemoptysis can be fatal and may be treated by surgery or transcatheter embolization *(18)*.

It has recently been reported that patients with heterozygote *CFTR* gene mutations who present with bronchiectasis and NTM infections are less likely to show improvement in the extent of their NTM infection when compared with the patients with normal genotypes *(20)*. Patients with heterozygote *CFTR* gene mutations showed no improvement in their bronchiectasis following antibiotic treatment

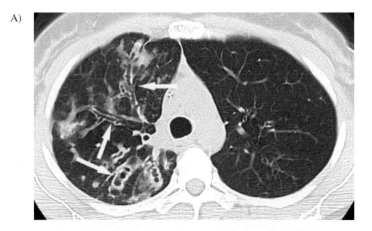

Fig. 6. *(Continued)*

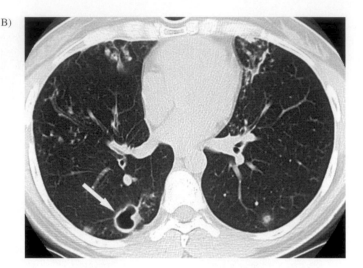

Fig. 6. (A) This is a young adult female with cystic fibrosis with upper lobe bronchiectasis, arrows, who also has MAC and *Mycobacterium abscessus* pulmonary infection. **(B)** This is the same patient as in Figure 6A and this axial multidetector-row CT image using 5-mm collimation shows a cavitating lesion in the right lower lobe, arrow. Cavity formation is more common in *M. abscessus* infection than in MAC infection.

for NTM infection on follow-up CT scans, but 35% of patients with either normal genotypes for CF and A1AD or heterozygote for A1AD showed improvement in their bronchiectasis *(20)*.

Recently, semi-quantitative analysis of HRCT scans has been shown to correlate better over a 2-year time frame with respiratory tract exacerbations (RTEs) in CF patients then did PFT testing *(21)*. The overall HRCT score, bronchiectasis score, and parenchymal lung disease score all correlated significantly with the number of RTEs, whereas pulmonary function tests, including the FEV1, did not correlate with the number of RTEs in this group of children with CF who were studied over a 2-year period of time *(21)*. The highest correlation was achieved with the HRCT bronchiectasis score, $r = 0.35$, $p = 0.005$ *(21)*.

9. NON-TUBERCULOUS MYCOBACTERIAL DISEASE INFECTION

Bronchiectasis is a common complication of MTB and NTM lung infections. The bronchiectasis in post-primary or re-infection MTB is usually focal and in areas of additional lung abnormalities most frequently involving the upper lobes and the superior segments of the lower lobes *(5)*. The additional findings include consolidation, cavity formation, cicatricial atelectasis and emphysema, branching type centrilobular nodule formation, and larger areas of calcified or non-calcified nodule formation.

The diagnosis of NTM-induced bronchiectasis can be a bit more challenging because of the different ways NTM infection can produce lung injury. *Mycobacterium avium* complex (MAC) is the most common NTM pulmonary pathogen *(22)*. *Mycobacterium kansasii*, *Mycobacterium xenopi*, and the rapid grower NTM organisms *Mycobacterium abscessus*, *Mycobacterium chelonai*, and *Mycobacterium fortuitum* are additional NTM pulmonary pathogens *(22)*. The presentation of MAC infection with low grade fever, productive cough, and fatigue coupled with the acid fast appearance of the organisms, which is indistinguishable from *Mycobacterium tuberculosis* on smear and the fact that the diagnosis must be made on cultures, which typically take 6 weeks to grow complicate the clinical diagnosis of MAC and at the same time enhances the diagnostic utilization of MDCT *(5)*.

There are three basic imaging presentations of patients with NTM infection *(5,23)*. The first NTM presentation is called "classic NTM infection" (Figs 7 and 8). This pattern of lung injury may be indistinguishable from secondary MTB infections, that is, upper lobe bronchiectasis associated with consolidation, cavity formation, cicatricial atelectasis and emphysema, branching-type centrilobular nodule formation, and larger areas of calcified or non-calcified nodule formation. These patients usually have underlying COPD and may initially be treated unsuccessfully for MTB infection (Fig. 8). In a recent report evaluating the chest radiographs and CT scans done on 26 immunocompetent patients with a culture-positive diagnoses of MAC, the classic NTM infection pattern indistinguishable from MTB infection was seen in 19% of the patients *(23)*.

The second NTM presentation is called "non-classical NTM infection" (Figs 9 and 10). Until relatively recently, it was not often believed that this represented true pulmonary infection and a condition that needed to be treated. Fortunately, this is no longer the case. These patients typically

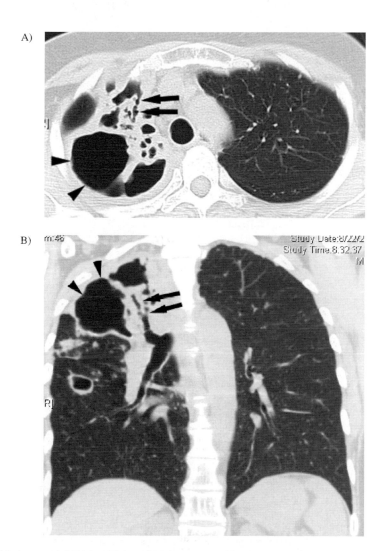

Fig. 7. (A) This is an axial 5-mm thick multidetector-row CT scan through the upper lobes in an older adult woman with the classic radiographic presentation of non-tuberculous mycobacterial infection do to MAC. There are large apical cavities in the right upper lobe, arrowheads, and bronchiectasis in the same area, arrows. **(B)** This is a coronal MPR image showing upper lobe cavities, arrowheads, and upper lobe bronchiectasis, arrows, in the same patient as in (A).

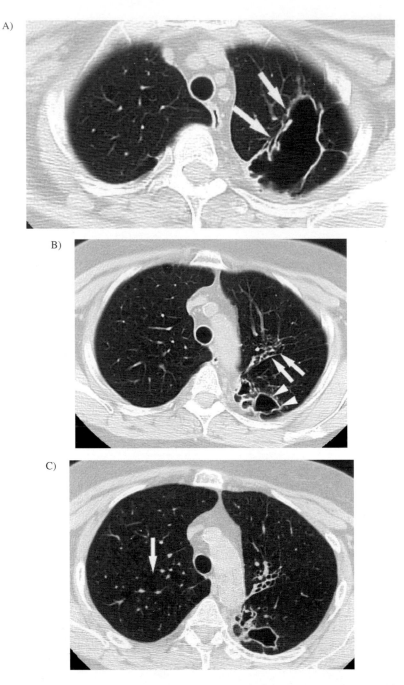

Fig. 8. (**A**) Adult female with *Mycobacterium kansasii* pulmonary infection. She has cavities in the apical-posterior segment of the left upper lobe, arrows, on this multidetector-row CT (MDCT) axial image using 5-mm collimation. This is the classic radiographic presentation of non-tuberculous mycobacterial (NTM) pulmonary infection. (**B**) This is the same patient as shown in Figure 8A. This axial MDCT image using 5mm collimation shows bronchiectasis in the left upper lobe, arrows, and cavity formation in the superior segment of the left lower lobe, arrowheads. (**C**) This high-resolution CT image using 1.25-mm collimation shows centrilobular emphysema, arrow, in the right upper lobe in the same patient shown in Figures 8A and 8B. The emphysema puts the patient at higher risk for developing the classic radiographic appearance of NTM pulmonary infection.

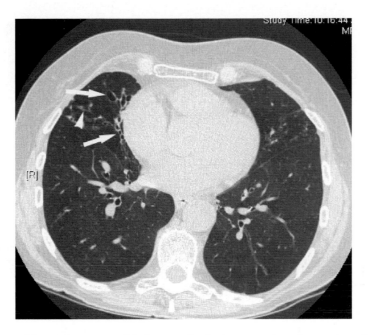

Fig. 9. This is an older adult woman with the non-classical presentation of non-tuberculous mycobacterial pulmonary infection secondary to MAC. There is evidence of both bronchiectasis in the right middle lobe, arrows, and tree-in-bud type centrilobular nodules, arrowhead, on this high-resolution CT axial image using 1.25-mm collimation.

present disease affecting the non-apical upper lobes, right middle lobe, lingula, and superior segments of the lower lobes. The imaging findings in this case include branching centrilobular nodule formation co-located with cylindrical, varicoid or cystic bronchiectasis, atelectasis, consolidation, larger nodule

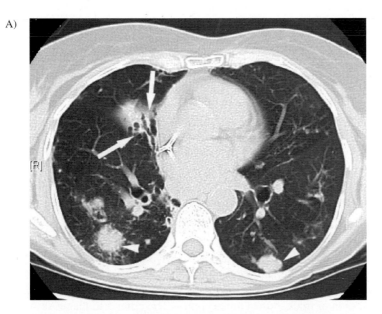

Fig. 10. *(Continued)*

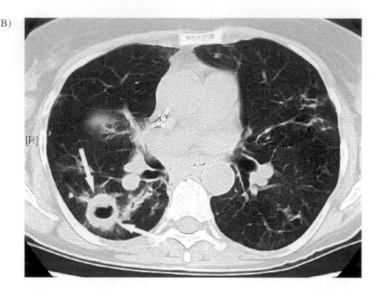

Fig. 10. (**A**) This is an multidetector-row CT (MDCT) axial image using 5-mm collimation showing extensive right middle lobe bronchiectasis, arrows, with associated atelectasis and consolidation in an adult woman with the non-classical radiographic presentation of non-tuberculous mycobacterial pulmonary infection secondary to *Mycobacterium abscessus*. There are several large nodular lesions, arrowheads, in the lower lobes. (**B**) This is the same MDCT study done on the same patient as in Figure 10A showing a cavitating lesion in the right lower lobe, arrows. The larger nodules and cavitary lesions are more common in *M. abscessus* infection than MAC infection.

formation, and cavity formation. Cicatricial atelectasis and emphysema are usually not seen in non-classical NTM infection. The patients are typically women with no pre-existing lung disease, that is, no COPD, no HIV-induced lung disease. In a recent report, this non-classical NTM infection pattern was seen in 77% of immunocompetent culture-positive MAC patients *(23)*.

The third category of NTM infection is the AIDS-associated NTM infection that occurs in AIDS patients with very low CD4 counts. These patients typically develop extensive consolidation, large pulmonary nodules, and hilar and mediastinal lymphadenopathy. AIDS patients with less severe CD4 lymphopenia may present with classical or non-classical NTM infection as well as other pulmonary infections.

A recent paper proposed an interesting hypothesis regarding the development of cavity formation in MAC *(24)*. The authors show that the peribronchial consolidation and centrilobular nodules first produces focal cystic bronchiectasis and the cystic bronchiectasis then progresses into the formation of a cavity on CT. They describe the "feeding bronchus" sign where an airway is seen going into the cavity. The traditional cavity that begins in the airspaces is seen to have the well-described "draining brochus" sign.

10. ALLERGIC BRONCHOPULMONARY ASPERGILLOSIS

ABPA or allergic bronchopulmonary mycosis (ABPM) is a hypersensitivity reaction, usually to a fungus, most commonly *Aspergillus fumigatus*, that occurs as a complication in patients with asthma and CF *(5)*. In ABPA, the airway lumen is overpopulated with fungal hyphae that results in large, impacted mucus plugs that dilate the airway producing cylindrical and varicoid bronchiectasis (Fig. 11). The clinical presentation includes fever, wheezing, eosinophilia, fleeting pulmonary opacities, expectoration of thick, brown mucus plugs. The criteria to diagnose ABPA includes airway hyperreactivity consistent with asthma, transient pulmonary infiltrates, type I immediate cutaneous

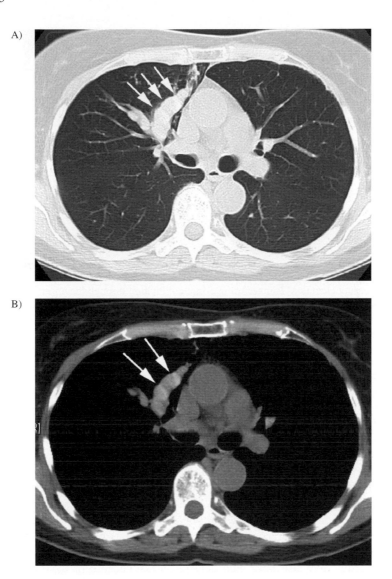

Fig. 11. (**A**) Multichannel CT image using 5-mm collimation in an adult woman with ABPA showing varicoid bronchiectasis in the right upper lobe with a large impacted mucus plug, arrows. Note the branching or "gloved finger" appearance of the large mucus plug. (**B**) This is the same CT image as Figure 11B but displayed with a mediastinal setting. It shows the increased X-ray attenuation of the ABPA mucus plug, arrows. The high attenuation is caused by the ABPA fungal hyphae.

hypersensitivity reaction to *A. fumigatus*, serum precipitins to *A. fumigatus*, peripheral eosinophilia, elevated immunoglobulin E and imaging evidence of central, multilobar varicoid, or cystic bronchiectasis, often with an upper lobe predominance *(5,25)*.

The typical MDCT findings of ABPA are central upper lobe varicoid and cystic bronchiectasis with mucoid impaction *(5)* (Fig. 11). MDCT is more sensitive than chest radiography in detecting bronchiectasis in patients with ABPA *(25,26)*. Central bronchiectasis is common in the diagnosis of ABPA, but it is not essential to the diagnosis *(5,26,27)*. Upper lobe-predominant bronchiectasis is the

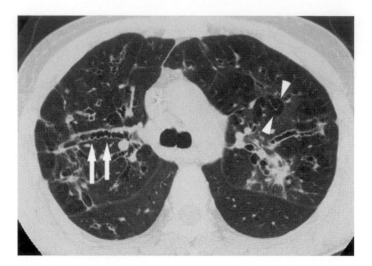

Fig. 12. This is a multichannel CT image using 5-mm collimation through the upper lobes in an adult woman with ZZ-type alpha-1 antitrypsin deficiency genotype. She also had a history of chronic pseudomonas airway infection. Note the varicoid bronchiectasis in the right upper lobe, arrows, and the centrilobular emphysema in the left upper lobe, arrowheads.

more common presentation of ABPA *(5,25,27)*. Cystic and varicoid bronchiectasis are more common in ABPA than cylindrical bronchiectasis *(5,17,25)*.

Mucoid impaction is a common finding in ABPA on MDCT and may have the so-called "gloved finger appearance" *(5)* (Fig. 11). The mucus plugs often have high attenuation values on MDCT secondary to the presence of fungal hyphae *(5)* (Fig. 11). Consolidation is also an important but non-specific finding on MDCT in ABPA, and these airspace opacities may not be associated bronchiectasis *(5)*. The differential diagnosis of the consolidative opacities in an asthmatic patient also includes infection, cryptogenic organizing pneumonia, Churg–Strauss syndrome *(5)*. Atelectasis is also another non-specific finding on MDCT in ABPA and is usually secondary to proximal bronchial mucoid impaction, and the atelectasis can be segmental, lobar, or involve an entire lung *(5)*.

In summary, the MDCT appearance of proximal cystic or varicoid bronchiectasis with upper lobe predominance involving one or more lobes, typically four or five, is highly suspicious for ABPA *(25)*. The airway plugs may also have high density on CT because of the large amount of fungal hyphae present in the mucus plugs.

11. ALPHA-1 ANTITRYPSIN DEFICIENCY

A1AD is a disorder where insufficient alpha-1 antitrypsin enzyme is transported out of the liver and available to neutrophils and macrophages in the lung. The inability to inactivate proteases that are secreted by neutrophils and macrophages in the normal host response to infectious and non-infectious antigens in the lung is believed to produce various lung injuries including emphysema and bronchiectasis (Fig. 12). The type and distribution of the emphysema has been typically described as panlobular emphysema with a lower lobe predominance.

The association of bronchiectasis with A1AD was reported in the Radiology literature in the early and mid 1990s *(28,29)* (Fig. 12). Guest and company *(29)* described the HRCT features of A1AD in 17 patients and noted not only the presence of emphysema but also the presence of bronchial wall thickening/bronchiectasis in seven patients with one patient having cystic bronchiectasis. King et al performed HRCT on 14 patients with A1AD to assess the presence of bronchiectasis and any clinical correlates. Six patients (43%) had bronchiectasis on HRCT scans. These patients with bronchiectasis had higher infection scores than those without bronchiectasis. Two of the patients had diffuse cystic bronchiectasis, and these two patients did not have any other disease known to predispose to bronchiectasis.

McMahon and colleagues *(30)* recently investigated the severity of bronchiectasis and associated emphysema with correlation to phenotype in patients with A1AD. They used a modified Ooi scoring system, which included the degree of bronchial dilatation and degree of emphysema *(30)*. All criteria were scored on a scale of 0–3. There were 26 patients with HRCT examinations included in the study. Nine patients were female and 17 were male. The median age was 56. Twenty-one patients had ZZ phenotype, three patients had MZ phenotype, and two patients had SZ phenotype. The mean percent predicted FEV1 was 43%. Of the 156 lung lobes that were analyzed, 38 (24%) had evidence of bronchiectasis. Fourteen of 26 patients had bronchiectasis. The overall median score for bronchiectasis was 2, and all patients had ZZ phenotype. The bronchiectasis more commonly affected the upper lobes. In the 17 ZZ phenotype patients with emphysema, 10 had bronchiectasis. There were four patients with ZZ phenotype who had bronchiectasis but did not have emphysema.

A1AD patients may be at some increased risk for developing NTM infections. It is important to consider this possibility in patients with the predominant findings of NTM infection or other infection.

12. IMMUNODEFICIENCIES

It has been known for some time that there is an increased incidence of bronchiectasis in patients with both primary and AIDS-related immunodeficiencies *(31,32)*.

Recently, it has been recognized that there is an increasing incidence of infectious bronchitis, bronchiolitis, and bronchiectasis in AIDS *(9,31,33)*. An aggressive form of bronchiectasis has been recently recognized *(9,31,33)*. This AIDS-related aggressive form of bronchiectasis is often preceded by a bronchitis or pneumonia from *Streptococcus*, *Haemophilus*, and *Pseudomonas*. HRCT demonstrates multi-lobar bronchiectasis with frequent symmetrical involvement of the lower lobes. Rapid development of bronchiectasis after a single episode of bronchitis or pneumonia is a defining feature of aggressive AIDS-related bronchiectasis. This form of bronchiectasis in AIDS is often associated with other HRCT features of bronchitis and bronchiolitis including bronchial wall thickening, tree in bud-type nodules, mucus plugging. CT scanning has been shown to be more sensitive in detecting bronchiectasis in AIDS patients than chest radiography *(31)*. CT scan detected 10 of 12 cases of bronchiectasis, and chest radiography detected 2 of 12 cases of bronchiectasis.

Bronchiectasis is a known complication of primary immunodeficiencies. A recent study looked at 22 patients with primary immunodeficiencies, 19 with B-cell disorders and 3 with T-cell disorders *(32)*. CT scanning was shown to be superior to chest radiography in detecting bronchiectasis in these disorders *(32)*. CT detected bronchiectasis in 15 of 19 patients with B-cell-type primary immunodeficiencies and in one of three patients with T-cell-type primary immunodeficiencies. In the 22 patients who had both CT scans and chest radiographs, CT detected bronchiectasis in 16 of 22 patients and chest radiography detected bronchiectasis in only 7 of 22 patients *(32)*.

Another recent study looked at the chest radiographic and CT findings in 46 patients with common variable immunodeficiency (CVID) *(34)*. It is known that CVID is associated with recurrent pneumonia and bronchiectasis, and also more recently with lymphoid interstitial pneumonia (LIP), other lymphoproliferative diseases, granulomatous disease, and organizing pneumonia *(34)*. In this study of CVID patients, three major patterns of disease were seen on CT, airway disease, nodules, and parenchymal opacification *(34)*. The airway pattern was believed to be caused mainly by recurrent airway infection (Fig. 13). The nodule pattern was believed to be caused mainly by LIP and granuloma formation. The parenchymal opacification pattern was believed to be caused mainly by LIP, organizing

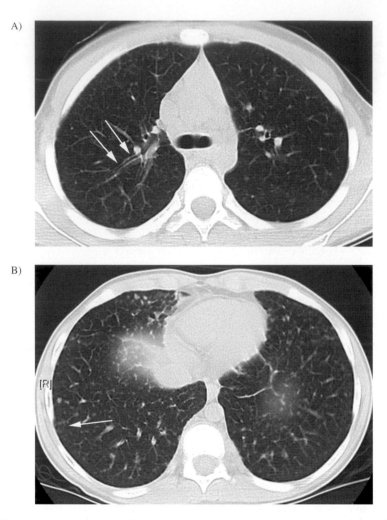

Fig. 13. (A) This is a multichannel CT image using 5-mm collimation of a young adult male with common variable immunodeficiency (CVID) and mild cylindrical bronchiectasis in the right upper lobe, arrows. **(B)** This is the same young adult male with CVID showing centrilobular nodules, arrow, in the right lower lobe. This case is an example of the airway CT pattern in CVID.

pneumonia, and LIP with non-necrotizing granulomas. Acute airspace pneumonia is also in the differential diagnosis in CVID patients with parenchymal opacification, but no infectious pneumonias were observed in this study *(34)*. Nodules (83%), ground glass opacities (60%), bronchiectasis (40%), and lymph node enlargement (53%) were the most common CT findings seen in these CVID patients *(34)*. Bronchiectasis was seen on chest radiography in 29% of patients and on CT in 40% of patients *(34)*. In the 13 patients with the airway pattern on CT, centrilobular micronodules (<3 mm) were present in all cases, bronchiectasis was seen in nine patients (69%), tree in bud pattern was seen in five cases (39%), and air trapping was seen in all three patients who had expiratory CT images *(34)*. Bronchiectasis was seen on CT in one of eight patients (13%) with the nodule pattern and in two of six patients (33%) with the parenchymal opacification pattern *(34)*. Among the 12 patients with CVID and CT evidence of bronchiectasis 11 patients had bronchectasis in more than one segment and one had bronchiectasis in only one segment. The distribution of the bronchiectasis was middle and lower lobe predominant in this study. In this same study, all CVID patients with CT evidence of bronchiectasis had involvement of the right middle lobe or lingula *(34)*. In four cases, the bronchiectasis involved all six zones of the lungs that were scored. The bronchiectasis was cylindrical in all patients in agreement with a previous report by Reiff *(17,34)*.

13. PRIMARY CILIARY DYSKINESIA

Primary ciliary dyskinesia is an autosomal recessive genetic disorder that affects the structure and/or function of ciliated epithelia. The most common ultrastructural defect of the cilia detected using electron microscopy is loss of the outer dynein arms *(5)*. The spectrum of ultrastructural abnormalities include loss of the inner dynein arms, loss of the central spokes, or complete absence of the cilia *(5)*. The epithelia in the tracheobronchial tree, nose, sinuses, and middle ear are affected *(5,35)*. The reduction or loss of normal cilia function results in bronchiectasis, middle ear infections, chronic sinusitus, nasal polyposis, and male infertility *(5,35)*. The diagnosis of primary ciliary dyskinesia can be made using electron microscopy and noting ultrastructural deficiencies in the cilia, the saccharin test, determination of ciliary beat frequency, and more recently with the measurement of nasal nitric oxide levels, which are markedly decreased in patients with primary ciliary dyskinesia *(5,35)*.

Kartagener's syndrome is the most dramatic manifestation of primary ciliary dyskinesia, (Fig. 14). It presents with complete thoracic and abdominal situs inversus, lower lobe predominant bronchiectasis (most often), and sinusitus. Chronic middle ear infections and infertility are frequently associated conditions. Kartagener's syndrome is a subset of primary ciliary dyskinesia. The normal left–right asymmetry or normal situs of the thorax, abdomen, and body is believed to result from the beating of the embryonic (Hensen's) node *(35)*. The normal ciliary function is required then during intrauterine fetal development for normal foregut rotation and the development of normal thoracic and abdominal situs. For this reason, half of patients with PCD have been believed to have complete situs inversus

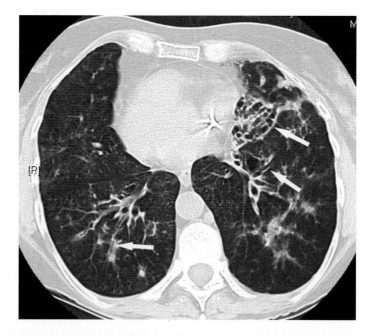

Fig. 14. Multi-channel CT scan using 5-mm collimation in an adult woman with PCD and Kartagener syndrome. Note the complete situs inversus and also the bronchiectasis in the left middle lobe and both lower lobes, arrows.

and half to have normal situs. There is in essence an equal chance of normal versus reversed foregut folding in PCD. The PCD patients with normal situs can share all the same maladies of Kartagener's syndrome minus the situs abnormality. However, recently, it has been noted that several of the ciliary deficiencies may not cause total immotility and all ultrastructural variants are not associated with situs inversus in 50% of cases *(35)*. PCD usually presents with lower lobe predominant bronchiectasis. It is associated with an increased risk of pulmonary infection secondary to poor airway clearance in the more dependent portions of the lung.

The bronchiectasis detected by MDCT in Kartagener's syndrome and other variants of primary ciliary dyskinesia is lower lobe predominant *(5,17)* (Fig. 14). The bronchiectasis is more likely to be cylindrical than varicoid or cystic *(5,17)*. There is no preferential involvement of the central or peripheral airways with bronchiectasis *(5,17)*.

REFERENCES

1. Reid LM. Reduction in bronchial subdivision in bronchiectasis. *Thorax* 1950;5(3):233–47.
2. King P, Holdsworth S, Freezer N, Holmes P. Bronchiectasis. *Int Med J* 2006;36(11):729–37.
3. Barker AF. Bronchiectasis. *N Engl J Med* 2002;346(18):1383–93.
4. King PT, Holdsworth SR, Freezer NJ, Villanueva E, Holmes PW. Characterization of the onset and presenting clinical features of adult bronchiectasis. *Respir Med* 2006;100(12):2183–39.
5. Newell JDJ, Chan ED, Martin RJ. Imaging of airway disease. In: Lynch DA, Newell JDJ, Lee JS, Eds. *Imaging of Diffuse Lung Disease*, 1 Ed. Hamilton: B.C. Deeker Inc; 2000:171–97.
6. King PT, Freezer NJ, Holmes PW, Holdsworth SR, Forshaw K, Sart DD. Role of CFTR mutations in adult bronchiectasis. *Thorax* 2004;59(4):357–58.
7. Divac A, Nikolic A, Mitic-Milikic M, et al. CFTR mutations and polymorphisms in adults with disseminated bronchiectasis: a controversial issue. *Thorax* 2005;60(1):85.
8. Sumikawa H, Johkoh T, Ichikado K, et al. Usual interstitial pneumonia and chronic idiopathic interstitial pneumonia: analysis of CT appearance in 92 patients. *Radiology* 2006;241(1):258–66.
9. Mcguinness G, Naidich DP. CT of airways disease and bronchiectasis. *Radiol Clin North Am* 2002;40(1):1–19.
10. Fraser RS, Muller NL, Colman N, Pare PD. Bronchiectasis and other bronchial abnormalities. In: Fraser RS, Muller NL, Colman N, Pare PD, Eds. *Diagnosis of Diseases of the Chest*, 4 Ed. Philadelphia: W.B. Saunders Company; 1999:2265–97.
11. Dodd JD, Souza CA, Muller NL. Conventional high-resolution CT versus helical high-resolution MDCT in the detection of bronchiectasis. *AJR* 2006;187(2):414–20.
12. Naidich DP, Mccauley DI, Khouri NF, Stitik FP, Siegelman SS. Computed tomography of bronchiectasis. *J Comput Assist Tomogr* 1982;6(3):437–44.
13. Brody AS, Kosorok MR, Li Z, et al. Reproducibility of a scoring system for computed tomography scanning in cystic fibrosis. *J Thor Imag* 2006;21(1):14–21.
14. Brody AS, Klein JS, Molina PL, Quan J, Bean JA, Wilmott RW. High-resolution computed tomography in young patients with cystic fibrosis: distribution of abnormalities and correlation with pulmonary function tests. *J Pediatr* 2004;145(1):32–38.
15. Sibtain NA, Ujita M, Wilson R, Wells AU, Hansell DM. Interlobular septal thickening in idiopathic bronchiectasis: a thin-section CT study of 94 patients. *Radiology* 2005;237(3):1091–96.
16. Hansell DM. Bronchiectasis. *Radiol Clin North Am* 1998;36(1):107–28.
17. Reiff DB, Wells AU, Carr DH, Cole PJ, Hansell DM. CT Findings in bronchiectasis: limited value in distinguishing between idiopathic and specific types. *AJR* 1995;165(2):261–67.
18. Fraser RS, Muller NL, Colman N, Pare PD. Cystic fibrosis. In: Fraser RS, Muller NL, Colman N, Pare PD, Eds. *Diagnosis of diseases of the chest*, 4 Ed. Philadelphia: W.B. Saunders Company; 1999:2298–315.
19. Mccolley SA. Cystic fibrosis lung disease: when does it start, and how can it be prevented? *J Pediatr* 2004;145(1):6–7.
20. Kim JS, Tanaka N, Newell JD, et al. Nontuberculous mycobacterial infection: CT scan findings, genotype, and treatment responsiveness. *Chest* 2005;128(6):3863–69.
21. Brody AS, Sucharew H, Campbell JD, et al. Computed tomography correlates with pulmonary exacerbations in children with cystic fibrosis. *Am J Respir Crit Care Med* 2005;172(9):1128–32.
22. Wickremasinghe M, Ozerovitch LJ, Davies G, et al. Non-tuberculous mycobacteria in patients with bronchiectasis. *Thorax* 2005;60(12):1045–51.
23. Wittram C, Weisbrod GL. Mycobacterium avium complex lung disease in immunocompetent patients: radiography-CT correlation. *Br J Radiol* 2002;75(892):340–44.

24. Kim TS, Koh WJ, Han J, et al. Hypothesis on the evolution of cavitary lesions in nontuberculous mycobacterial pulmonary infection: thin-section CT and histopathologic correlation. *AJR* 2005;184(4):1247–52.

25. Mitchell TA, Hamilos DL, Lynch DA, Newell JD. Distribution and severity of bronchiectasis in allergic bronchopulmonary aspergillosis (ABPA). *J Asthma* 2000;37(1):65–72.

26. Angus RM, Davies ML, Cowan MD, Mcsharry C, Thomson NC. Computed tomographic scanning of the lung in patients with allergic bronchopulmonary aspergillosis and in asthmatic patients with a positive skin test to *Aspergillus fumigatus*. *Thorax* 1994;49(6):586–89.

27. Neeld DA, Goodman LR, Gurney JW, Greenberger PA, Fink JN. Computerized tomography in the evaluation of allergic bronchopulmonary aspergillosis. *Am Rev Respir Dis* 1990;142(5):1200–05.

28. King MA, Stone JA, Diaz PT, Mueller CF, Becker WJ, Gadek JE. Alpha 1-antitrypsin deficiency: evaluation of bronchiectasis with CT. *Radiology* 1996;199(1):137–41.

29. Guest PJ, Hansell DM. High resolution computed tomography (HRCT) in emphysema associated with alpha-1-antitrypsin deficiency. *Clin Radiol* 1992;45(4):260–66.

30. Mcmahon MA, O'Mahony MJ, O'Neill SJ, Mcelvaney NG, Logan PM. Alpha-1 antitrypsin deficiency and computed tomography findings. *J Comput Assist Tomogr* 2005;29(4):549–53.

31. Mcguinness G, Naidich DP, Garay S, Leitman BS, Mccauley DI. AIDS Associated bronchiectasis: CT features. *J Comput Assist Tomogr* 1993;17(2):260–66.

32. Obregon RG, Lynch DA, Kaske T, Newell JD, Jr., Kirkpatrick CH. Radiologic findings of adult primary immunodeficiency disorders. Contribution of CT. *Chest* 1994;106(2):490–95.

33. Mcguinness G, Gruden JF, Bhalla M, Harkin TJ, Jagirdar JS, Naidich DP. AIDS-related airway disease. *AJR* 1997;168(1):67–77.

34. Tanaka N, Kim JS, Bates CA, et al. Lung diseases in patients with common variable immunodeficiency: chest radiographic and computed tomographic findings. *J Comput Assist Tomogr* 2006;30(5):828–38.

35. Carlen B, Stenram U. Primary ciliary dyskinesia: a review. *Ultrastruct Pathol* 2005;29(3–4):217–20.

III Small Airways

10

Asthma

Philippe A. Grenier, Catherine Beigelman-Aubry, and Pierre-Yves Brillet

Summary

The clinical indications for CT in patients with asthma include detection of bronchiectasis in patients with suspicion of allergic bronchopulmonary aspergillosis; documentation of the presence and extent of emphysema in smokers with asthma; and identification of conditions, such as hypersensitivity pneumonitis, that may be confused with asthma. However, high-resolution volumetric helical acquisition using MDCT and improvement image analysis techniques have made possible accurate and reproducible quantitative assessment of airway wall and lumen areas and lung density. This may permit the in vivo assessment of the degree of airway wall remodeling and the extent of small airway obstruction. These parameters should become accepted biomarkers for assessing effect of treatments in clinical trials and ultimately in the clinical management of individual patients.

Key Words: Asthma; air trapping; airway wall remodeling; small airway obstruction; bronchial wall thickening.

1. INTRODUCTION

Asthma is a chronic inflammatory condition involving the airways. This inflammation causes a generalized increase in existing bronchial hyperresponsiveness to various stimuli. This feature is commonly used in practice to confirm the clinical diagnosis of asthma. In susceptible individuals, this inflammation induces recurrent episodes of wheezing, chest tightness, breathlessness, and coughing usually associated with widespread but variable airflow obstruction that is often reversible either spontaneously or with treatment. The chronic inflammation process leads to structural changes, such as new vessel formation, airway smooth muscle (ASM) thickening, and fibrosis, which may result in irreversible airway narrowing.

In cases of mild persistent asthma, the current therapy is based on an inhaled corticosteroid as a controller (anti-inflammatory) medication. When necessary, bronchodilator (β2 agonist) used for additional symptomatic relief. For moderate persistent asthma, additional treatment may include a long-acting beta agonist, a leukotriene receptor antagonist or theophylline. For severe persistent asthma, in addition to the above, anti-immunoglobulin E therapy and/or oral steroids may be considered. Additional therapeutic impact can be achieved by allergen immunotherapy and by evaluation and treatment for sinusitis and gastroesophageal reflux.

CT is not commonly indicated in the routine assessment of patients with asthma. However, it is sometimes used particularly when complications of asthma such as allergic bronchopulmonary aspergillosis (ABPA) are suspected (1) or in documenting the presence and extent of emphysema

From: *Contemporary Medical Imaging: CT of the Airways*
Edited by: P. M. Boiselle and D. A. Lynch © Humana Press, Totowa, NJ

in smokers with asthma *(2,3)*. ABPA is associated with more severe bronchial dilation than that typically seen in patients with uncomplicated asthma. CT may also be helpful to identify conditions that may be confused with asthma, such as hypersensitivity pneumonitis *(4)*.

Beyond these classical indications, the real current challenge for CT in asthma is to visualize and quantify the lung attenuation and the airway lumen and wall to assess the extent of airway obstruction, the degree of inflammatory changes in small airways, and to evaluate in vivo the degree of airway wall remodeling. This has been used for getting better insights in pathophysiology of asthma, and it will become crucial in the monitoring of current and future therapy.

2. CT FINDINGS

Bronchial dilatation, bronchial wall thickening, mucoïd impaction, centrilobular bronchiolar abnormalities, patchy areas of mosaic perfusion, and regional air trapping on expiratory scans may be identified on high-resolution CT (HRCT) in patients with uncomplicated asthma. On the whole, the severity of these abnormalities correlates with the severity of asthma measured by pulmonary function tests. In one study, forced expiratory volume in 1 s (FEV1) values were inversely correlated with bronchial wall thickening, hyperlucency, mucoid impaction, linear shadows, centrilobular prominence, and bronchial dilation *(5)*. The prevalence of these thin-section CT abnormalities increases with increasing severity of symptoms *(6)*. Considerable variation exists however in the reported frequency of abnormalities. This variation is related to differences in diagnostic criteria and patient selection. Smoking may influence the type of airway inflammation observed in asthma and its response to therapy. On HRCT, airway and parenchymal abnormalities have proven to be more common in smoking asthma patients than in non-smokers *(7)*. The presence and frequency of airway and parenchymal abnormalities on HRCT in elderly asthmatic patients are related to the duration of asthma. In a study of 68 clinically stable asthmatic patients aged 60 years or more, those with early-onset asthma (disease duration ≥ 5 years) had significantly higher frequency of focal or diffuse area of lung hypoattenuation, bronchial dilatation, and bronchial wall thickening than late-onset asthmatic patients (disease duration <5 years) *(8)*.

Only few of the published studies compared the frequency of the findings observed in asthmatics with a control group *(9–12)*. Park et al. *(12)* demonstrated that only three findings were significantly more frequent in asthmatic patients than in normal individuals: bronchial wall thickening, bronchial dilatation, and expiratory air trapping.

2.1. Bronchial Wall Thickening

Bronchial wall thickening has been reported in 16–92% of patients *(9–12)* a discrepancy that cannot be ascribed to the effects of smoking: although nearly half of the subjects in the study of Lynch et al. *(10)* were smokers, only 12 of 50 asthmatic individuals in the study of Grenier et al. *(9)* were current or ex-smokers. On all these studies, there is a tendency for the degree of bronchial wall thickening to correlate with the severity of disease *(13–15)* (Figs 1 and 2).

2.2. Bronchial Dilatation

Identification of bronchiectasis in patients with asthma but without ABPA is plausible because bronchiectatic changes are seen at autopsy in patients who have died with long-standing asthma. The true prevalence of bronchiectasis or bronchial dilation in patients with uncomplicated chronic asthma however remains unclear *(9–11,16)*. In a study by Lynch et al., 77% of asthmatic patients and 153 (36%) of 429 bronchi assessed in asthmatic patients were associated with a bronchial–pulmonary arterial diameter ratio greater than 1 *(10)*. In a study by Grenier et al. *(9)*, bronchial dilatation was found in 28.5% of the asthmatic subjects, primarily involving subsegmental and distal bronchi (Fig. 2). Takemura et al. *(16)* found at least one dilated bronchus in 62% of 23 asthmatics and in 2 of 10 (2%) controls. Mild cylindrical bronchial dilation, based on a mild elevation of the bronchoarterial

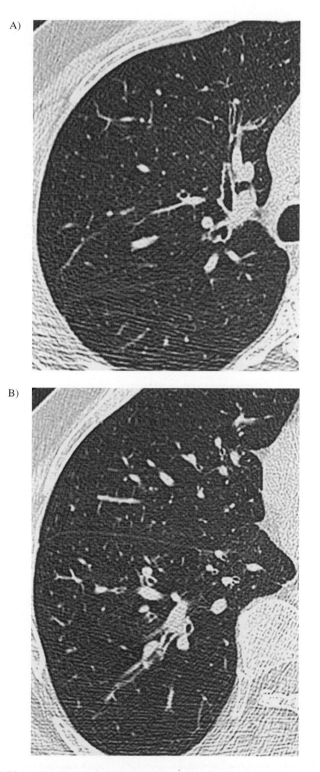

Fig. 1. HRCT (**A** and **B**) scans targeted on the right lung in a patient with severe persistent asthma. There is diffuse bronchial wall thickening with some irregularities in bronchial wall contours.

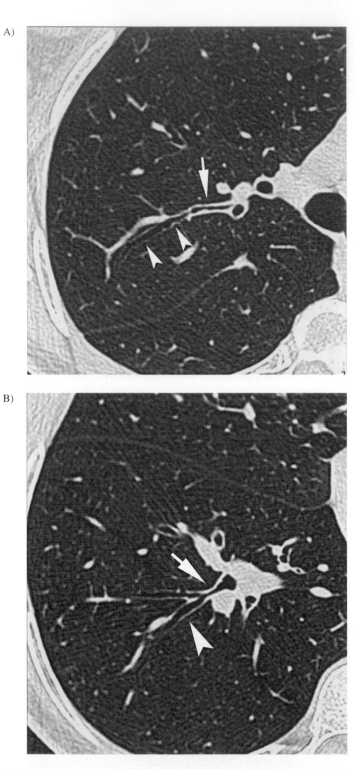

Fig. 2. Patient with moderate persistent asthma. (**A**) HRCT scan targeted on the right upper lobe shows bronchial wall thickening that reduces the bronchial lumen of a subsegmental bronchus (arrow), associated with distal bronchial dilatation (arrowhead). (**B**) HRCT scan targeted on the right lower lobe shows bronchial wall thickening (arrow) and slight dilatation of the distal bronchi (arrowhead) in the laterobasal segment.

ratio, may occur in patients with asthma because of hypoxic pulmonary vasoconstriction related to localized areas of air trapping *(4)*. Because of a visual illusion, thick-walled bronchi will appear larger than the adjacent vessel, even if their internal diameters are the same. Therefore, mild cylindrical bronchiectasis should be diagnosed with caution in patients with asthma and should not be the sole criterion for suggesting the diagnosis of ABPA in these patients.

2.3. Mucoid Impaction

Mucoid impaction has been reported in as many as 21% of asthmatic patients; this abnormality may clear following treatment *(11)*. Linear bands reflecting subsegmental atelectasis are sometimes observed; they have been proven to be reversible. Branching or nodular centrilobular opacities have been reported to be present in as many as 10–21% of patients, sometimes manifested as a tree-in-bud appearance. These likely reflect bronchiolar wall thickening or inflammation, with or without mucoid impaction. However, this finding is absent or tends to be inconspicuous in most patients with asthma.

2.4. Decreased Lung Attenuation

Focal or diffuse hyperlucency has been observed on inspiratory scans in 18–31% of patients *(9,10,12,17)*, undoubtedly owing to small airway obstruction, air trapping, and mosaic perfusion (Fig. 3). Laurent et al. compared the inspiratory and expiratory thin-section CT findings of 22 patients classified with moderate asthma, with 22 healthy volunteers (10 smokers and 12 non-smokers). Mosaic perfusion was found in 23% of the asthmatics, 5% of the smokers, and 0% of the non-smokers. A significant positive correlation was found between physiologic findings of small airways obstruction and the HRCT mosaic perfusion score *(17)*. In a study by Newman et al. *(18)*, the extent of air trapping, quantified on expiratory CT, correlated with the physiologic severity of asthma.

In severe persistent asthma, diffuse decreased lung attenuation and expiratory air trapping make the pattern difficult to distinguish from that of obliterative bronchiolitis *(19)*, although bronchial dilatation, vascular attenuation, and decreased lung attenuation are significantly more prevalent and more extensive in obliterative bronchiolitis than in asthma *(20)*.

A)

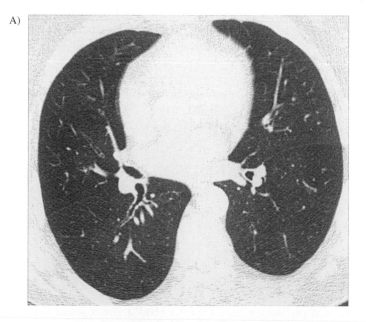

Fig. 3. *(Continued)*

B)

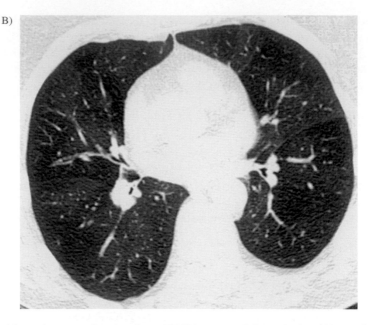

Fig. 3. Patient with moderate persistent asthma. HRCT scans at full inspiration (**A**) and full expiration (**B**). There are bilateral areas of decreased lung attenuation with mosaic perfusion pattern, present on the inspiratory HRCT scan, and accentuated on expiratory HRCT because of air trapping.

2.5. Expiratory Air Trapping

Expiratory CT scan shows evidence of patchy air trapping in asthmatic patients even in the absence of morphologic abnormalities visible on inspiratory scans *(12,17,21)* (Fig. 4). In a study by Park et al., air trapping involving more than one segment was seen in 50% of asthmatic patients. Air-trapping scores were significantly higher in the asthmatics than in non-smoking control subjects, but not in smokers *(12)*. In the study by Laurent et al. *(17)*, air-trapping scores were significantly higher in the asthmatic patients than in the normal controls. Both FEV1 and reversibility of small airway

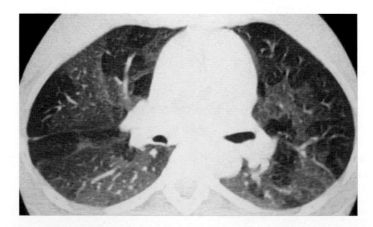

Fig. 4. Patient with mild persistent asthma. Expiratory HRCT shows patchy areas of air trapping in both lungs. Inspiratory HRCT scan was normal.

obstruction correlated with air-trapping scores *(17)*. In a series of children with mild-to-moderate asthma, air trapping on expiratory HRCT scans expressed as pixel index defined by the percentage of pixels in lung fields below—910 HU correlated with the ratio of FEV1 to forced vital capacity and with the percentage predicted forced expiratory flow between 25 and 75% *(22)*.

3. AIRWAY HYPERRESPONSIVENESS AND SMALL AIRWAY INFLAMMATION

CT analysis of lung attenuation and airway dimension in asthma may provide additional data to that derived from traditional measures of lung function. Some investigators have used CT to evaluate airway hyperresponsiveness in asthmatics.

3.1. Bronchial Hyperresponsiveness

Okasawa et al. measured the luminal area of bronchi in asthmatics and controls at full inspiration before and after methacholine challenge. They showed that there was no difference in the pattern of airway narrowing in the asthmatics as opposed to the normal subjects. However, the same degree of narrowing was achieved using a much lower dose of methacholine in the asthmatics *(23)*. In another study by King et al. *(24)*, airway narrowing after bronchial challenge was heterogeneous in the large airways of asthmatics, and this heterogeneity was larger than in control subjects. Brown et al. demonstrated that deep inspiration dilated the airways to a comparable degree in asthmatics and normal subjects at baseline. They also showed that after inhaling methacholine, deep inspiration caused further bronchial narrowing in asthmatics as opposed to substantial bronchodilatation in normal individuals. The authors suggested that this phenomenon indicated abnormality in the smooth muscle response to stretch in the asthmatic subjects *(25)*.

Beigelman-Aubry et al. *(26)* demonstrated that patients with mild intermittent asthma present with baseline bronchoconstriction compared with normal subjects when examined with CT performed at a controlled lung volume lower than total lung capacity (TLC) (65% of TLC), following a deep inspiration. This was confirmed by the fact that inhalation of salbutamol after methacholine challenge increased the bronchial cross-sectional area of asthmatic airways, to a level greater than the baseline value, and comparable to the bronchial area of the control group (Fig. 5). This suggests that bronchoconstriction in asthmatic patients is due to an increased baseline tone or an impaired stretching. In the same study, the degree of change in bronchial cross-section area after methacholine challenge was similar in asthmatics and in normal subjects. Conversely, in the same patients, the presence of expiratory air trapping induced by methacholine challenge and partly reversible after salbutamol inhalation confirmed that the methacholine-induced bronchoconstriction involves mainly or exclusively the smallest airways *(26)* (Fig. 6).

3.2. Small Airway Hyperresponsiveness

Mitsunobi et al. *(27)* have shown mean lung density on inspiratory CT scans decreased during exacerbation of asthma, because of the constriction of small airways. In a study by Gückel et al., thin-section CT was performed at suspended inspiration immediately and 30 min after methacholine bronchoprovocation in 22 asthmatic subjects, who were randomly assigned to breathe room air, oxygen through nasal prongs at 5 L/min and oxygen through facemask at 12 L/min. In induced bronchoconstriction, the appearance of mosaic attenuation on inspiratory CT was decreased with administration of oxygen, suggesting that hypoxic vasoconstriction, rather than changes in lung inflation, largely accounts for this phenomenon *(28)*.

Air trapping assessed on expiratory CT has also been used to quantify hyperresponsiveness of small airways. To measure air trapping in asthmatics before and after bronchial challenge, Goldin et al. assessed the distribution of lung attenuation values at residual volume at baseline after inhalation

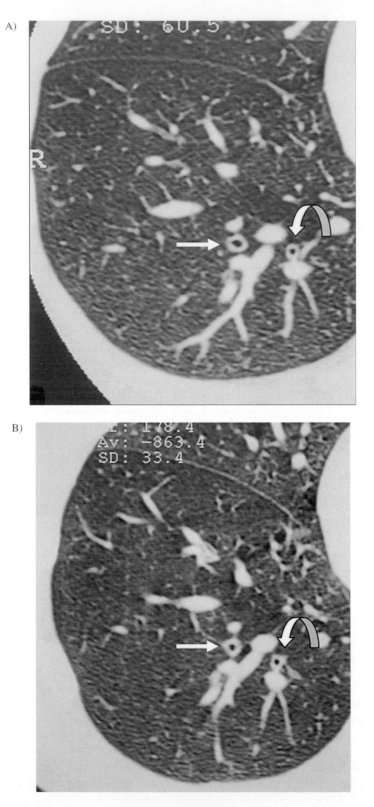

Fig. 5. *(Continued)*

C)
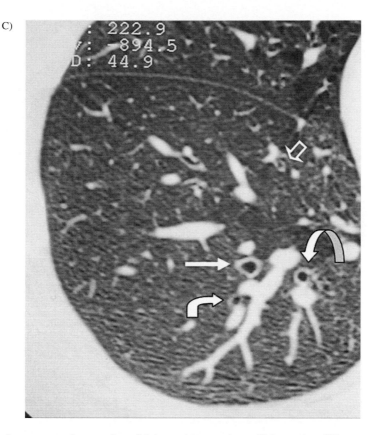

Fig. 5. Airway hyperresponsiveness in mild intermittent asthma. Thin-section CT scans targeted on the right lower lobe at 65% of total lung capacity controlled by spirometrical triggering (**A**) at baseline, (**B**) after methacholine inhalation, and (**C**) 10 mm after salbutamol inhalation. The cross-section of two thick-walled subsegmental bronchi of the posterobasal segment of the right lower lobe (white arrows) demonstrate moderate bronchoconstriction after methacholine (**B**). After salbutamol (**C**), the bronchial lumens are dilated and appear larger than before challenge. Other small bronchial lumens (open arrows) not previously visible have dilated sufficiently to be visible after salbutamol. Figure reprinted with permission from Grenier et al. New frontiers in CT imaging of airway diseases. *Eur Radiol* 2002;12:1022–1044.

of methacholine in mild asthmatic patients. They showed significant leftward shifts in the frequency distribution of lung parenchymal attenuation values after methacholine challenge. This effect returned to normal after the administration of albuterol *(29)*. The same authors used this functional imaging technique to compare the relative efficacy of two different medications on small airway hyperreactivity and regional air trapping in mild and moderate asthma. The difference between both medications was essentially the size of inhaled particles (0.8–1.2 µm vs. 3.5–4 µm). In a double-blind randomized parallel group pilot study, the authors performed HRCT at residual volume before and after methacholine challenge test before and after 4 weeks of treatment. The HFA-Beclomethasone group (small-size particles) showed the significantly more improvement in air trapping than CFC-Beclomethasone group *(30)*. This study was the first example of quantitative CT assessment of airway responsiveness used as a biomarker of small airway inflammation in a clinical trial.

Quantitative image analysis of HRCT performed at residual volume, before and after methacholine, was also used to assess the response to therapy targeted to the small airways. Zeidler et al. hypothesized that treatment with montelukast, an oral anti-leukotriene that reaches the small airways through the

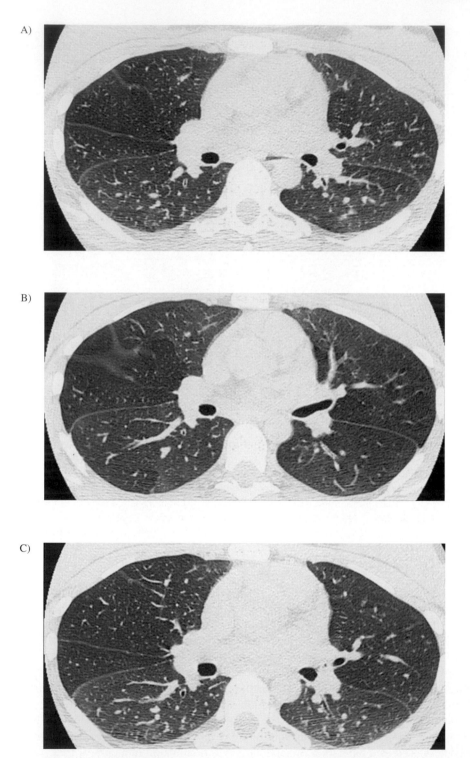

Fig. 6. Mild intermittent asthmatic. HRCT scans at full expiration obtained before (**A**) and after (**B**) inhalation of methacholine and then salbutamol (**C**). Bilateral extensive areas of air trapping (lower, attenuation lung) were observed after methacholine inhalation. Air trapping disappeared completely after salbutamol inhalation.

circulation, would lead to improved small airway patency. They performed a double-blind crossover study comparing the effect of montelukast versus placebo for 4 weeks in 16 mild-to-moderate steroid naïve asthmatics. Montelukast treatment resulted in significantly less regional air trapping on HRCT on the pre-methacholine images, when compared with placebo, as well as improvement in total quality-of-life scores and symptoms subscores. This improvement of distal airway disease assessed with HRCT was not detected with conventional physiological studies *(31)*.

3.3. Small Airway Inflammation

Measuring lung attenuation at controlled lung volume has also been used to assess indirectly the degree of inflammation in small airways. Beigelman-Aubry et al. measured lung attenuation and anteroposterior attenuation gradient at 65% TLC lung volume monitored by pneumotachography in mild intermittent asthmatics and normal subjects. They found significantly higher values in asthmatics and hypothesized that the peribronchial and small airway inflammation occurring in asthma was responsible for the change in elastic properties of the lung explained the attenuation and gradient increases *(26)*. The observation that these increased attenuation values were not affected by methacholine and salbutamol challenges supports the hypothesis that bronchoconstriction played only a small or no role in attenuation changes and that distal inflammation was a more likely contender. Brillet et al. assessed quantitative airway dimensions using volumetric high-resolution MDCT acquisition during a single breath hold at 65% TLC volume controlled by pneumotachography in 12 mild or moderate asthmatics before and after 12 weeks of inhaled treatment by salmeterol/fluticasone 150/50 disks. Image data analysis showed significant shortening in length of subsegmental bronchi and decrease in attenuation of the non-dependent areas of lung parenchyma. This indicates both decrease in resistance linked to change in pulmonary elastic recoil and decrease in small airway inflammation *(32)*.

4. AIRWAY WALL REMODELING AND AIRFLOW OBSTRUCTION

4.1. Pathologic and Functional Findings

Airway remodeling is an established pathologic feature of asthma. Examinations of autopsied or resected lungs have enabled detailed morphologic and morphometric studies and have provided fundamental knowledge of airway remodeling in asthma. However, such materials are only accidentally available. Bronchial mucosa biopsy has been widely used since the 1980s and has contributed substantially to basic investigations of inflammation and remodeling. More recently, Benayoun et al. performed bronchial biopsies in control subjects ($n = 10$), intermittent asthmatics ($n = 10$), mild-to-moderate persistent asthmatics ($n = 15$), and COPD patients. They showed that higher number of fibroblasts ($p < 0.001$), increase in collagen type III deposition ($p < 0.002$), large mucous gland ($p < 0.04$), larger ASM areas ($p < 0.001$), augmented ASM cell size ($p < 0.001$), and myosin light-chain kinase expression ($p < 0.005$) distinguished patients with severe persistent asthma from patients with mild disease or with COPD *(33)*. These structural changes in the airways, particularly smooth muscle hypertrophy and hyperplasia, are thought to be responsible for progressive and persistent airflow obstruction and explain why the progressive decrease of FEV1 over time is higher and faster in asthmatics than in controls *(34)*. However, biopsy specimens are limited in size and depth, limited to central airways, and the procedure may be too invasive to be repeated.

4.2. CT Assessment

CT has recently been utilized to assess airway remodeling in asthma *(35)* (Figs 2, 7, and 8). Ito et al. showed in a short series of 10 never smokers with stable asthma that air trapping at expiratory CT remained unchanged after bronchodilator inhalation, although significant reversibility of FEV1

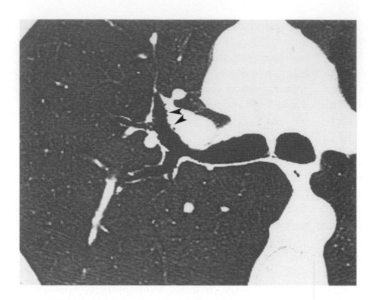

Fig. 7. Minimum intensity projection on a 5-mm thick axial slab after thin collimation MDCT acquisition in a severe persistent asthmatic patient. Small air collections (arrowheads) in the bronchial wall reflect dilatation of the mucous glands.

was observed. In addition, air-trapping scores correlated significantly with airway wall thickening, suggesting that air trapping is irreversible and represents structural remodeling of small airways *(36)*. Awadh et al. measured the ratio of airway wall thickness to the outer airway diameter (i.e., T/D) in normal subjects and in asthmatic patients with varying severity of disease. The mean T/D was significantly higher (0.27) in patients with an episode of near-fatal asthma, as compared to those with mild asthma (0.25) or normal (0.23) *(13)*.

Little et al. performed HRCT in 49 optimally controlled asthmatic patients and measured total airway cross-sectional area and airway wall thickness to airway diameter ratio and demonstrated statistically significant positive association between these parameters and asthma severity, and an inverse association with gas-transfer coefficient *(14)*. Kasahara showed a strong-positive correlation between the epithelial reticular basement membrane (Rbm) of the airway wall thickness determined in biopsy specimen and whole airway wall thickness determined by HRCT scanning in patients with asthma. Furthermore, this thickening was correlated with deterioration in respiratory function *(37)*. This study suggested that Rbm thickening appears simultaneously with hypertrophy and hyperplasia of other components of the airway wall that may cause respiratory function deterioration in patients with asthma. The relationship between Rbm thickening and airway wall area assessed on HRCT found in adults with asthma however does not appear so clear in children. De Blic et al. *(38)* in a series of 37 children with severe asthma demonstrated a significant correlation between bronchial wall-thickening score and Rbm thickening, and alveolar nitric oxide concentration, a marker of airway inflammation, whereas in the Saglani et al. *(39)* series of 27 children with difficult asthma, there was no relationship between Rbm thickness and bronchial wall thickening.

In adults, bronchial wall thickening measured at CT has proven to be more prominent in patients with more severe asthma. Niimi et al., by measuring wall area on HRCT scans at the apical and subsegmental bronchus of the right upper lobe in 81 asthmatics and 28 healthy controls, showed that, as compared with controls, wall area, and wall area corrected for body surface area were increased in patients with mild, moderate, and severe persistent asthma and not in intermittent asthma. In addition, they demonstrated that these parameters correlated with the duration and severity of

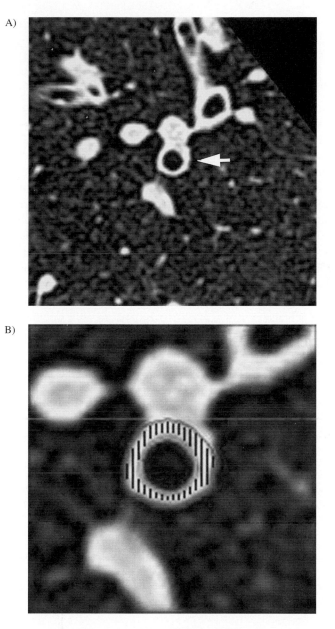

Fig. 8. A bronchial cross-section of the posterior and segmental bronchus of the right upper lobe (arrow) in a mild persistent asthmatic was reformatted perpendicular to the central airway axis after thin collimation volumetric helical MDCT acquisition (**A**). The results of automatic segmentation of outer and inner contours of the bronchial cross-section (**B**) allow measurement of the wall area.

asthma and the degree of airflow obstruction at pulmonary function tests *(40)*. Gono et al. studied 24 asymptomatic asthmatics who had been optimally treated with inhaled and/or oral corticosteroids for longer than 6 months. All patients were given an inhaled bronchodilator 20–30 min before the HRCT examination. Airway wall thickness and air trapping were significantly greater for the 14 asthmatics with non-reversible airflow obstruction than for the 10 asthmatics with normal spirometry and normal controls *(41)*. These observations support the concept that quantitative assessment of bronchial wall area at CT could be used to assess airway wall remodeling in asthmatic patients for longitudinal studies to evaluate the effects of new therapies *(42)*.

4.3. Effect of Treatment

Niimi et al. *(43)* in another study evaluated the effect of corticosteroids on airway wall thickening measured on helical CT images of the right upper lobe apical segmental bronchus in 45 corticosteroid naïve patients with persistent asthma and 28 healthy controls. Before treatment, airway wall areas even when adjusted for body surface area were greater in asthma than in controls ($p < 0.001$). Treatment with 800 μg of inhaled beclomethasone daily for 12 weeks led to a significant decrease (11%, $p < 0.001$) in the wall area, reflecting an overall reduction in airway inflammation in asthmatics. This decrease did not return airway dimensions to those in the age-matched asymptomatic control group ($p < 0.001$), suggesting that these unresponsive components reflected structural changes leading to airflow obstruction. In patients with long-standing asthma, airway wall thickness was reduced less, and airway wall thickening after treatment was more prominent *(43)*. The same authors in another study investigated the relationship between airway wall thickness as assessed by helical CT and airway responsiveness in patients with stable asthma *(44)*. Airway reactivity was negatively correlated with airway wall thickness in patients with and without inhaled steroid treatment, suggesting that airway wall thickening attenuates airway reactivity in patients with asthma *(44)*.

All these preliminary studies suggest that CT assessment of air trapping and airway wall dimensions may be a more sensitive endpoint than physiology in clinical trials and ultimately in the clinical management of individual patients. Because important questions remain to be answered in this common disease, further use of CT in research setting seems to be justified.

REFERENCES

1. Neeld DA, Goodman LR, Gurney JW, Greenberger PA, Fink JN. Computerized tomography in the evaluation of allergic bronchopulmonary aspergillosis. *Am Rev Respir Dis* 1990;142:1200–1205.
2. Kinsella M, Muller NL, Staples C, Vedal S, Chan-Yeung M. Hyperinflation in asthma and emphysema. Assessment by pulmonary function testing and computed tomography. *Chest* 1988;94:286–289.
3. Kondoh Y, Taniguchi H, Yokoyama S, Taki F, Takagi K, Satake T. Emphysematous change in chronic asthma in relation to cigarette smoking. Assessment by computed tomography. *Chest* 1990;97:845–849.
4. Lynch DA. Imaging of asthma and allergic bronchopulmonary mycosis. *Radiol Clin North Am* 1998;36:129–142.
5. Harmanci E, Kebapci M, Metintas M, Ozkan R. High-resolution computed tomography findings are correlated with disease severity in asthma. *Respiration* 2002;69:420–426.
6. Paganin F, Seneterre E, Chanez P, et al. Computed tomography of the lungs in asthma: influence of disease severity and etiology. *Am J Respir Crit Care Med* 1996;153:110–114.
7. Boulet LP, Lemiere C, Archambault F, Carrier G, Descary MC, Deschesnes F. Smoking and asthma: clinical and radiologic features, lung function, and airway inflammation. *Chest* 2006;129:661–668.
8. Yilmaz S, Ekici A, Ekici M, Keles H. High-resolution computed tomography findings in elderly patients with asthma. *Eur J Radiol* 2006;59:238–243.
9. Grenier P, Mourey-Gerosa I, Benali K, et al. Abnormalities of the airways and lung parenchyma in asthmatics: CT observations in 50 patients and inter- and intraobserver variability. *Eur Radiol* 1996;6:199–206.
10. Lynch DA, Newell JD, Tschomper BA, Cink TM, Newman LS, Bethel R. Uncomplicated asthma in adults: comparison of CT appearance of the lungs in asthmatic and healthy subjects. *Radiology* 1993;188:829–833.
11. Paganin F, Trussard V, Seneterre E, et al. Chest radiography and high resolution computed tomography of the lungs in asthma. *Am Rev Respir Dis* 1992;146:1084–1087.
12. Park CS, Muller NL, Worthy SA, Kim JS, Awadh N, Fitzgerald M. Airway obstruction in asthmatic and healthy individuals: inspiratory and expiratory thin-section CT findings. *Radiology* 1997;203:361–367.
13. Awadh N, Muller NL, Park CS, Abboud RT, FitzGerald JM. Airway wall thickness in patients with near fatal asthma and control groups: assessment with high resolution computed tomographic scanning. *Thorax* 1998;53:248–253.
14. Little SA, Sproule MW, Cowan MD, et al. High resolution computed tomographic assessment of airway wall thickness in chronic asthma: reproducibility and relationship with lung function and severity. *Thorax* 2002;57:247–253.

15. Park JW, Hong YK, Kim CW, Kim DK, Choe KO, Hong CS. High-resolution computed tomography in patients with bronchial asthma: correlation with clinical features, pulmonary functions and bronchial hyperresponsiveness. *J Investig Allergol Clin Immunol* 1997;7:186–192.

16. Takemura M, Niimi A, Minakuchi M, et al. Bronchial dilatation in asthma: relation to clinical and sputum indices. *Chest* 2004;125:1352–1358.

17. Laurent F, Latrabe V, Raherison C, Marthan R, Tunon-de-Lara JM. Functional significance of air trapping detected in moderate asthma. *Eur Radiol* 2000;10:1404–1410.

18. Newman KB, Lynch DA, Newman LS, Ellegood D, Newell JD, Jr. Quantitative computed tomography detects air trapping due to asthma. *Chest* 1994;106:105–109.

19. Jensen SP, Lynch DA, Brown KK, Wenzel SE, Newell JD. High-resolution CT features of severe asthma and bronchiolitis obliterans. *Clin Radiol* 2002;57:1078–1085.

20. Copley SJ, Wells AU, Muller NL, et al. Thin-section CT in obstructive pulmonary disease: discriminatory value. *Radiology* 2002;223:812–819.

21. Arakawa H, Webb WR. Air trapping on expiratory high-resolution CT scans in the absence of inspiratory scan abnormalities: correlation with pulmonary function tests and differential diagnosis. *AJR Am J Roentgenol* 1998;170: 1349–1353.

22. Jain N, Covar RA, Gleason MC, Newell JD, Jr., Gelfand EW, Spahn JD. Quantitative computed tomography detects peripheral airway disease in asthmatic children. *Pediatr Pulmonol* 2005;40:211–218.

23. Okazawa M, Muller N, McNamara AE, Child S, Verburgt L, Pare PD. Human airway narrowing measured using high resolution computed tomography. *Am J Respir Crit Care Med* 1996;154:1557–1562.

24. King GG, Carroll JD, Muller NL, et al. Heterogeneity of narrowing in normal and asthmatic airways measured by HRCT. *Eur Respir J* 2004;24:211–218.

25. Brown RH, Scichilone N, Mudge B, Diemer FB, Permutt S, Togias A. High-resolution computed tomographic evaluation of airway distensibility and the effects of lung inflation on airway caliber in healthy subjects and individuals with asthma. *Am J Respir Crit Care Med* 2001;163:994–1001.

26. Beigelman-Aubry C, Capderou A, Grenier PA, et al. Mild intermittent asthma: CT assessment of bronchial cross-sectional area and lung attenuation at controlled lung volume. *Radiology* 2002;223:181–187.

27. Mitsunobu F, Ashida K, Hosaki Y, et al. Decreased computed tomographic lung density during exacerbation of asthma. *Eur Respir J* 2003;22:106–112.

28. Guckel C, Wells AU, Taylor DA, Chabat F, Hansell DM. Mechanism of mosaic attenuation of the lungs on computed tomography in induced bronchospasm. *J Appl Physiol* 1999;86:701–708.

29. Goldin JG, McNitt-Gray MF, Sorenson SM, et al. Airway hyperreactivity: assessment with helical thin-section CT. *Radiology* 1998;208:321–329.

30. Goldin JG, Tashkin DP, Kleerup EC, et al. Comparative effects of hydrofluoroalkane and chlorofluorocarbon beclomethasone dipropionate inhalation on small airways: assessment with functional helical thin-section computed tomography. *J Allergy Clin Immunol* 1999;104:S258–267.

31. Zeidler MR, Kleerup EC, Goldin JG, et al. Montelukast improves regional air-trapping due to small airways obstruction in asthma. *Eur Respir J* 2006;27:307–315.

32. Brillet PY, Becquemin MH, Beigelman-Aubry C, et al. Assessment by multidetector CT (MDCT) of bronchi dimensions in mild to moderate asthmatics following 12 weeks treatment by salmeterol/fluticasone 50/250 Dickus bd (SFC). *Proc Am Thorac Soc*; 2006; 3:A64.

33. Benayoun L, Druilhe A, Dombret MC, Aubier M, Pretolani M. Airway structural alterations selectively associated with severe asthma. *Am J Respir Crit Care Med* 2003;167:1360–1368.

34. Lange P, Parner J, Vestbo J, Schnohr P, Jensen G. A 15-year follow-up study of ventilatory function in adults with asthma. *N Engl J Med* 1998;339:1194–1200.

35. Niimi A, Matsumoto H, Takemura M, Ueda T, Nakano Y, Mishima M. Clinical assessment of airway remodeling in asthma: utility of computed tomography. *Clin Rev Allergy Immunol* 2004;27:45–58.

36. Ito R, Yokoyama A, Hamada H, Yasuhara Y, Kohno N, Higaki J. Effect of inhaled bronchodilators on air trapping in patients with stable asthma. *J Asthma* 2006;43:125–129.

37. Kasahara K, Shiba K, Ozawa T, Okuda K, Adachi M. Correlation between the bronchial subepithelial layer and whole airway wall thickness in patients with asthma. *Thorax* 2002;57:242–246.

38. de Blic J, Tillie-Leblond I, Emond S, Mahut B, Dang Duy TL, Scheinmann P. High-resolution computed tomography scan and airway remodeling in children with severe asthma. *J Allergy Clin Immunol* 2005;116:750–754.

39. Saglani S, Papaioannou G, Khoo L, et al. Can HRCT be used as a marker of airway remodelling in children with difficult asthma? *Respir Res* 2006;7:46.

40. Niimi A, Matsumoto H, Amitani R, et al. Airway wall thickness in asthma assessed by computed tomography. Relation to clinical indices. *Am J Respir Crit Care Med* 2000;162:1518–1523.

41. Gono H, Fujimoto K, Kawakami S, Kubo K. Evaluation of airway wall thickness and air trapping by HRCT in asymptomatic asthma. *Eur Respir J* 2003;22:965–971.

42. Mitsunobu F, Tanizaki Y. The use of computed tomography to assess asthma severity. *Curr Opin Allergy Clin Immunol* 2005;5:85–90.
43. Niimi A, Matsumoto H, Amitani R, et al. Effect of short-term treatment with inhaled corticosteroid on airway wall thickening in asthma. *Am J Med* 2004;116:725–731.
44. Niimi A, Matsumoto H, Takemura M, Ueda T, Chin K, Mishima M. Relationship of airway wall thickness to airway sensitivity and airway reactivity in asthma. *Am J Respir Crit Care Med* 2003;168:983–988.

11

Infectious Small Airways Diseases and Aspiration Bronchiolitis

Kyung Soo Lee

Summary

Infectious bronchiolitis, as a sole component or more frequently as a constellation of histologic findings related to diseases of more proximal airways or alveolated parenchyma, can be caused by respiratory syncytial virus (RSV), *Mycoplasma pneumoniae*, *Chlamydia pneumoniae*, *Streptococcus pneumoniae*, *Hemophilus influenzae*, tuberculous and nontuberculous mycobacterial organisms, and *Aspergillus* species. Infectious bronchiolitis and diffuse aspiration bronchiolitis (DAB) most commonly appear on high-resolution CT (HRCT) scans as centrilobular nodules and branching linear structures in the secondary pulmonary lobules or areas of air trapping.

Key Words: Aspiration; bronchiolar diseases; foreign body reaction; high-resolution CT; pulmonary infection; small airways disease.

1. INTRODUCTION

The term "small airway" refers to airways of <3 mm in diameter, the vast majority of which represent bronchioles. Therefore, small airways disease is often used as synonymous with bronchiolitis. Bronchiolitis refers to an inflammatory lung disease primarily affecting the small conducting airways. It is caused by various conditions and has variable clinical courses, histologic appearances, and imaging findings *(1,2)*.

Bronchiolitis may be an isolated pathologic finding, although it is often a secondary consequence of diseases affecting other parts of the conducting apparatus (e.g., bronchiectasis) or pulmonary acinus (e.g., pneumonia). Divergent causes of bronchiolitis may have similar microscopic findings. Histologically, most examples of bronchiolitis demonstrate acute inflammation, usually corresponding to viral infection *(3,4)*.

The most common high-resolution CT (HRCT) findings of bronchiolitis are centrilobular nodules and branching linear structures in the secondary pulmonary lobules or areas of air trapping. These findings can be helpful in suggesting the presence of bronchiolitis. However, they are nonspecific because there are overlapping features among various kinds of bronchiolitis *(1–3)*.

2. INFECTIOUS BRONCHIOLITIS

Acute bronchiolitis is a term most often used to describe an illness in infants and children characterized by acute wheezing with concomitant signs of respiratory viral infection *(5,6)*. Respiratory syncytial virus (RSV) is the etiologic agent in the majority of patients, but other viruses (adenovirus, influenza, and parainfluenza) and nonviral pathogens (Mycoplasma, Chlamydia) can cause a similar syndrome *(5–7)*. Acute infectious bronchiolitis is occasional in adults. Because small airways in

From: *Contemporary Medical Imaging: CT of the Airways*
Edited by: P. M. Boiselle and D. A. Lynch © Humana Press, Totowa, NJ

adults contribute less to total pulmonary resistance, acute infectious bronchiolitis may spare adults the severe symptoms characteristic of the bronchiolitis in infants. Infectious bronchiolitis in adults, which is usually reversible, may be caused by RSV, *Mycoplasma pneumoniae, Chlamydia pneumoniae, Hemophilus influenzae, Streptococcus pneumoniae*, mycobacterial organisms, and *Aspergillus* species. Constrictive bronchiolitis has been reported in adults as a result of infectious bronchiolitis *(8)*.

3. CAUSES OF NONINFECTIOUS BRONCHIOLITIS

Viral bronchiolitis—RSV pneumonia
Mycoplasmal bronchiolitis
Chlamydia pneumonia
Bacterial bronchiolitis
Bronchiolitis due to granulomatous disease
Bronchiolitis due to *Aspergillus* infection

3.1. Respiratory Syncytial Virus Pneumonia

Worldwide, RSV is the leading viral pathogen responsible for lower respiratory tract infection in children requiring hospitalization. Premature infants and children with chronic lung and congenital heart disease are at greater risk of severe RSV infection. RSV has also been associated with severe respiratory illness not only in the elderly or immunocompromised patients but also in previously healthy adults *(9)*. The spectrum of RSV disease ranges from mild upper respiratory tract infection, lower respiratory infection, to respiratory failure. Primary RSV infection is almost always symptomatic; up to 70% of infants who are first exposed to the virus developed RSV-associated pneumonia (10–30%) or bronchiolitis (50–90%) *(10)*.

Pathology shows acute and chronic inflammation of the bronchioles with associated epithelial necrosis and sloughing. There may be associated edema as well as inflammatory exudates and mucus in the bronchiolar lumen (Fig. 1). In RSV bronchiolitis, respiratory epithelial cells respond to viral infection by producing several chemokines, which recruit and activate neutrophils, lymphocytes, macrophages, eosinophils, and natural killer cells at the site of infection. In addition, chemokine receptor may contribute to mucus production and airway hyperreactivity associated with RSV bronchiolitis *(11,12)*.

A)

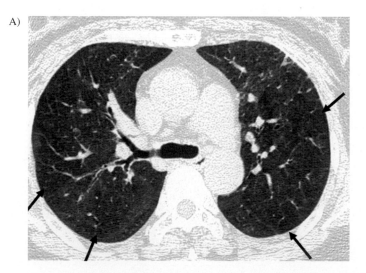

Fig. 1. *(Continued)*

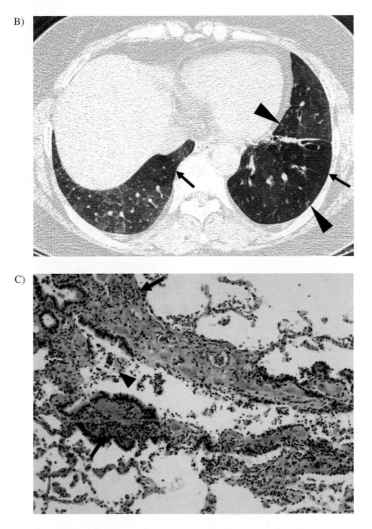

Fig. 1. Infectious bronchiolitis caused by respiratory syncytial virus (RSV) in a 54-year-old woman. (**A**) Transverse lung-window CT (1.0-mm section thickness) scan obtained at the level of right upper lobar bronchus shows multifocal areas (arrows) of mosaic perfusion in both lungs. (**B**) CT scan obtained at the level of liver dome shows patchy areas of mosaic perfusion (arrows). Also note bronchiectasis and tree-in-bud opacities (arrowheads) in left lung. (**C**) Photomicrograph from lung biopsy specimen demonstrates membranous bronchiole thickened with cellular infiltration (arrows). Also note intraluminal desquamated bronchiolar epithelium and inflammatory exudates (arrowhead). (H & E, ×100)

Chest radiography typically demonstrates hyperinflation only *(13)*. Tiny nodules, linear opacities, patchy ground-glass opacities or consolidation, and atelectasis may sometimes be seen. HRCT shows small, ill-defined centrilobular nodules representing bronchioles impacted with inflammatory material and peribronchiolar inflammation; branching linear opacities corresponding to inflamed airway walls; and focal areas of consolidation due to bronchopneumonia. Air trapping is secondary to bronchiolitis *(1–3,14)*.

3.2. Mycoplasma pneumoniae Pneumonia

Mycoplasma pneumoniae is a common cause of community-acquired pneumonia *(15,16)*. Although only 3–10% of patients with *M. pneumoniae* infection develop pneumonia, up to 30% of all pneumonias in general population may be caused by *M. pneumoniae (15–17)*. *M. pneumoniae* infection is typically a disease of children and young adults; however, it is estimated to cause more than 15% of pneumonias in patients >40 years *(17)*. *M. pneumoniae* pneumonia usually has a good prognosis *(15,18)*, but it may occasionally be complicated by adult respiratory distress syndrome, massive pleural effusion, bacterial superinfection, pulmonary fibrosis, or bronchiolitis obliterans *(15)*.

Histologically, *M. pneumoniae* infection is characterized by the presence of acute cellular bronchiolitis, which may progress to bronchopneumonia. The bronchiolitis is characterized by edematous and ulcerative lesions of the bronchiolar walls and by peribronchiolar inflammation containing lymphocytes, plasma cells, and macrophages *(1,19)*. The alveoli surrounding involved bronchioles contain a mononuclear cell infiltration. Parenchymal involvement consists of bronchopneumonia with a lobular distribution. The inflammatory processes are typically bounded by interlobular septae, involving some secondary pulmonary lobules while sparing others. In severe cases, diffuse alveolar damage with fibrinous exudates and hyaline membrane formation may develop *(1,19)*.

The patterns of presentation of *M. pneumoniae* infection on chest radiography are nonspecific, consisting of patchy areas of airspace consolidation, reticular interstitial infiltrates (Fig. 2), or both *(15,16)*. The most distinct abnormality seen on CT consisted of poorly defined centrilobular nodules or tree-in-bud opacities, consistent with bronchiolitis (Figs 2 and 3). The areas of patchy airspace consolidation or ground-glass attenuation frequently had a lobular distribution, a characteristic histologic feature of bronchopneumonia. Although the main abnormalities were in the airspaces, thickening of the axial interstitium and interlobular septa was commonly seen *(20)* (Fig. 3).

3.3. *Chlamydia pneumoniae* Pneumonia

Chlamydia pneumoniae accounts for 6–12% of cases of community-acquired pneumonia and is the third most common pathogen following *S. pneumoniae* and *M. pneumoniae (21,22)*. Chlamydia species, together with *Mycoplasmae*, is known as atypical pneumonia, which is characterized clinically by a nonproductive cough or a mildly elevated or normal white blood cell count. The diagnosis

A)

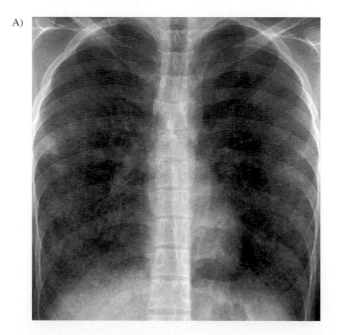

Fig. 2. *(Continued)*

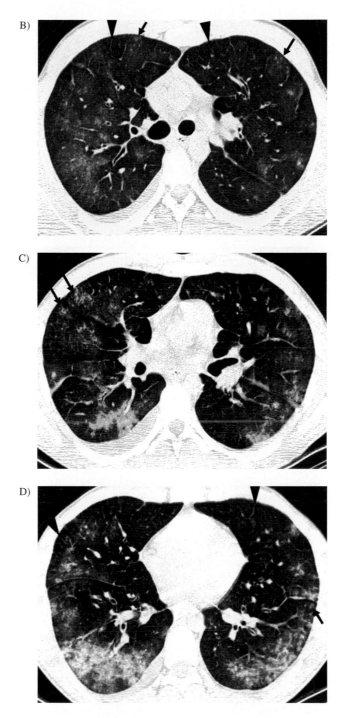

Fig. 2. *Mycoplasma pneumoniae* pneumonia in a 20-year-old man. (**A**) Chest radiograph shows bilateral reticulonodular opacities in both lungs. (**B**) Transverse lung-window CT (1.0-mm section thickness) scan obtained at the level of main bronchi shows poorly defined centrilobular nodules or branching structures (arrows), septal thickening (arrowheads), and patchy ground-glass opacities in both lungs. (**C**) CT scan obtained at the level of bronchus intermedius demonstrates poorly defined tree-in-bud opacities (arrows), lobular opacity (arrowhead), and patchy ground-glass opacities in both lungs. (**D**) CT scan obtained at basal segmental bronchi demonstrates poorly defined tree-in-bud opacities (arrows), septal thickening (arrowheads), and patchy ground-glass opacities in both lungs.

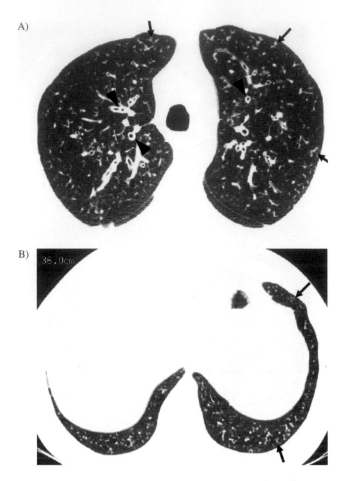

Fig. 3. *Mycoplasma pneumoniae* pneumonia in a 55-year-old man. (**A, B**) Transverse lung-window CT (1.5-mm section thickness) scans obtained at the levels of aortic arch and liver dome, respectively, show tree-in-bud opacities (arrows) and bronchial wall thickening (arrowheads) in both lungs.

of *C. pneumoniae* pneumonia depends on serologic test results, for which we should wait for several days. *C. pneumoniae* often leads to reinfection or chronic infection in patients who carry *C pneumoniae* antibodies and occasionally require a prolonged course of medication to eradicate the disease. *C. pneumoniae* has been noted to be associated with coronary artery disease. Patients with *C. pneumoniae* pneumonia are older in their ages than those with *M. pneumoniae* pneumonia *(23)*.

    Chlamydia pneumoniae pneumonia demonstrates a wide spectrum of HRCT findings including consolidation, bronchovascular bundle thickening, centrilobular small nodules, and airway dilatation that are similar to those of *S. pneumoniae* pneumonia and *M. pneumoniae* pneumonia. Centrilobular nodules and branching linear structures, indicative of bronchiolitis, are seen in about 38% of patients. Airway dilatation and bronchovascular thickening are significantly more frequent in patients with *C pneumoniae* pneumonia than those with *S. pneumoniae* or *M. pneumoniae* pneumonia *(23)* (Fig. 4).

3.4. Bacterial Bronchiolitis

Streptococcus pneumoniae is the most common pathogen in community-acquired pneumonia and accounts for approximately 35% of identified organisms. *H. influenzae* holds 2–8% of identified organisms *(21)*. Although most common patterns are lobar pneumonia (60–70%) for *S. pneumoniae*

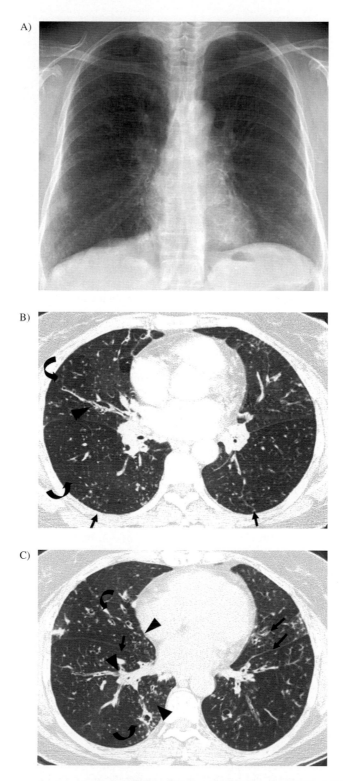

Fig. 4. *(Continued)*

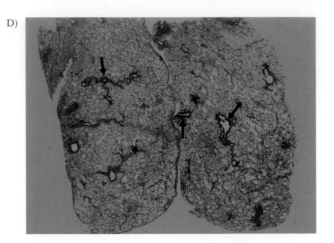

Fig. 4. *Chlamydia pneumoniae* pneumonia in a 58-year-old woman. (**A**) Chest radiograph shows reticulonodular opacities in entire right lung and in the left lower lung zone. (**B, C**) Transverse lung-window CT (1.5-mm section thickness) scans obtained at levels of basal trunk (**B**) and inferior pulmonary veins (**C**), respectively, show tree-in-bud opacities (arrows), bronchial dilatation and wall thickening (arrowheads), and multifocal areas of mosaic perfusion (curved arrows) in both lungs. (**D**) Photomicrograph of biopsy specimen shows cellular bronchiolitis with bronchiolar wall thickening and intraluminal inflammatory cell plugs (arrows) (H & E, ×1).

infection and bronchopneumonia (50–60%) for *H. influenzae*, these organisms may occasionally cause bronchiolitis pattern of disease, by itself or in combination with airspace consolidation *(21,24)*. Bacterial bronchiolitis is more commonly observed in patients with impaired airway defenses. Immunocompromised patients, especially HIV-positive patients and patients with AIDS, are highly susceptible to the more common gram-positive (*Staphylococcus*, *Streptococcus*) and gram-negative (*H. influenzae*, *E. coli*, *Klebsiella*, *Pseudomonas*) bacteria *(25)*. Most inflammatory bronchiolar diseases due to pyogenic infections are diagnosed by noninvasive means and do not require lung biopsy. It is characterized histologically by an active cellular bronchiolitis with mononuclear cell inflammation of the respiratory bronchioles and the presence of an inflammatory exudate and mucus in the bronchiolar lumina.

HRCT findings in pyogenic bronchiolitis consist of a tree-in-bud pattern characterized by small, ill-defined centrilobular lesions and branching linear opacities, and focal areas of consolidation due to bronchopneumonia (Fig. 5). In pyogenic airway infection of AIDS, bronchitis, bronchiolitis, and bronchiectasis are often seen in conjunction and, when pronounced, may be suggested by characteristic chest radiographic findings. When this constellation of combined small and large airways disease is symmetric and is distributed through the lower lobe, it usually suggests a bacterial or less commonly a viral cause. Although similar changes may be seen in patients with mycobacterial infections, these agents far more characteristically cause focal rather than diffuse and symmetric abnormalities. The inflammatory changes in the small airways are reversible in the majority of cases; however, recurrent and persistent infections my lead to bronchiolectasis *(14,25)*.

3.5. Bronchiolitis Due to Granulomatous Disease

Post-primary tuberculosis initially presents as a localized granulomatous inflammatory lesion in the upper lung zone. Caseation necrosis is followed by liquefaction necrosis and is accompanied by formation of cavities and later bronchogenic spread to other parts of the lung or lobe. Bronchogenic spread of tuberculosis appears as tree-in-bud opacity, whereas initial focus of infection manifests as constellation of CT findings of airspace consolidation, cavitation, scattered centrilobular nodules, and

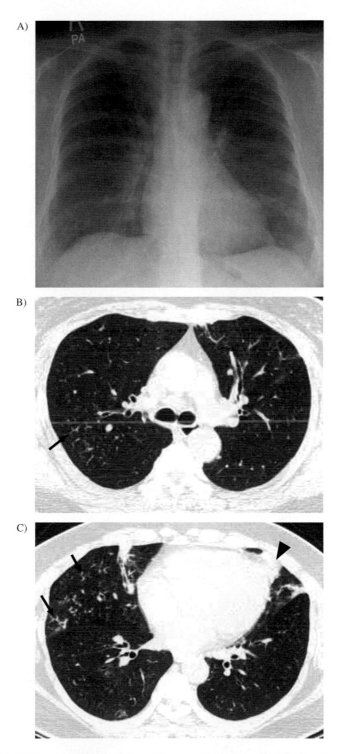

Fig. 5. *Hemophilus influenzae* pneumonia in a 50-year-old woman. (**A**) Chest radiograph shows multiple small nodular densities in both lungs. (**B, C**) Transverse lung-window CT (1.5-mm section thickness) scans obtained at levels of azygos arch and inferior pulmonary veins, respectively, show tree-in-bud opacities (arrows) and lobular (arrowhead) and triangular subpleural consolidation in both lungs.

branching structures (Fig. 6). The tree-in-bud opacity represents a kind of tuberculous bronchiolitis, which is comprised histologically of necrosis and granulomatous inflammation within and immediately adjacent to bronchioles *(26)*.

Nontuberculous mycobacterial (NTM) pulmonary infection in immunocompetent hosts has two distinct radiologic manifestations: an upper lobe cavitary form and a nodular bronchiectatic form *(27)*. The nodular bronchiectatic form usually occurs in middle-aged women without underlying lung disease. The radiologic features of the nodular bronchiectatic form are bronchiectasis and branching

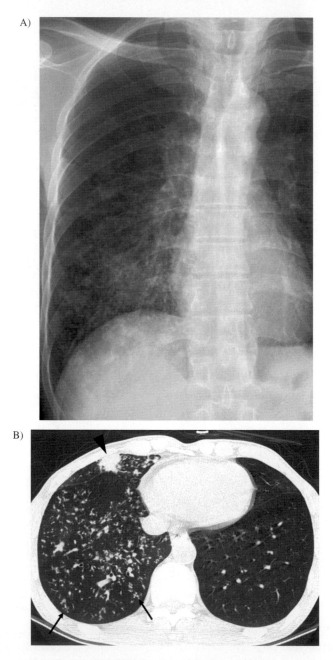

Fig. 6. *(Continued)*

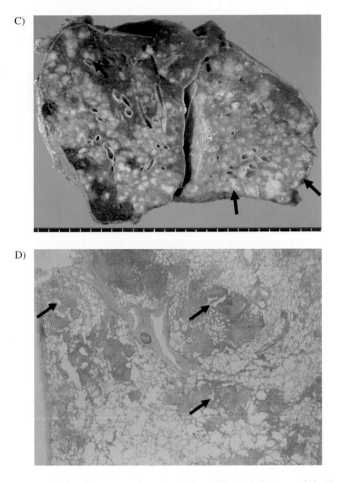

Fig. 6. Bronchogenic spread of pulmonary tuberculosis in a 49-year-old man. (**A**) Chest radiograph shows small nodular lesions in right middle and lower lung zones. (**B**) Transverse lung-window (1.0-mm section thickness) scan obtained at level of suprahepatic inferior vena cava demonstrates tree-in-bud opacities (arrows) in right lower lobe. Also note lobular consolidation (arrowhead) in right middle lobe. (**C**) Photograph of right pneumonectomy pathologic specimen from a different patient demonstrates small nodules of centrilobular location and nodular branching lesions (arrows) which manifested as tree-in-bud opacities on high-resolution CT (HRCT) scans. (**D**) Photomicrograph obtained from branching centrilobular nodules demonstrates relatively well defined lesions, adjacent to small membranous bronchioles (arrows). (H & E, ×40)

centrilobular nodules (tree-in-bud pattern), which are most severe in the lingula and in the right middle lobe (Fig. 7). The tree-in-bud pattern in NTM pulmonary infection, like tuberculous bronchiolitis, again represents NTM granulomas and caseous materials within or around the terminal or respiratory bronchioles. The radiologic findings can be bilateral and extensive and may show no specific lobar predominance *(27,28)*.

3.6. Bronchiolitis Due to Aspergillus Infection

Airway invasive aspergillosis accounts for about 15–30% of cases of invasive pulmonary *Aspergillus* infection *(29)*. It is characterized histologically by liquefactive necrosis and a neutrophilic infiltrate that is centered about membranous and respiratory bronchioles. Its most common radiographic presentation consists of patchy unilateral or bilateral areas of consolidation. HRCT demonstrates

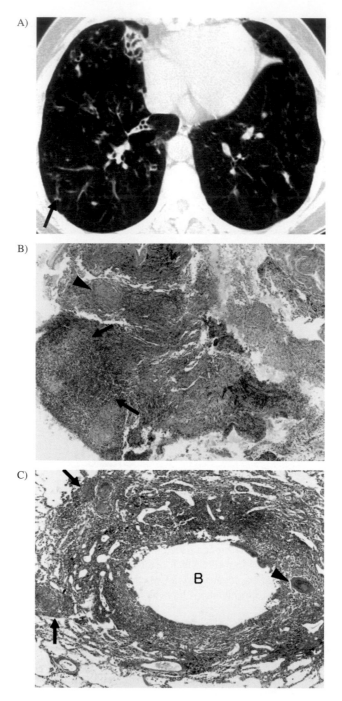

Fig. 7. Nontuberculous mycobacterial (*Mycobacterium avium-intracellulare* complex) pulmonary infection in a 58-year-old woman. (**A**) Transverse lung-window CT (2.5-mm section thickness) scan obtained at the level of suprahepatic inferior vena cava shows varicose bronchiectasis with volume loss, tree-in-bud opacities (arrows) in right middle lung lobe, lingular division of left upper lobe, and both lower lobes. (**B**) Photomicrograph shows infiltration of lymphocytes with mural granulomas (arrows) at the bronchiolar wall. A small granuloma (arrowhead) in the peribronchiolar interstitium also is shown (H & E, ×40). (**C**) Photomicrograph obtained from different area from B demonstrates well-defined granulomas (arrows) around inflamed bronchiole (B). Also note the Langhans-type giant cells (arrowhead) (H & E, ×100) (from ref. *27*, with permission).

centrilobular nodules and branching linear opacities (tree-in-bud pattern), and patchy areas of consolidation often with a peribronchial distribution (Fig. 8). These findings histologically correspond to foci of necrotizing bronchitis and bronchiolitis, typically associated with a neutrophilic inflammatory reaction. In such situations, *Aspergillus* organisms can be observed to have infiltrated airway walls and immediately adjacent parenchyma *(29)*.

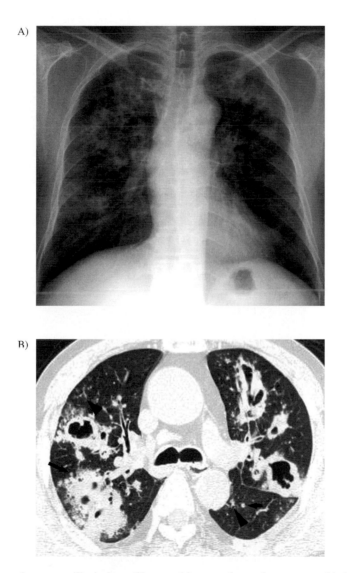

Fig. 8. Airway invasive aspergillosis in a 59-year-old man who underwent steroid therapy for arthritis. **(A)** Chest radiograph shows bronchial dilatation and wall thickening along with peribronchial consolidation in bilateral upper and middle lung zones. **(B)** Transverse lung-window CT (1.0-mm section thickness) scan obtained at the level of main bronchi shows bronchial dilatation, wall thickening, peribronchial consolidation and ground-glass opacity, and cavity formation in both lungs. Also note accompanying centrilobular nodules (arrows) and tree-in-bud opacities (arrowheads) in both lungs. (Courtesy of Dr. Yeon Joo Jeong, Department of Radiology, Pusan National University Hospital, Pusan, Korea)

4. ASPIRATION BRONCHIOLITIS

Diffuse aspiration bronchiolitis (DAB) is characterized by a chronic inflammatory reaction of the bronchioles to recurrently aspirated foreign particles *(30)*. Oropharyngeal dysphagia is observed in half of the patients with DAB, and two-thirds of patients with DAB are bedridden. The onset of DAB is more insidious than aspiration pneumonia, and in half of the patients with DAB, episodes of aspiration are unrecognized. Neurologic disorders and dementia are commonly associated disease (52 and 48%, respectively) *(30,31)*.

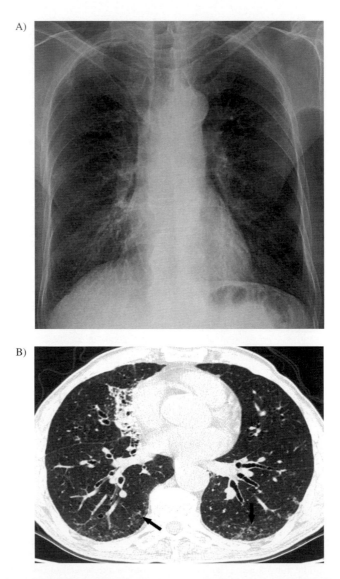

Fig. 9. Aspiration bronchiolitis in a 66-year-old man with gastroesophageal reflux disease. (**A**) Chest radiograph shows reticulonodular densities in both lungs. (**B**) Transverse lung-window CT (1.0-mm section thickness) scan obtained at the level of inferior pulmonary veins demonstrates bronchiectasis and volume decrease in right middle lobe and tree-in-bud opacities (arrows) in both lower lobes.

The cut surface of gross pathologic specimen of DAB lung shows diffusely scattered small yellowish nodules that resemble those of diffuse panbronchiolitis. Histologic findings of DAB are characterized by localization of chronic mural inflammation with foreign body reaction on bronchioles. Recurrence of small amounts of aspiration may play a role in the pathogenesis of DAB *(30)*.

Radiograph shows small, 1- to 3-mm nodular opacities, although nodules as large as 1 cm in diameter have been observed *(32,33)*. On HRCT, DAB manifests as centrilobular nodules, some with the tree-in-bud configuration *(32,33)* (Fig. 9). In patients with these findings, the tree-in-bud pattern reflects the presence of bronchiolar impaction with secretions. A granulomatous pneumonitis caused by aspiration of leguminous vegetables is known as lentil aspiration pneumonia, which manifests as small poorly defined nodules up to 10 mm in diameter on radiographs and CT scans *(32)*.

5. CONCLUSION

Small airways disease, which refers to an inflammatory lung disease primarily affecting the small conducting airways, is often used as synonymous with bronchiolitis. Bronchiolitis is pathologically defined as any inflammatory process that involves air-conducting passages measuring <2 mm in diameter. Bronchiolitis often represents one component in a constellation of histologic findings related to diseases of more proximal airways or alveolated parenchyma. As an isolated microscopic finding, it is etiologically nonspecific and thus should be interpreted in the context of clinical presentation and radiographic features. Infectious bronchiolitis can be caused by RSV, *M. pneumoniae*, *C. pneumoniae*, *S. pneumoniae*, *H. influenzae*, tuberculous and nontuberculous mycobacterial organisms, and *Aspergillus* species. Infectious bronchiolitis and DAB most commonly appear on HRCT scans as centrilobular nodules and branching linear structures in the secondary pulmonary lobules or areas of air trapping.

REFERENCES

1. Müller NL, Miller RR. Diseases of the bronchioles: CT and histopathologic findings. *Radiology* 1995;196:3–12.
2. Franquet T, Müller NL. Disorders of the small airways: high-resolution computed tomographic features. *Semin Respir Crit Care Med* 2003;24:437–444.
3. Ryu JH, Myers JL, Swensen SJ. Bronchiolar disorders. *Am J Respir Crit Care Med* 2003;168:1277–1292.
4. Visscher DW, Myers JL. Bronchiolitis: the pathologist's perspective. *Proc Am Thorac Soc* 2006;3:41–47.
5. Hall CB. Respiratory syncytial virus and parainfluenza virus. *N Engl J Med* 2001;344:1917–1928.
6. Andersen P. Pathogenesis of lower respiratory tract infections due to *Chlamydia*, *Mycoplasma*, *Legionella* and viruses. *Thorax* 1998;53:302–307.
7. Myers JL, Colby TV. Pathologic manifestations of bronchiolitis, constrictive bronchiolitis, cryptogenic organizing pneumonia, and diffuse panbronchiolitis. *Clin Chest Med* 1993;14:611–622.
8. Penn CC, Liu C. Bronchiolitis following infection in adults and children. *Clin Chest Med* 1993;14:645–654.
9. Mejias A, Chavez-Bueno S, Ramilo O. Respiratory syncytial virus pneumonia: mechanisms of inflammation and prolonged airway hyperresponsiveness. *Curr Opin Infect Dis* 2005;18:199–204.
10. Psarras S, Papadopoulos NG, Johnston SL. Pathogenesis of respiratory syncytial virus bronchiolitis-related wheezing. *Paediatr Respir Rev* 2004;5:S179–S184.
11. Harrison AM, Bonville CA, Rosenberg HF, Domachowske JB. Respiratory syncytical virus-induced chemokine expression in the lower airways: eosinophil recruitment and degranulation. *Am J Respir Crit Care Med* 1999;159:1918–1924.
12. Miller AL, Strieter RM, Gruber AD, Ho SB, Lukacs NW. CXCR2 regulates respiratory syncytial virus-induced airway hyperreactivity and mucus overproduction. *J Immunol* 2003;170:3348–3356.
13. Coffin SE. Bronchiolitis: in-patient focus. *Pediatr Clin North Am* 2005;52:1047–1057.
14. Franquet T, Stern EJ. Bronchiolar inflammatory diseases: high-resolution CT findings with histologic correlation. *Eur Radiol* 1999;9:1290–1303.
15. Mansel JK, Rosenow EC, Smith TF. *Mycoplasma pneumoniae* pneumonia. *Chest* 1989;95:639–646.
16. Tanaka N, Matsumoto T, Kuramitsu T, et al. High resolution CT findings in community-acquired pneumonia. *J Comput Assist Tomogr* 1996;20:600–608.
17. Talkington DF, Thacker WL, Keller DW, et al. Diagnosis of *Mycoplasma pneumoniae* infection in autopsy and open-lung biopsy tissues by nested PCR. *J Clin Microbiol* 1998;4:1151–1153.

18. Moine P, Vercken JB, Chevret S, Chastang C, Gajdos P. Severe community-acquired pneumonia. Etiology, epidemiology, and prognosis factors. French Study Group for Community-Acquired Pneumonia in the Intensive Care Unit. *Chest* 1994;105:1487–1495.

19. Worthy SA, Müller NL. Small airway diseases. *Radiol Clin North Am* 1998;36:163–173.

20. Reittner P, Müller NL, Heyneman L, et al. *Mycoplasma pneumoniae* pneumonia: radiographic and high-resolution CT features in 28 patients. *AJR Am J Roentgenol* 2000;174:37–41.

21. Ruiz M, Ewig S, Marcos MA, et al. Etiology of community-acquired pneumonia: impact of age, comorbidity, and severity. *Am J Respir Crit Care Med* 1999;160:397–405.

22. Kuo CC, Jackson LA, Campbell LA, Grayston JT. *Chlamydia pneumoniae* (TWAR). *Clin Microbiol Rev* 1995;8:451–461.

23. Nambu A, Saito A, Araki T, et al. Chlamydia pneumoniae: comparison with findings of Mycoplasma pneumoniae and Streptococcus pneumoniae at thin-section CT. *Radiology* 2005;238:330–338.

24. Pearlberg J, Haggar AM, Saravolatz L, et al. *Hemophilus influenzae* pneumonia in the adult. Radiographic appearance with clinical correlation. *Radiology* 1984;151:23–26.

25. McGuinness G, Gruden JF, Bhalla M, Harkin TJ, Jagirdar JS, Naidich DP. AIDS-related airway disease. *AJR Am J Roentgenol* 1997;168:67–77.

26. Lee JY, Lee KS, Jung K-J, et al. Pulmonary tuberculosis: CT-pathologic correlation. *J Comput Assist Tomogr* 2000;24:691–698.

27. Jeong YJ, Lee KS, Koh WJ, Han J, Kim TS, Kwon OJ. Nontuberculous mycobacterial pulmonary infection in immunocompetent patients: comparison of thin-section CT and histopathologic findings. *Radiology* 2004;231:880–886.

28. Koh WJ, Lee KS, Kwon OJ, Jeong YJ, Kwak SH, Kim TS. Bilateral bronchiectasis and bronchiolitis at thin-section CT: diagnostic implications in nontuberculous mycobacterial pulmonary infection. *Radiology* 2005;235:282–288.

29. Logan PM, Primack SL, Miller RR, Müller NL. Invasive aspergillosis of the airways: radiographic, CT, and pathologic findings. *Radiology* 1994;193:383–388.

30. Matsuse T, Oka T, Kida K, Fukuchi Y. Importance of diffuse aspiration bronchiolitis caused by chronic occult aspiration in the elderly. *Chest* 1996;110:1289–1293.

31. Teramoto S, Yamamoto H, Yamaguchi Y, et al. Diffuse aspiration bronchiolitis due to achalasia. *Chest* 2004;125:349–350.

32. Marom EM, McAdams HP, Sporn TA, Goodman PC. Lentil aspiration pneumonia: radiographic and CT findings. *J Comput Assist Tomogr* 1998;22:598–600.

33. Janoski MM, Raymond GS, Puttagunta L, Man GC, Barrie JR. Psyllium aspiration causing bronchiolitis: radiographic, high-resolution CT, and pathologic findings. *AJR Am J Roentgenol* 2000;174:799–801.

Noninfectious Inflammatory Small Airways Diseases

David A. Lynch

Summary

Multiple noninfectious diseases should be considered in the differential diagnosis of noninfectious small airways diseases. Diffuse panbronchiolitis, most commonly seen in Asian individuals, shows typical features of inflammatory bronchiolitis, with tree in bud pattern, bronchiolectasis, and associated bronchiolectasis and sinusitis. Follicular bronchiolitis is typically seen in Sjögren's syndrome or immunodeficiency. Inflammatory bronchiolitis may be seen after acute inhalation injury, with chronic exposure to burning biomass fuels, and in pneumoconioses. CT features of inflammatory bronchiolitis may also be found with diffuse lung disease such as hypersensitivity pneumonitis, sarcoidosis, or Langerhans histiocytosis, and with collagen vascular disease or inflammatory bowel disease.

Key Words: Diffuse panbronchiolitis; follicular bronchiolitis; Sjögren's syndrome; toxic fume inhalation; bronchocentric granulomatosis.

1. CLASSIFICATION OF NONINFECTIOUS SMALL AIRWAYS DISEASE

While most inflammatory small airways disease is due to infection or aspiration, noninfectious entities should also be considered in the differential diagnosis of the CT appearances of inflammatory small airways disease. These noninfectious entities are listed in Table 1. Diffuse Panbronchiolitis will be discussed first because its CT appearances are prototypic.

2. DIFFUSE PANBRONCHIOLITIS

Diffuse panbronchiolitis (DPB) is an idiopathic transmural inflammation of the respiratory bronchioles which occurs primarily in East Asia, particularly in Japanese adults. Though most widely recognized in Japan, it has now been described in most parts of the world, including the USA *(1–3)*, South America *(4)*, Turkey *(5)*, and Scandinavia *(6)*. Indeed, it may be under-recognized in non-Asian people *(1)*. The higher prevalence of this disease in Asia is likely related to genetic predisposition, as panbronchiolitis is associated with several genes that are more prevalent in Asians *(7)*. In Japanese patients, it appears to be associated with the human leukocyte antigen (HLA) Bw54, whereas in Koreans it appears to be associated with HLA A11 *(8)*. More detailed genetic linkage analysis suggests that an HLA-associated major susceptibility gene for DPB is probably located in the class I region, 300 kb telomeric of the HLA-B locus on the chromosome 6p21.3 *(9)*. Additionally, panbronchiolitis is associated with a polymorphism of the *MUC5B* gene *(10)*.

DPB may be associated with various underlying diseases. Patients infected by human T-cell lymphotropic virus type 1 (HTLV-1) may develop a bronchiolitis that is clinically and pathologically similar to DPB, though it may respond less well to treatment *(11)*. Because HTLV-1 may

From: *Contemporary Medical Imaging: CT of the Airways*
Edited by: P. M. Boiselle and D. A. Lynch © Humana Press, Totowa, NJ

Table 1
Noninfectious Inflammatory Small Airways Diseases

Inhalational lung disease
  Respiratory bronchiolitis related to cigarette smoking
  Acute toxic inhalation
  Hut lung
  Hypersensitivity pneumonitis
  Pneumoconiosis
    Asbestosis
    Silicosis
    Flock
Bronchiolitis associated with bronchiectasis
Bronchiolitis occurring as component of diffuse lung diseases
  Hypersensitivity pneumonitis
  Sarcoidosis
Bronchiolitis associated with systemic diseases
  Collagen vascular disease
  Inflammatory bowel disease
Miscellaneous
  Diffuse panbronchiolitis
  Follicular bronchiolitis
  Eosinophilic bronchiolitis
  Bronchocentric granulomatosis

be associated with T-cell leukemia, patients with this condition may also suffer from panbronchiolitis *(12)*. There is an association between DPB and thymoma *(13,14)* (Fig. 1); these patients may also have hypogammaglobulinemia *(15,16)*. As discussed below, patients with rheumatoid arthritis or inflammatory bowel disease may also develop DPB.

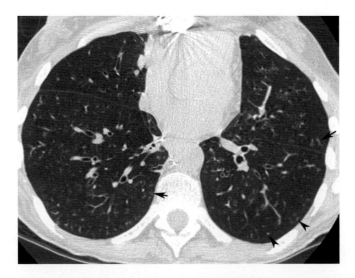

Fig. 1. Panbronchiolitis pattern in 44-year-old woman with history of resection of thymoma. Thin-section CT shows widespread centrilobular nodularity with tree in bud pattern and mild cylindric bronchiectasis. Pseudomonas grew from culture.

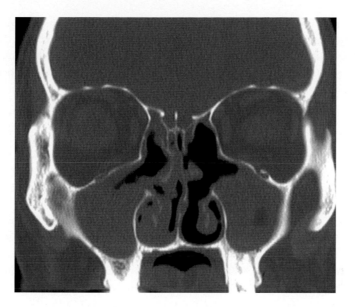

Fig. 2. Panbronchiolitis in a 52-year-old Caucasian man. Sinus CT shows evidence of previous surgery and extensive mucosal thickening due to sinusitis.

Patients with DPB typically present with subacute onset of cough productive of purulent sputum, dyspnea, and physiologic evidence of airway obstruction. On physical examination, coarse crackles are usually found. Physiologic evaluation reveals evidence of airway obstruction, sometimes associated with restriction, and hypoxia is common. Often these patients acquire the clinical label of chronic obstructive pulmonary disease (COPD), but most are nonsmokers. Organisms characteristically found in the sputum include *Hemophilus influenzae, Streptococcus pneumoniae,* and, typically in more advanced disease, *Pseudomonas aeruginosa (17).* Associated sinusitis is found in more than 80% of cases (Fig. 2) *(17–19).* The disease is typically found in adults, with a mean age of onset of 40 years *(17),* though it has been described in childhood *(20).* As the disease progresses, progressive airway obstruction occurs, complicated by recurrent acute bacterial infections, and may culminate in respiratory failure *(1).* The Japanese Ministry of Health and Welfare has published diagnostic criteria for DPB (Table 2) *(21).*

The most important reason to make the diagnosis of DPB is that it typically responds well to long-term treatment with macrolide antibiotics such as erythromycin or clarithromycin *(22).* This treatment effect may be due in part to antibacterial action but seems to be primarily due to other properties,

Table 2
Diagnostic Criteria for Diffuse Panbronchiolitis *(21)*

All of the following:
Persistent cough, sputum, and exertional dyspnea
Past history of or current sinusitis
Bilateral diffuse small nodular shadows on chest radiograph,
or centrilobular nodular shadows on chest CT scans
At least two of the following:
Bilateral coarse crackles on physical examination
FEV1/FVC ratio <70% and PaO$_2$ <80 mm Hg
Cold agglutinin titers $\geq$64

---

including attenuation of biofilm formation *(23)* and suppression of production of pro-inflammatory cytokines such as interleukin-8 *(24)*. Discovery of these effects in patients with DPB has led to the use of the macrolide antibiotics in other inflammatory small airways diseases, including bronchiolitis related to lung transplantation *(25)* and cystic fibrosis *(23)*. Macrolides have also been used in asthma, but data are inadequate to recommend their widespread use *(26)*.

2.1. Imaging Features

The chest radiographic findings in DPB are of obstructive lung disease, with hyperinflation, associated with fine nodular abnormalities in the lower lungs (Fig. 3). In more advanced disease, ring shadows of bronchiectasis or bronchiolectasis may become radiographically visible. Less commonly, bullae may be seen, and pneumothorax may occur.

High-resolution CT (HRCT) findings are pivotal in the diagnosis of DPB, and indeed chest CT may provide the initial suspicion of this diagnosis. The CT features include centrilobular nodules, tree in bud pattern, cystic bronchiolar dilation, and bronchiectasis (Fig. 4). Mosaic attenuation may be seen, and air trapping may be seen on expiratory images. The abnormalities almost always predominate in the lower lobes. When correlated with pathology, the centrilobular nodules correlate with inflamed bronchioles, tree in bud pattern correlates with secretion-filled bronchioles, and the cystic structures represent dilated bronchioles and bronchi *(27)*. Other imaging findings may include patchy consolidation (perhaps indicating Pseudomonas pneumonia), mucoid impaction in bronchi, and segmental atelectasis *(28)*.

The initial CT descriptions of panbronchiolitis *(29,30)*, and associated radiologic–pathologic correlation *(27)*, were most helpful in improving understanding of the secondary pulmonary lobule and its role in diagnosing small airways disease. An early paper by Akira et al. *(29)* developed an imaging-based classification of panbronchiolitis: Type I centrilobular nodules, Type II centrilobular nodules connected by branching lines, Type III bronchiolectasis, and Type IV bronchiectasis. Classification of panbronchiolitis in this way correlated with the clinical stage of disease and with the pathologic severity of disease.

CT may be very helpful in monitoring the course of patients with DPB. On serial evaluation in untreated patients, centrilobular nodules are found to progress with development of bronchiolectasis and bronchiectasis; conversely, in patients treated with erythromycin, the nodules decrease in size and number, though areas of decreased attenuation may persist (Fig. 4) *(31,32)*. Bronchiolectasis also improves on treatment, but bronchiectasis does not significantly change *(33)*. Improvement in the extent of centrilobular nodules on treatment correlates with physiologic evidence of decreased air trapping *(33)*.

2.2. Differential Diagnosis

There appears to be a form of chronic small airways disease that does not have the characteristic histologic findings of DPB but has clinical and imaging features similar to DPB *(34,35)*: some of these cases may have underlying HTLV-1 infection *(11)* or rheumatoid arthritis. These patients tend to respond less well to macrolide treatment than those with DPB. Other differential diagnostic considerations include chronic infection (particularly mycobacterial infection), cystic fibrosis, ciliary dysmotility, immune deficiency, and chronic aspiration.

In a review of the CT findings of 320 carriers of HTLV-1 *(36)*, 98 subjects had abnormal chest CT scans—almost all of these had centrilobular nodules, whereas thickening of bronchovascular bundles, ground-glass abnormality, and bronchiectasis were each seen in about 50% of cases, and interlobular septal thickening was seen in 29%. Lymph node enlargement was seen in only about 5% of patients.

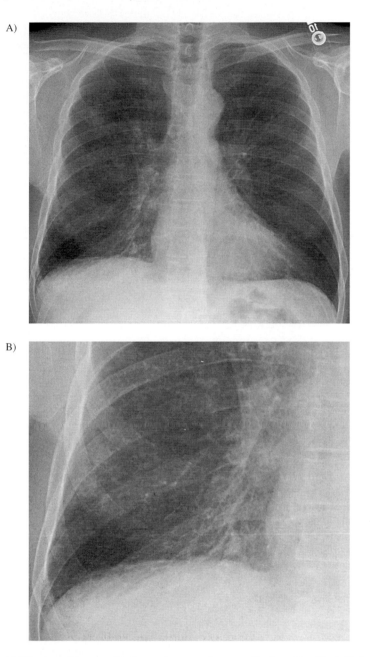

Fig. 3. Panbronchiolitis in a 52-year-old Caucasian man (same patient as Fig. 2). Initial chest radiograph (**A**) shows mild hyperinflation and diffuse airway wall thickening. Focal consolidation in the right upper lobe was due to Pseudomonas pneumonia. (**B**) Detail view of right lower lobe shows a diffuse fine irregular nodular pattern.

On radiologic–pathologic correlation, centrilobular nodules corresponded to lymphocytic infiltration along respiratory bronchioles. Among 46 patients who were treated with erythromycin, centrilobular nodules improved in only 7, remained unchanged in 35, and progressed in 4. In 20 untreated patients who received followup scans, centrilobular nodules progressed in 7.

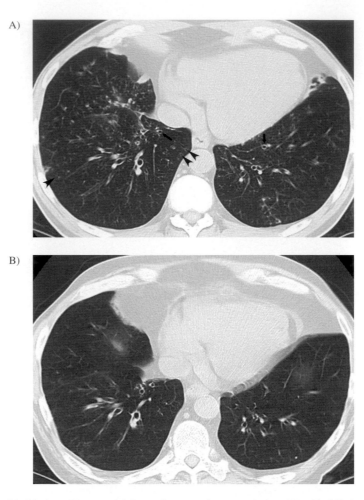

Fig. 4. Panbronchiolitis in a 52-year-old Caucasian man (same patient as Fig. 2). (**A**) CT through the lower lungs shows moderate cylindric bronchiectasis and extensive tree in bud pattern. (**B**) CT obtained 4 months later, following treatment with erythromycin, shows substantial clearing of tree in bud pattern, but persistent bronchiectasis.

3. FOLLICULAR BRONCHIOLITIS

Follicular bronchiolitis is a pathologic entity defined by the presence of abundant hyperplastic lymphoid follicles with germinal centers, distributed along the bronchioles *(37,38)*. The lymphoid population is polyclonal. Within the spectrum of pulmonary lymphoproliferative disease, follicular bronchiolitis is usually regarded as being a form of reactive lymphoid hyperplasia *(39)*. Although the peribronchiolar predominance of the abnormality in follicular bronchiolitis is distinct from the diffuse homogenous lymphocytic infiltration found in lymphoid interstitial pneumonia, there may be some overlap in the histologic and imaging appearances of these reactive disorders. Identification of follicular bronchiolitis may be important because it may respond to treatment with macrolide antibiotics *(40)*.

Although follicular bronchiolitis may be idiopathic, it is frequently associated with underlying collagen vascular disease (especially Sjögren's syndrome and rheumatoid arthritis) and immunodeficiency states including acquired immunodeficiency syndrome *(39)*. It has also been described as the

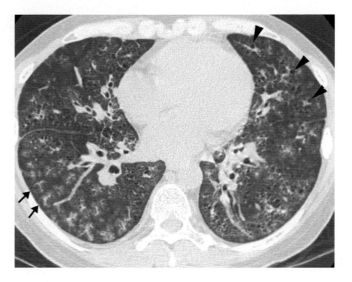

Fig. 5. Follicular bronchiolitis in patient with Sjögren's syndrome. CT shows profuse centrilobular ground-glass abnormality, with tree in bud pattern (arrows). Numerous peribronchial cysts (arrowheads) are thought to be due to bronchiolar obstruction. Similar cysts may be seen in lymphoid interstitial pneumonia.

salient lesion in workers exposed to nylon or polyethylene flock (see Section 4.3) *(41,42)*. Histologic follicular bronchiolitis may also be seen as a subsidiary finding in patients with chronic infections or bronchiectasis *(37)*: the radiologist may have an important role in identifying these conditions when follicular bronchiolitis is seen on biopsy.

On CT scanning of patients with follicular bronchiolitis, centrilobular nodules are universally present and are usually the predominant feature (Fig. 5) *(37,38)*. They may be associated with tree-in-bud pattern. While the nodules are typically small (less than 3 mm), larger nodules measuring up to 10 mm may also be seen. Peribronchial nodules are common, being found in 3 of 6 cases in one study *(37)* and in 5 of 12 patients in another study *(38)*. Ground-glass abnormality is more variable, being seen in 1 of 6 and 9 of 12 patients in these two studies. The presence of ground-glass abnormality is probably indicative of histologic interstitial inflammation, in addition to the peribronchiolar abnormalities.

4. INHALATIONAL LUNG DISEASE

4.1. Toxic Inhalation

Acute or chronic injury to the bronchioles may be caused by a wide variety of inhaled substances (Table 3). Acute bronchiolar injury is generally due to a substantial inhalation of noxious gas or fumes. These agents may also cause lung injury edema. The clinical manifestations of this type of injury probably depends on multiple factors including the type of agent, the concentration, the duration of exposure, and underlying host issues. Acute toxic inhalation injury may cause injury at one or several levels in the respiratory tract, including the upper airway, larynx, trachea, bronchi, bronchioles, and lung parenchyma: the site of maximal injury may depend on the physical characteristics of the inhaled substance, including particle size and water solubility. Typically, inhaled particles greater than 10 μm will be deposited in the upper airway, whereas particles between 0.5 and 10 μm can reach the bronchioles, and those less than 0.5 μm may be exhaled without deposition *(43)*. Irritant gases that are highly water-soluble (e.g., ammonia, sulfur dioxide, hydrogen chloride) tend to dissolve in the upper airways, causing immediate symptoms of conjunctivitis and rhinorrhea. However, less water-soluble

Table 3
Causes of Inhalational Lung Injury

Acute
   Ammonia
   Chlorine
   Hydrogen chloride
   Oxides of nitrogen
   Ozone
   Phosgene
   Smoke
   Sulfur dioxide
   Cocaine
Chronic
   Cigarette smoke
   Particulate matter
   Inhaled dusts
      Silica
      Coal dust
      Asbestos
   Diacetyl
Acute or chronic
   Hypersensitivity pneumonitis

gases such as oxides of nitrogen may cause less immediate symptoms and may penetrate more deeply into the airway tree. For example, in inhalational injury due to burns, sooty particles tend to be deposited in the upper airway and trachea, whereas chemicals from burning plastics may be inhaled deep into the bronchial tree.

The clinical course of acute inhalational injury has been well characterized in individuals with silo-fillers' lung, caused by inhalation of oxides of nitrogen accumulating in a partially filled silo, just above the surface of the grain. Significant exposure typically results in the development of cough, dyspnea, and fever after a latent period of 3–24 h. Bronchospasm is common, with wheezing on examination. Initial chest radiograph is often normal, but noncardiac pulmonary edema may develop. CT may show ground-glass abnormality due to edema, or evidence of bronchiolitis (Fig. 6). Following recovery from the acute phase of lung injury, some patients develop a relapse of symptoms within 3–6 weeks, characterized by severe, progressive airway obstruction, with histologic and imaging findings of bronchiolitis obliterans (Fig. 7).

In addition to the syndromes of acute bronchiolitis and subsequent bronchiolitis obliterans described above, a third consequence of toxic inhalation may be reactive airways dysfunction syndrome (RADS). This syndrome, which begins within 24 h of exposure to a high concentration of respiratory irritant such as chlorine gas, is characterized by airflow obstruction, with increased sensitivity of the airways to bronchoconstrictor agents such as methacholine *(44)*. The imaging features of this syndrome are similar to those of asthma (Fig. 8).

4.2. Anthracosis Related to Biomass Fuels

One of the commonest forms of inhalational lung injury worldwide is related to inhalation of burning biomass fuels. Biomass fuels include wood, hay, straw, and dried dung: in the developing world, these are often burned in enclosed, poorly ventilated huts for cooking and heating. On combustion, they release large quantities of carbon (soot) particles, which are inhaled by inhabitants (Fig. 9). Consequences of lung-term inhalation of these particulate materials are not well documented

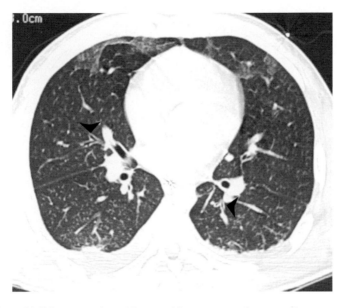

Fig. 6. Cellular bronchiolitis pattern in a 17-year-old man exposed to an unknown toxin in an automobile body shop. Thin-section CT shows marked diffuse airway wall thickening and widespread tree in bud pattern. Ground-glass abnormality in the anterior lung is presumed to represent lung injury edema.

but may include symptoms of recurrent respiratory infections and symptomatic chronic bronchitis or COPD. Patients may develop anthracotic bronchial plaques *(45)*. They are probably at increased risk of development of lung cancer. In a 2002 WHO report, the global burden of disease attributed to indoor air pollution from biomass combustion accounted for 2.7% of all worldwide disability adjusted life-years lost, placing indoor smoke as the second largest environmental contributor to poor health, behind unsafe water and sanitation *(46)*. Indoor smoke was said to account for 4–5% of global mortality, with 56% of these deaths related to childhood acute lower respiratory infections and the remainder due to COPD and lung cancer, primarily in women.

The term "hut lung" has been applied to the domestically acquired particulate lung disease related to inhalation of burning biomass fuels *(47,48)*. Some individuals with radiographic evidence of hut lung may be asymptomatic *(47,49)*. When symptoms are present, cough (productive or nonproductive) is most common *(48)*, followed by dyspnea on exertion. Symptoms typically persist after removal from exposure *(48)*. Chronic hypoxia may lead to cor pulmonale. Physical examination may show wheezes or crackles. Histologically, the most common finding is anthracosis, either involving the bronchi or the around the bronchioles in the lung parenchyma *(47,48)*. A similar anthracotic condition has been described in a charcoal worker *(48)*, and we have seen a similar condition in an individual exposed to burning diesel oil (Fig. 9).

The imaging features of hut lung and related anthracotic conditions have been evaluated in several case reports and two series *(45,47–49)*. In the initial description of 25 patients by Grobbelaar et al. *(47)*, the findings on chest radiographs were similar to those of silicosis, with features ranging from a fine nodular pattern to a pattern of progressive massive fibrosis. Indeed, some of these patients had previously been assumed to have silicosis from grinding grain ("Transkei silicosis"). On CT scanning, the nodules may be centrilobular *(48)*, or may be distributed along the bronchovascular bundle *(45)*. Septal thickening and lymphadenopathy may also be seen *(45)*.

In a study from Turkey, Kara et al. compared the HRCT findings in 32 asymptomatic women exposed to biomass fuels, 30 symptomatic biomass-exposed women, and 30 asymptomatic unexposed

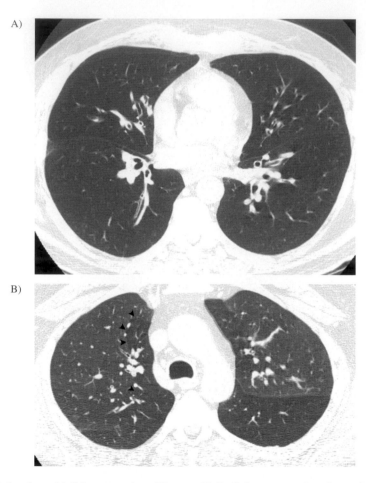

Fig. 7. Constrictive bronchiolitis pattern in a 53-year-old firefighter exposed to fumes in a burning home. Initial chest CT was normal. (**A**) CT obtained 4 weeks later shows diffuse airway wall thickening and decreased lung attenuation. (**B**) Expiratory CT at a higher level shows marked patchy air trapping.

controls *(49)*. The most common findings in the asymptomatic exposed were ground-glass abnormality, fibrotic bands, and irregular pleural interfaces. Surprisingly, nodules and peribronchovascular thickening were relatively uncommon, being seen in only about 25% of cases, and were almost equally prevalent in the symptomatic and asymptomatic exposed groups. Whereas ground-glass abnormality and irregular pleural interfaces were less common in the symptomatic exposed group than in the asymptomatic subjects, pleural thickening (often associated with calcification), mosaic attenuation, bullae, and bronchiectasis (largely traction bronchiectasis) were more common in the symptomatic group. The findings of this and other studies suggest that in individuals with biomass exposure, the presence of nodules on chest radiograph or chest CT is often not associated with symptoms: the presence of fibrosis, with bullae and traction bronchiectasis, and associated pleural thickening is more commonly associated with symptoms.

4.3. Flock Lung

Flock is a fine nylon fiber that is applied to backing to produce the plush material used in luxury upholstery, wallpaper, greeting cards, and many other products. The manufacture of this product may result in a dust of tiny respirable fibers that can reach the alveoli. Some flock workers develop a

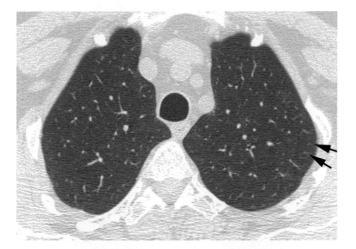

Fig. 8. Reactive airways dysfunction syndrome (RADS) in a 53-year-old woman following exposure to ammonia. CT shows subtle centrilobular thickening (arrows).

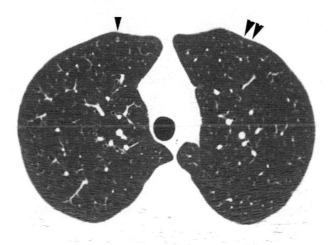

Fig. 9. Anthracosis in a 38-year-old man who developed cough and physiologic impairment following occupational exposure to burning diesel fuel. CT shows centrilobular nodularity (arrowheads). Biopsy confirmed peribronchiolar anthracosis.

respiratory illness called flockworkers' lung, characterized pathologically by a pattern of lymphocytic bronchiolitis and peribronchiolitis with lymphoid hyperplasia *(50)*. On HRCT scanning, flockworkers' lung is characterized by a combination of ground-glass attenuation (Fig. 10) and centrilobular nodularity, sometimes appearing similar to the findings in hypersensitivity pneumonitis or respiratory bronchiolitis *(51)*. HRCT may identify similar findings in symptomatic patients who do not meet current criteria for flockworkers' lung. In a study of 43 workers exposed to flock, 30 had an abnormal CT scan, including 19 who did not meet clinical criteria for the disease *(51)*. Among the 11 workers with clinical flock workers lung, 10 had ground-glass abnormality, while 9 had micronodules. Reticular opacity, consolidation, traction bronchiectasis, and septal thickening were seen in a minority of these individuals. Among 32 exposed workers who did not meet clinical criteria for disease, micronodules were most common finding, being seen in 16, while ground-glass abnormality was seen in 13

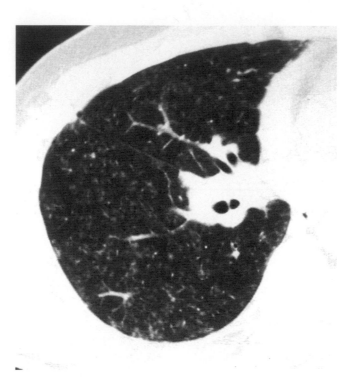

Fig. 10. Flockworkers' lung in a 28-year-old man. CT shows profuse, poorly defined centrilobular nodules with tree in bud pattern. Biopsy showed lymphocytic bronchiolitis.

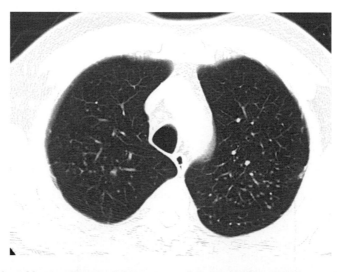

Fig. 11. Silicosis in a 66-year-old man. CT shows centrilobular nodules, best seen in the posterior left upper lobe. Coalescence of nodules along the left lateral chest wall results in "pseudoplaques."

individuals. Most of these workers were symptomatic and likely had mild disease. In the individuals with flock workers lung, the abnormalities tend to improve after withdrawal from exposure.

4.4. Pneumoconioses

Bronchiolitis is described as part of the pathology in most of the pneumoconioses, including coal workers' pneumoconiosis, silicosis, and asbestosis *(52)*. Centrilobular nodularity and tree in bud pattern may sometimes be the predominant manifestation of any of these entities (Fig. 11). In a review of the CT findings in workers with pneumoconiosis, Akira et al. found centrilobular nodules and branching opacities, often associated with centrilobular emphysema, in all 55 patients who were classified as having type p opacities by the ILO classification system *(53)*.

5. BRONCHIOLITIS ASSOCIATED WITH DIFFUSE LUNG DISEASES

Several diffuse lung diseases are characterized by bronchiolar or peribronchiolar involvement as a major or minor component and must therefore be considered in the differential diagnosis of bronchiolitis.

5.1. Hypersensitivity Pneumonitis

Bronchiolitis is a characteristic pathologic feature of hypersensitivity pneumonitis, being seen on biopsy in over 50% of cases of chronic hypersensitivity pneumonitis *(54)* and even more commonly in acute or subacute hypersensitivity pneumonitis. Airway obstruction is commonly found on physiologic evaluation of individuals with hypersensitivity pneumonitis. The centrilobular nodules commonly identified on CT in this condition reflect peribronchiolar inflammation, whereas mosaic attenuation and expiratory air trapping reflect bronchiolar obstruction (Fig. 12). Tree in bud pattern may be seen in some cases of hypersensitivity pneumonitis.

5.2. Sarcoidosis

Because of the perilymphatic distribution of sarcoid granulomas, the granulomas often cluster around large and small airways, and airway obstruction is a common physiologic finding in this condition. On CT scanning, centrilobular nodules and air trapping may be seen (Fig. 13).

5.3. Langerhans Cell Histiocytosis

The characteristic granulomas and stellate scars of Langerhans cell histiocytosis are typically centered on the bronchiole. The nodules of this condition are typically centrilobular, and the characteristic cysts are thought to be related to distal bronchiolar obstruction. This condition is more fully discussed in Chapter 14.

6. BRONCHIOLITIS ASSOCIATED WITH SYSTEMIC DISEASES

6.1. Collagen Vascular Disease

Rheumatoid arthritis is associated with several types of bronchiolitis. Constrictive bronchiolitis (discussed in Chapter 13) appears to be the most common. Follicular bronchiolitis *(38,40,55–57)* and panbronchiolitis *(58–61)* may also be found.

6.2. Inflammatory Bowel Disease

Ulcerative colitis and Crohn's disease are associated with a wide variety of uncommon pulmonary complications. These complications may precede the diagnosis of inflammatory bowel disease or may present many years after the initial diagnosis, and even after complete colectomy for ulcerative colitis

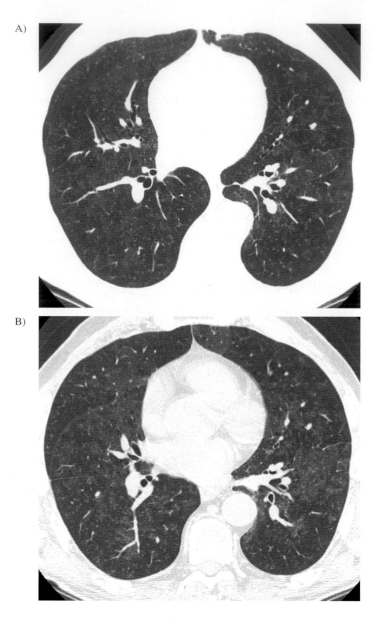

Fig. 12. Hypersensitivity pneumonitis related to *Mycobacterium avium* complex in a 70-year-old man with an indoor swimming pool. (**A**) Inspiratory CT shows profuse poorly defined centrilobular nodules and ground-glass abnormality. (**B**) Expiratory CT shows moderate air trapping.

(62). Both conditions can be associated with an intense tracheobronchitis, sometimes associated with subglottic, tracheal, or bronchial stenosis *(63,64)*. Bronchiectasis may also occur (Fig. 14). Small airway involvement can have a histologic pattern of panbronchiolitis *(65)* or, in Crohn's disease, of granulomatous bronchiolitis *(66)*.

In a series of seven patients with inflammatory airway disease related to ulcerative colitis, *(64)* all had bronchial wall thickening, six had bronchiectasis, and three had airway stenosis. Four patients had evidence of small airways disease with a pattern similar to that of panbronchiolitis. A more recent

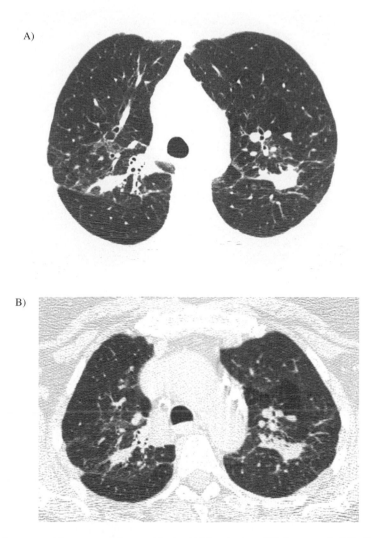

Fig. 13. Fifty-five-year old woman with sarcoidosis. (**A**) Inspiratory CT shows typical findings of sarcoidosis, with centrilobular nodules, septal thickening, ground-glass abnormality, peribronchovascular conglomeration, and bronchial distortion. (**B**) Expiratory CT shows multifocal air trapping.

case series by Mahadeva and coworkers included 3 symptomatic patients with Crohn's disease and 14 with ulcerative colitis *(62)*. Among the three patients with Crohn's disease, one had bronchiectasis with tree in bud pattern (Fig. 14), one had bronchiectasis alone, and one had marked air trapping. In the 14 patients with ulcerative colitis, 4 had bronchiectasis with tree in bud pattern (Fig. 15) and 7 had bronchiectasis without tree in bud pattern. Eight patients had air trapping.

7. BRONCHOCENTRIC GRANULOMATOSIS

This uncommon condition, first described by Liebow in 1973, *(67)* differs from Wegener granulomatosis in that it is localized to the lung, and centered around airways (bronchocentric) rather than vessels (angiocentric). Pathologically, small airways and bronchioles are filled and replaced

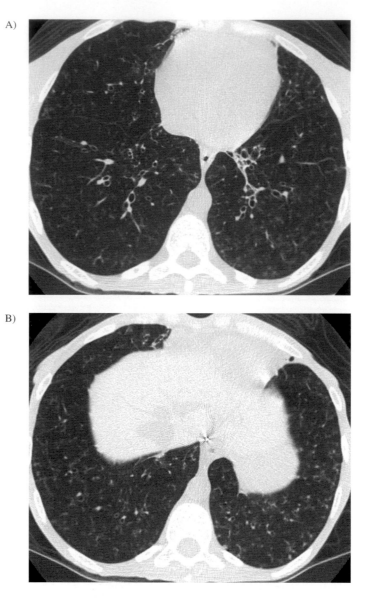

Fig. 14. Panbronchiolitis related to Crohn's disease in 30-year-old female. (**A, B**) CT images show basal predominant cylindrical bronchiectasis and widespread tree in bud pattern.

by cellular debris and necrotic granulomas surrounded by palisaded epithelioid cells. Large airways may show mucoid impaction, and the distal lung is often consolidated by an eosinophilic or obstructive pneumonitis. Vasculitic changes appear to be minor and incidental. There is evidence that bronchocentric granulomatosis in asthmatics is etiologically different from that seen in nonasthmatics. In asthmatics, the major part of the cellular infiltrate is made up of eosinophils, whereas in nonasthmatics the plasma cell is dominant *(68)*. In many asthmatics, there is histological, serological, and microbiological evidence that bronchocentric granulomatosis is caused by *Aspergillus* and forms part of the spectrum of allergic bronchopulmonary aspergillosis *(69,70)*. In nonasthmatics, the cause

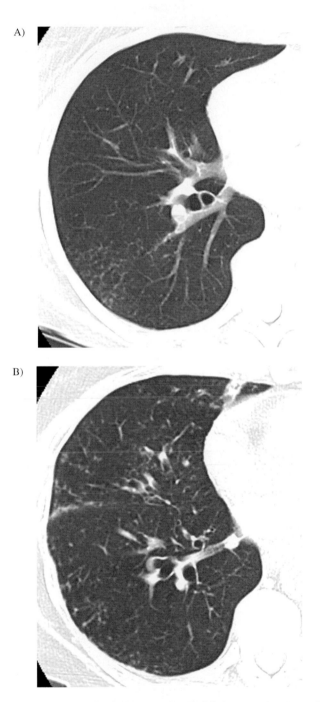

Fig. 15. Diffuse panbronchiolitis related to ulcerative colitis. (**A**) Baseline CT shows focal tree in bud pattern in the right lower lobe. (**B**) Followup 3 years later shows substantial progression of tree in bud pattern, associated with diffuse cylindrical bronchiectasis.

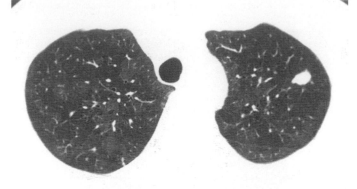

Fig. 16. Bronchocentric granulomatosis. CT through the upper lobes shows a focal left upper lobe nodule, associated with diffuse mosaic attenuation. (Courtesy of Dr Lawrence Goodman, Medical College of Wisconsin)

is generally obscure though recently cases have been reported associated with tuberculosis and a variety of fungi *(69)*.

Only four series of patients with bronchocentric granulomatosis have been recorded *(68,71–73)*, representing a total of 60 cases. However, there have been many additional case reports. Patients commonly present in their forties, but there is a wide age range (9–76 years) and a tendency for asthmatics to present at a younger age (mean age, 22 years) than nonasthmatics (mean age, 50 years) *(68)*. The incidence in both sexes is equal. Sixteen (29%) of 55 patients in the described series were asthmatic *(68,71–73)*. Symptoms may be absent or minor. About 50% of patients have a blood eosinophilia, a finding that appears to be limited to asthmatics *(68,72)*.

On the chest radiograph *(68,71,72,74)*, two major patterns are seen: consolidation or nodules/ masses. Consolidation may be lobar or sublobar, may be associated with volume loss, and tends to be more common in the upper zones *(68,74)*. Nodules or masses (Fig. 16) are commonly solitary, but can be multiple. They are considered to represent a mass of necrotic tissue with surrounding granulomatous or organizing pneumonitis. They vary in size from 2 to 15 cm *(75)* and are often not particularly well defined. Occasionally they cavitate *(68,75,76)*. Adenopathy and pleural disease are not seen *(76)*. In a study of five patients with bronchocentric granulomatosis *(73)*, CT showed spiculated mass lesions in three cases and consolidation in two. Extensive mucoid impaction was seen in two patients. The imaging findings were felt to be due to granuloma formation with or without proximal airway obstruction.

The prognosis of bronchocentric granulomatosis is good. Lesions may clear spontaneously or with steroids and generally do not recur following surgical removal.

REFERENCES

1. Krishnan P, Thachil R, Gillego V. Diffuse panbronchiolitis: a treatable sinobronchial disease in need of recognition in the United States. *Chest* 2002;121:659–61.
2. Fisher MS Jr, Rush WL, Rosado-de-Christenson ML, Goldstein ER, Tomski SM, Wempe JM, et al. Diffuse panbronchiolitis: histologic diagnosis in unsuspected cases involving North American residents of Asian descent. *Arch Pathol Lab Med* 1998;122:156–60.
3. Fitzgerald JE, King TE Jr, Lynch DA, Tuder RM, Schwarz MI. Diffuse panbronchiolitis in the United States. *Am J Respir Crit Care Med* 1996;154:497–503.
4. Souza R, Kairalla RA, Santos Ud Ude P, Takagaki TY, Capelozzi VL, Carvalho CR. Diffuse panbronchiolitis: an underdiagnosed disease? Study of 4 cases in Brazil. *Rev Hosp Clin Fac Med Sao Paulo* 2002;57:167–74.
5. Gulhan M, Erturk A, Kurt B, Gulhan E, Ergul G, Unal P, et al. Diffuse panbronchiolitis observed in a white man in Turkey. *Sarcoidosis Vasc Diffuse Lung Dis* 2000;17:292–6.

6. Naalsund A, Foerster A, Aasebo U, Kearney M, Boe J. [An answer to an inquiry on diffuse panbronchiolitis. Now it has found its way here!]. *Lakartidningen* 1995;92:3119–21.

7. Keicho N, Tokunaga K, Nakata K, Taguchi Y, Azuma A, Bannai M, et al. Contribution of HLA genes to genetic predisposition in diffuse panbronchiolitis. *Am J Respir Crit Care Med* 1998;158:846–50.

8. Park MH, Kim YW, Yoon HI, Yoo CG, Han SK, Shim YS, et al. Association of HLA class I antigens with diffuse panbronchiolitis in Korean patients. *Am J Respir Crit Care Med* 1999;159:526–9.

9. Keicho N, Ohashi J, Tamiya G, Nakata K, Taguchi Y, Azuma A, et al. Fine localization of a major disease-susceptibility locus for diffuse panbronchiolitis. *Am J Hum Genet* 2000;66:501–7.

10. Kamio K, Matsushita I, Hijikata M, Kobashi Y, Tanaka G, Nakata K, et al. Promoter analysis and aberrant expression of the MUC5B gene in diffuse panbronchiolitis. *Am J Respir Crit Care Med* 2005;171:949–57.

11. Kadota J, Mukae H, Fujii T, Seki M, Tomono K, Kohno S. Clinical similarities and differences between human T-cell lymphotropic virus type 1-associated bronchiolitis and diffuse panbronchiolitis. *Chest* 2004;125:1239–47.

12. Ono K, Shimamoto Y, Matsuzaki M, Sano M, Yamaguchi T, Kato O, et al. Diffuse panbronchiolitis as a pulmonary complication in patients with adult T-cell leukemia. *Am J Hematol* 1989;30:86–90.

13. Xie G, Li L, Liu H, Xu K, Zhu Y. Diffuse panbronchiolitis complicated with thymoma: a report of 2 cases with literature review. *Chin Med J (Engl)* 2003;116:1723–7.

14. Okano A, Sato A, Suda T, Suda I, Yasuda K, Iwata M, et al. [A case of diffuse panbronchiolitis complicated by malignant thymoma and Sjogren's syndrome]. *Nihon Kyobu Shikkan Gakkai Zasshi* 1991;29:263–8.

15. Tsuburai T, Ikchara K, Suzuki S, Shinohara T, Mishima W, Tagawa A, et al. [Hypogammaglobulinemia associated with thymoma (Good syndrome) similar to diffuse panbronchiolitis]. *Nihon Kokyuki Gakkai Zasshi* 2003;41:421–5.

16. Chijimatsu Y, Nakazato Y, Homma H, Mizuguchi K [A case report of Good syndrome complicated by diffuse panbronchiolitis]. *Nihon Kyobu Shikkan Gakkai Zasshi* 1982;20:803–8.

17. Poletti V, Casoni G, Chilosi M, Zompatori M. Diffuse panbronchiolitis. *Eur Respir J* 2006;28:862–71.

18. Chen Y, Kang J, Li S. Diffuse panbronchiolitis in China. *Respirology* 2005;10:70–5.

19. Fitzgerald JE, King TJ, Lynch DA, Tuder RM, Schwarz MI. Diffuse panbronchiolitis in the United States. *Am J Respir Crit Care Med* 1996;154:497–503.

20. Aslan AT, Ozcelik U, Talim B, Haliloglu M, Dogru D, Dalgic F, et al. Childhood diffuse panbronchiolitis: a case report. *Pediatr Pulmonol* 2005;40:354–7.

21. Azuma A, Kudoh S. Diffuse panbronchiolitis in East Asia. *Respirology* 2006;11:249–61.

22. Irwin RS, Baumann MH, Bolser DC, Boulet LP, Braman SS, Brightling CE, et al. Diagnosis and management of cough executive summary: ACCP evidence-based clinical practice guidelines. *Chest* 2006;129:1S–23S.

23. Schultz MJ. Macrolide activities beyond their antimicrobial effects: macrolides in diffuse panbronchiolitis and cystic fibrosis. *J Antimicrob Chemother* 2004;54:21–8.

24. Amsden GW. Anti-inflammatory effects of macrolides—an underappreciated benefit in the treatment of community-acquired respiratory tract infections and chronic inflammatory pulmonary conditions? *J Antimicrob Chemother* 2005;55:10–21.

25. Shitrit D, Bendayan D, Gidon S, Saute M, Bakal I, Kramer MR. Long-term azithromycin use for treatment of bronchiolitis obliterans syndrome in lung transplant recipients. *J Heart Lung Transplant* 2005;24:1440–3.

26. Richeldi L, Ferrara G, Fabbri LM, Lasserson TJ, Gibson PG. Macrolides for chronic asthma. *Cochrane Database Syst Rev* 2005:CD002997.

27. Nishimura K, Kitaichi M, Izumi T, Itoh H. Diffuse panbronchiolitis: correlation of high-resolution CT and pathologic findings. *Radiology* 1992;184:779–85.

28. Sueyasu Y. Diffuse panbronchiolitis—a thin-section CT scoring system. *Kurume Med J* 1996;43:63–71.

29. Akira M, Kitatani J, Yong-Sik L, Kita N, Yamamoto S, Higashihara T, et al. Diffuse panbronchiolitis: evaluation with high-resolution CT. *Radiology* 1988;168:433–8.

30. Murata K, Itoh H, Senda M, et al. Stratified impairment of pulmonary ventilation in "diffuse panbronchiolitis": PET and CT studies. *J Comput Assist Tomogr* 1989;13:48–53.

31. Akira M, Higashihara T, Sakatani M, Hara H. Diffuse panbronchiolitis: follow-up CT examination. *Radiology* 1993;189:559–62.

32. Ichikawa Y, Hotta M, Sumita S, Fujimoto K, Oizumi K. Reversible airway lesions in diffuse panbronchiolitis. Detection by high-resolution computed tomography. *Chest* 1995;107:120–5.

33. Yamada G, Igarashi T, Itoh E, Tanaka H, Sekine K, Abe S. Centrilobular nodules correlate with air trapping in diffuse panbronchiolitis during erythromycin therapy. *Chest* 2001;120:198–202.

34. Poletti V, Zompatori M, Boaron M, Rimondi M, Baruzzi G. Cryptogenic constrictive bronchiolitis imitating imaging features of diffuse panbronchiolitis. *Monaldi Arch Chest Dis* 1995;50:116–7.

35. Kadota J, Mukae H, Mizunoe S, Kishi K, Tokimatsu I, Nagai H, et al. Long-term macrolide antibiotic therapy in the treatment of chronic small airway disease clinically mimicking diffuse panbronchiolitis. *Intern Med* 2005;44:200–6.

36. Okada F, Ando Y, Yoshitake S, Yotsumoto S, Matsumoto S, Wakisaka M, et al. Pulmonary CT findings in 320 carriers of human T-lymphotropic virus type 1. *Radiology* 2006;240:559–64.

37. Romero S, Barroso E, Gil J, Aranda I, Alonso S, Garcia-Pachon E. Follicular bronchiolitis: clinical and pathologic findings in six patients. *Lung* 2003;181:309–19.
38. Howling SJ, Hansell DM, Wells AU, Nicholson AG, Flint JD, Muller NL. Follicular bronchiolitis: thin-section CT and histologic findings. *Radiology* 1999;212:637–42.
39. Exley CM, Suvarna SK, Matthews S. Follicular bronchiolitis as a presentation of HIV. *Clin Radiol* 2006;61:710–3.
40. Hayakawa H, Sato A, Imokawa S, Toyoshima M, Chida K, Iwata M. Bronchiolar disease in rheumatoid arthritis. *Am J Respir Crit Care Med* 1996;154:1531–6.
41. Boag AH, Colby TV, Fraire AE, Kuhn C, 3rd, Roggli VL, Travis WD, et al. The pathology of interstitial lung disease in nylon flock workers. *Am J Surg Pathol* 1999;23:1539–45.
42. Eschenbacher WL, Kreiss K, Lougheed MD, Pransky GS, Day B, Castellan RM. Nylon flock-associated interstitial lung disease. *Am J Respir Crit Care Med* 1999;159:2003–8.
43. Weiss SM, Lakshminarayan S. Acute inhalation injury. *Clin Chest Med* 1994;15:103–16.
44. Nowak D. Chemosensory irritation and the lung. *Int Arch Occup Environ Health* 2002;75:326–31.
45. Diaz JV, Koff J, Gotway MB, Nishimura S, Balmes JR. Case report: a case of wood-smoke-related pulmonary disease. *Environ Health Perspect* 2006;114:759–62.
46. Bruce N, Perez-Padilla R, Albalak R. Indoor air pollution in developing countries: a major environmental and public health challenge. *Bull World Health Organ* 2000;78:1078–92.
47. Grobbelaar JP, Bateman ED. Hut lung: a domestically acquired pneumoconiosis of mixed aetiology in rural women. *Thorax* 1991;46:334–40.
48. Gold JA, Jagirdar J, Hay JG, Addrizzo-Harris DJ, Naidich DP, Rom WN. Hut lung. A domestically acquired particulate lung disease. *Medicine (Baltimore)* 2000;79:310–7.
49. Kara M, Bulut S, Tas F, Akkurt I, Seyfikli Z. Evaluation of pulmonary changes due to biomass fuels using high-resolution computed tomography. *Eur Radiol* 2003;13:2372–7.
50. Kern DG, Crausman RS, Durand KT, Nayer A, Kuhn C, 3rd. Flock worker's lung: chronic interstitial lung disease in the nylon flocking industry. *Ann Intern Med* 1998;129:261–72.
51. Weiland DA, Lynch DA, Jensen SP, Newell JD, Miller DE, Crausman RS, et al. Thin-section CT findings in flock worker's lung, a work-related interstitial lung disease. *Radiology* 2003;227:222–31.
52. Hwang JH, Kim TS, Lee KS, Choi YH, Han J, Chung MP, et al. Bronchiolitis in adults: pathology and imaging. *J Comput Assist Tomogr* 1997;21:913–9.
53. Akira M, Higashihara T, Yokoyama K, Yamamoto S, Kita N, Morimoto S, et al. Radiographic type p pneumoconiosis: high-resolution CT. *Radiology* 1989;171:117–23.
54. Ryu JH. Classification and approach to bronchiolar diseases. *Curr Opin Pulm Med* 2006;12:145–51.
55. Hakala M, Paakko P, Huhti E, Tarkka M, Sutinen S. Open lung biopsy of patients with rheumatoid arthritis. *Clin Rheumatol* 1990;9:452–60.
56. Kinoshita M, Higashi T, Tanaka C, Tokunaga N, Ichikawa Y, Oizumi K. Follicular bronchiolitis associated with rheumatoid arthritis. *Intern Med* 1992;31:674–7.
57. Athreya BH, Doughty RA, Bookspan M, Schumacher HR, Sewell EM, Chatten J. Pulmonary manifestations of juvenile rheumatoid arthritis. A report of eight cases and review. *Clin Chest Med* 1980;1:361–74.
58. Yamanishi Y, Maeda H, Hiyama K, Ishioka S, Yamakido M. Rheumatoid arthritis associated with diffuse panbronchiolitis. *Intern Med* 1998;37:338–41.
59. Homma S, Kawabata M, Kishi K, Tsuboi E, Narui K, Nakatani T, et al. Diffuse panbronchiolitis in rheumatoid arthritis. *Eur Respir J* 1998;12:444–52.
60. Sugiyama Y, Saitoh K, Kano S, Kitamura S. An autopsy case of diffuse panbronchiolitis accompanying rheumatoid arthritis. *Respir Med* 1996;90:175–7.
61. Sugiyama Y, Ohno S, Kano S, Maeda H, Kitamura S. Diffuse panbronchiolitis and rheumatoid arthritis: a possible correlation with HLA-B54. *Intern Med* 1994;33:612–4.
62. Mahadeva R, Walsh G, Flower CD, Shneerson JM. Clinical and radiological characteristics of lung disease in inflammatory bowel disease. *Eur Respir J* 2000;15:41–8.
63. Camus P, Piard F, Ashcroft T, Gal AA, Colby TV. The lung in inflammatory bowel disease. *Medicine (Baltimore)* 1993;72:151–83.
64. Garg K, Lynch DA, Newell JD. Inflammatory airways disease in ulcerative colitis: CT and high-resolution CT features. *J Thorac Imaging* 1993;8:159–63.
65. Desai SJ, Gephardt GN, Stoller JK. Diffuse panbronchiolitis preceding ulcerative colitis. *Chest* 1989;95:1342–4.
66. Casey MB, Tazelaar HD, Myers JL, Hunninghake GW, Kakar S, Kalra SX, et al. Noninfectious lung pathology in patients with Crohn's disease. *Am J Surg Pathol* 2003;27:213–9.
67. Liebow AA. The J. Burns Amberson lecture—pulmonary angiitis and granulomatosis. *Am Rev Respir Dis* 1973;108:1–18.
68. Katzenstein AL, Liebow AA, Friedman PJ. Bronchocentric granulomatosis, mucoid impaction, and hypersensitivity reactions to fungi. *Am Rev Respir Dis* 1975;111:497–537.

69. Katzenstein A-L. *Katzenstein and Askin's Surgical Pathology of Non-Neoplastic Lung Disease*. 3 ed. Philadelphia: WB Saunders; 1997.

70. Hanson G, Flor N, Wells I, Novey H, Galant S. Bronchocentric granulomatosis: a complication of allergic bronchopulmonary aspergillosis. *J Allergy Clin Immunol* 1977;59:83–90.

71. Saldana M. Bronchocentric granulomatosis: clinicopathologic observations in 17 patients. *Lab Invest* 1979;40:281–2.

72. Koss MN, Robinson RG, Hochholzer L. Bronchocentric granulomatosis. *Hum Pathol* 1981;12:632–8.

73. Ward S, Heyneman LE, Flint JD, Leung AN, Kazerooni EA, Muller NL. Bronchocentric granulomatosis: computed tomographic findings in five patients. *Clin Radiol* 2000;55:296–300.

74. Robinson RG, Wehunt WD, Tsou E, Koss MN, Hochholzer L. Bronchocentric granulomatosis: roentgenographic manifestations. *Am Rev Respir Dis* 1982;125:751–6.

75. Berendsen HH, Hofstee N, Kapsenberg PD, van Reesema DR, Klein JJ. Bronchocentric granulomatosis associated with seropositive polyarthritis. *Thorax* 1985;40:396–7.

76. Frazier AA, Rosado-de-Christenson ML, Galvin JR, Fleming MV. Pulmonary angiitis and granulomatosis: radiologic-pathologic correlation. *Radiographics* 1998;18:687–710.

13

Obliterative Bronchiolitis

C. Isabela S. Silva and Nestor L. Müller

Summary

Obliterative bronchiolitis (OB) is a condition characterized by inflammation and fibrosis of the bronchiolar walls resulting in narrowing or obliteration of the bronchiolar lumen. The most common causes are childhood lower respiratory tract infection, hematopoietic stem cell or lung and heart-lung transplantation, and toxic fume inhalation. The most frequent clinical manifestations are progressive dyspnea and dry cough. Pulmonary function tests demonstrate airflow obstruction and air trapping. Radiographic manifestations include reduction of the peripheral vascular markings, increased lung lucency, and overinflation. The chest radiograph, however, is often normal. High-resolution CT is currently the imaging modality of choice in the assessment of patients with suspected or proven OB. The characteristic findings on high-resolution CT consist of areas of decreased attenuation and vascularity (mosaic perfusion pattern) on inspiratory scans and air trapping on expiratory scans. Other CT findings of OB include bronchiectasis and bronchiolectasis, bronchial wall thickening, small centrilobular nodules, and three-in-bud opacities. Recent studies suggest that hyperpolarized [3]He-enhanced magnetic resonance imaging may allow earlier recognition of obstructive airway disease and therefore may be useful in the diagnosis and follow-up of patients with OB.

Key Words: Bronchiolitis; bronchiolitis obliterans; bronchiolitis obliterans syndrome; constrictive bronchiolitis; computed tomography; obliterative bronchiolitis; small airways disease.

1. INTRODUCTION

Bronchiolitis is a generic term applied to various inflammatory and fibrosing diseases that affect the small airways, which by definition are airways that measure less than 2 mm in diameter (i.e., primarily membranous and respiratory bronchioles) *(1,2)*. Bronchiolitis is common and occurs in various clinical settings *(1–5)*. Several classification schemes have been proposed based on histologic features, etiology, or computed tomography (CT) findings *(1–3,6,7)*. Although none of these classification schemes is widely accepted and there is controversy about the classification of some of the subtypes of bronchiolitis, there is overall agreement on the histologic, radiologic, and clinical features of obliterative bronchiolitis (OB).

2. DEFINITION AND TERMINOLOGY

Obliterative bronchiolitis, also known as *constrictive bronchiolitis*, *bronchiolitis obliterans*, or *cicatricial bronchiolitis*, is a condition characterized by inflammation and fibrosis of the bronchiolar walls and contiguous tissues resulting in narrowing and, in some cases, complete obliteration of the bronchiolar lumen *(1,2,8)*. OB may result from a large number of acute and chronic processes and may occasionally be idiopathic (Table 1).

From: *Contemporary Medical Imaging: CT of the Airways*
Edited by: P. M. Boiselle and D. A. Lynch © Humana Press, Totowa, NJ

Table 1
Most Common Conditions Associated with Obliterative Bronchiolitis

Childhood respiratory infection, most commonly adenovirus, respiratory syncytial virus, and *Mycoplasma pneumoniae* bronchiolitis and bronchopneumonia

Chronic rejection following lung and heart-lung transplantation

Chronic graft-versus-host disease following allogeneic hematopoietic stem-cell transplantation

Postinhalational

    Nitrogen dioxide (Silo filler's disease), ammonia, chlorine, fire smoke, hydrogen bromide, hydrogen selenide, sulfur dioxide, thionyl chloride, and diacetyl (2,3-butanedione)

Ingested toxins

    Sauropus androgynus (vegetable alleged to help weight control)

Connective tissue disorders, most commonly rheumatoid arthritis. Occasionally, Sjögren's syndrome, systemic lupus erythematosus, and scleroderma

Drugs

    D-penicillamine, lamustine, and gold therapy

Inflammatory bowel diseases

    Ulcerative colitis and Crohn's disease

Cryptogenic (idiopathic)

Other conditions

    Diffuse idiopathic neuroendocrine cell hyperplasia with multiple carcinoid tumorlets

    Eosinophilic fasciitis

    Stevens–Johnson syndrome and paraneoplastic pemphigus

    Asthma

    Bronchiectasis

    Cystic fibrosis

    Hypersensitivity pneumonitis

    Sarcoidosis

There has been historical confusion between the term "bronchiolitis obliterans" as it refers to OB and the term "bronchiolitis obliterans organizing pneumonia" (BOOP) *(9–11)*. The histologic hallmark of BOOP is the presence of buds of loose granulation tissue, termed Masson bodies, within alveolar ducts and air spaces, that is, organizing pneumonia *(1,2,12)*. The patients may or may not have granulation polyps within terminal and respiratory bronchioles, but they rarely have fibrosis within the bronchiolar walls or peribronchiolar tissues, that is, they do not have OB. Because the predominant clinical, histologic, and radiologic manifestations of BOOP are those of organizing pneumonia, the American Thoracic Society and European Respiratory Society multidisciplinary consensus classification recommended that the term BOOP be replaced by the term organizing pneumonia and idiopathic BOOP by cryptogenic organizing pneumonia *(12)*. Organizing pneumonia may result from various causes or underlying pathologic processes including pulmonary infection, aspiration, collagen vascular disorders, drugs, radiation, inhalational injury, and hypersensitivity pneumonitis. Cryptogenic organizing pneumonia is currently classified as a form of idiopathic interstitial pneumonia *(12,13)* and is beyond the scope of this chapter. We will limit our discussion to the histologic, clinical, and radiologic findings of OB.

3. CLINICAL FEATURES

The most common clinical manifestations of OB consist of progressive dyspnea, nonproductive cough, and airflow obstruction, which usually progress over weeks to months. Associated symptoms may include chest pain, respiratory distress, and cyanosis *(14)*. Auscultation of the chest may reveal crackles and midinspiratory squeaks. Occasionally, patients may present with pneumothorax or pneumomediastinum *(15–17)*. In many cases, OB is first detected on CT in patients with no apparent symptoms or with symptoms secondary to associated conditions such as bronchiectasis or asthma.

A presumptive diagnosis of OB can often be made with a high degree of confidence based on a clinical history of persistent symptoms of obstructive pulmonary disease, demonstration of airflow obstruction on pulmonary function tests, and characteristic findings on high-resolution CT. However, the clinical diagnosis of OB requires exclusion of other causes of chronic airway obstruction, including emphysema, chronic bronchitis, and asthma *(18,19)*.

4. PULMONARY FUNCTION TESTS

The functional manifestations of OB are those of airflow obstruction, and air trapping with reduction in forced expiratory volume in 1 s (FEV_1), increased residual volume (RV) and RV to total lung capacity (TLC) ratio, and no significant response to bronchodilators *(8,18)*. The TLC is often normal until the late stages of the disease, which accounts for the usually normal lung volumes on the chest radiograph. Lung diffusion as measured by the carbon monoxide diffusing capacity (DLCO) is typically within normal limits, which allows distinction from emphysema.

5. HISTOLOGIC FINDINGS

Obliterative bronchiolitis is characterized histologically by concentric or, less commonly eccentric, thickening of terminal and respiratory bronchiolar walls by submucosal collagenous fibrosis resulting in progressive narrowing and distortion of the bronchiolar lumen. Associated features include epithelial metaplasia, smooth muscle hyperplasia, bronchiolectasis with mucous stasis, and patchy chronic inflammation (cellular bronchiolitis) (Fig. 1) *(1,2)*. Severe fibrosis may result in complete obliteration of the bronchiolar lumen, the bronchiole being replaced by scar tissue (Fig. 2). In such cases, the diagnosis may be difficult to make histologically, the obliterated bronchiole being misinterpreted as being a small scar.

The pathogenesis of OB is not well known. The initial event is believed to be bronchiolar inflammation, with resulting epithelial necrosis. The inflammation can involve the mucosa, submucosa, and peribronchiolar parenchyma and be followed by the development of fibrous connective tissue that compromises the bronchiolar lumen. Significant involvement of the interstitium is uncommon. OB may be classified as "active" when an inflammatory component is present or "inactive" when inflammation is absent *(20)* .

Definitive diagnosis of OB requires lung biopsy. The patchy distribution of the disease and inadequate tissue sampling result in a large percentage of false-negative diagnosis on transbronchial biopsy specimens *(21–26)*. It should be noted that even on surgical biopsy specimens, subtle changes or completely distorted and scarred bronchioles may be missed on routine hematoxylin-eosin stains. Optimal assessment requires the use of elastic tissue stains (Fig. 3) *(2,14)*. Because of the subtlety of the histologic findings, lung biopsies in patients with BO may occasionally be read as normal or near-normal. In such patients, the presence of typical imaging findings should prompt a request for review, re-staining, or re-sectioning of the biopsy specimen.

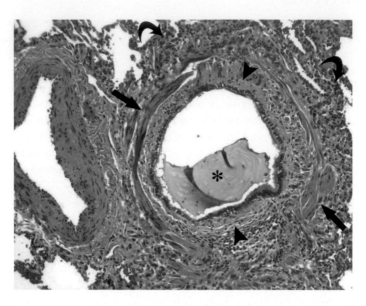

Fig. 1. Obliterative bronchiolitis. Surgical lung biopsy specimen shows small bronchiole with submucosal fibrosis (arrowheads), muscle hypertrophy (straight arrows), peribronchiolar inflammation (curved arrows), and associated mucostasis (asterix). The findings are characteristic of mild obliterative bronchiolitis (H and E, intermediate magnification) (Courtesy of Dr. Thomas Colby, Mayo Clinic, Scottsdale).

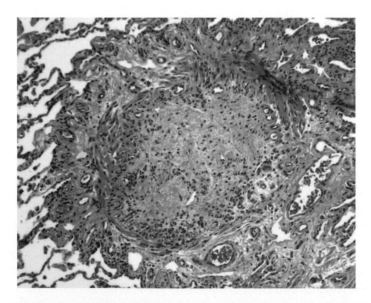

Fig. 2. Obliterative bronchiolitis. Surgical lung biopsy specimen demonstrates complete obliteration of bronchiolar lumen by fibrous tissue (H and E, intermediate magnification). (Courtesy of Dr. Thomas Colby, Mayo Clinic, Scottsdale).

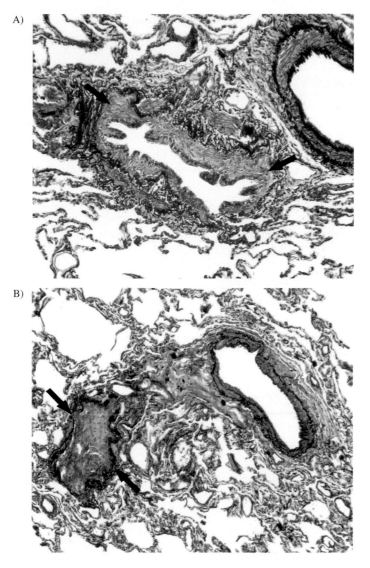

Fig. 3. Obliterative bronchiolitis. Surgical lung biopsy specimen shows bronchiole with concentric submucosal scarring (arrows, **A**), and completely obliterated bronchiole (**B**) in which the preexisting elastica is highlighted with elastic tissue stain (arrows) (elastic tissue stain, intermediate magnification) (Courtesy of Dr. Thomas Colby, Mayo Clinic, Scottsdale).

6. IMAGING FINDINGS

The most common imaging modalities used in the assessment of patients with suspected or proven OB are chest radiography and high-resolution CT. Scintigraphy plays a limited role. Ventilation/perfusion scans generally reveal diminished ventilation in the lung periphery; perfusion abnormalities may also be present, but these are usually much milder than the ventilation abnormalities *(27,28)*. Recently, it has been shown that magnetic resonance (MR) allows functional imaging of pulmonary ventilation and perfusion with the additional benefit of lack of radiation *(29)*. Hyperpolarized [3]He-enhanced MR may allow earlier recognition of obstructive airway disease and therefore be useful in the early recognition and follow-up of patients with OB *(30,31)*. Although potentially useful, functional MR imaging is only available at a very small number of centers and remains an investigational tool.

6.1. Chest Radiography

In patients with mild-to-moderate OB, the chest radiograph is often normal. The earliest manifestations, which are often quite subtle, consist of increased lung lucency and reduction of the peripheral vascular markings. Severe disease results in hyperinflation detected by the overall increase in lung volumes, flattening of the diaphragm, and increase in the retrosternal airspace (Fig. 4). Other findings include increased bronchial markings, bronchiectasis, and, occasionally, nodular or reticulonodular opacities *(9,32–36)* (Table 2).

There is poor correlation between the radiographic findings and the clinical and functional severity of disease *(37)* and considerable inter-observer and intra-observer variability in interpretation of findings *(38)*. The chest radiograph therefore plays a limited role in the diagnosis and follow-up of patients with OB.

6.2. Computed Tomography Findings

High-resolution CT is currently the imaging modality of choice in the assessment of patients with suspected or proven small airways disease, being superior to chest radiography in demonstrating the presence and extent of abnormalities *(39)*. Because the bronchiolar wall is too thin to be visualized on high-resolution CT, even in patients with OB, the analysis of the CT images is limited to assessment

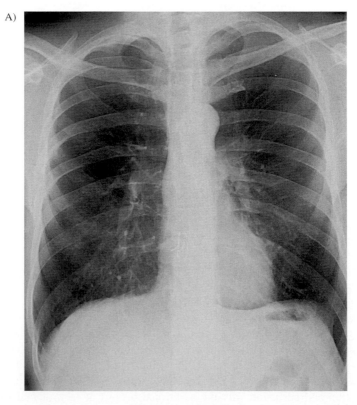

A)

Fig. 4. *(Continued)*

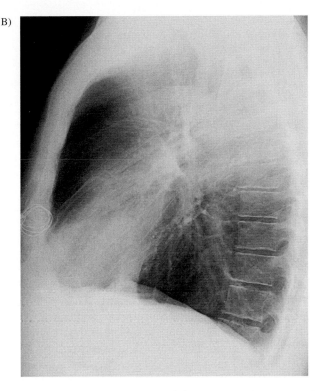

Fig. 4. Obliterative bronchiolitis on chest radiography. (**A**) Posteroanterior chest radiograph show increased lung volumes and reduction of the peripheral vascular markings. (**B**) Lateral view shows increased retrosternal airspace and flattening of the diaphragm. The patient was a 44-year-old man with obliterative bronchiolitis following bilateral lung transplantation for cystic fibrosis.

of secondary signs related to the small airway obstruction. The main CT finding of OB on CT scans performed at end-inspiration is a geographic inhomogeneity of lung attenuation (mosaic attenuation pattern), seen in 40–80% of patients *(40–47)* (Table 3). This pattern consists of patchy lobular, segmental or, occasionally, lobar regions of decreased attenuation and vascularity and blood flow redistribution to relatively normal lung resulting in areas of normal or increased attenuation and

Table 2
Radiographic Findings of Obliterative Bronchiolitis

Chest radiograph may be normal in mild to moderate disease
Common findings
    Increased lung lucency
    Reduction of peripheral vascular markings
Late findings
    Hyperinflation
    Flattening of the diaphragm
    Increased retrosternal airspace
Ancillary findings
    Prominent bronchial markings, bronchiectasis, and nodular or reticulonodular opacities

Table 3
High-Resolution CT Findings of Obliterative
Bronchiolitis

Common findings

    Decreased attenuation and vascularity
    Mosaic perfusion pattern
    Air trapping at expiratory images

Ancillary findings

    Bronchiectasis and bronchiolectasis
    Bronchial wall thickening
    Centrilobular nodules
    Tree-in-bud opacities

---

increased vascularity (mosaic perfusion pattern) (Fig. 5) *(6,8,46)*. The areas of decreased attenuation result from decreased perfusion of hypoventilated alveoli distal to obstructed bronchioles. The abnormalities may be subtle on inspiratory images. The presence of airflow obstruction and air trapping is usually easier to detect on CT scans performed during maximal expiration or at end-expiration *(48–51)*. Regions with airflow obstruction because of OB show no decrease in volume or less decrease in volume than the adjacent uninvolved lung and therefore remain lucent while the remaining lung increases in attenuation. This results in increased contrast between areas with airflow obstruction and normal lung facilitating recognition of air trapping on high-resolution CT (Fig. 6). Expiratory CT images may demonstrate air trapping in patients with normal findings on inspiratory scans (Fig. 7) *(48,50,52–55)*. The extent of air trapping on expiratory CT in patients with OB correlates with severity of airflow obstruction and air trapping on pulmonary function tests *(18)*. CT performed during maximal expiratory maneuver or at end-expiration therefore plays an important role and is recommended in the initial evaluation and follow-up of patients with OB *(50,52)*.

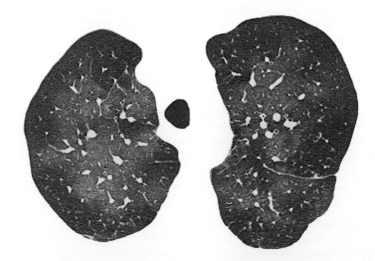

Fig. 5. Mosaic perfusion pattern. High-resolution CT image demonstrates geographic areas of decreased attenuation and vascularity interspersed with areas of increased attenuation that contain enlarged vessels, reflecting pulmonary blood flow redistribution. The patient was 48-year-old man with obliterative bronchiolitis.

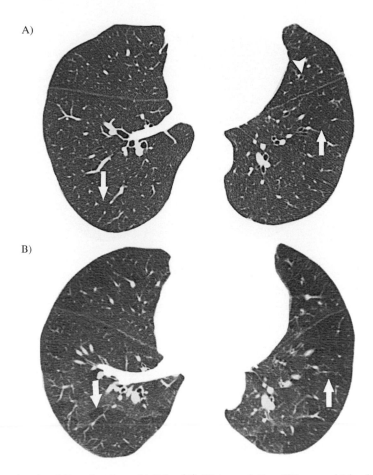

Fig. 6. Air trapping in obliterative bronchiolitis. (**A**) High-resolution CT scan obtained at end-inspiration shows subtle areas of decreased attenuation (straight arrows). Also noted is mild bronchiectasis in the lingula and anteromedial basal segment of the left lower lobe (arrowhead). (**B**) High-resolution CT scan performed at the end of maximal expiration demonstrates air trapping (arrows). The patient was a 66-year-old woman with cryptogenic obliterative bronchiolitis.

Several studies have suggested that post-processing of high-resolution CT images particularly with the use of minimum intensity projection (MinIP) reconstructions improves the detection of subtle areas of low attenuation encountered in patients with emphysema and small airways disease (Fig. 8). *(56–61)* These techniques may be particularly helpful in patients with high clinical suspicion for OB and otherwise apparently normal CT findings.

Ancillary high-resolution CT findings of OB include central and peripheral bronchial dilatation (bronchiectasis), bronchiolectasis, and bronchial wall thickening, findings that have been reported in 20–90% of patients (Fig. 9). *(18,40,43,46,47,62)* Less common CT findings of OB include small centrilobular nodules and tree-in-bud opacities representing thick-walled bronchioles with or without intraluminal debris, seen in up to 30% of patients (Fig. 10) (see Table 3) *(47)*.

In the appropriate clinical setting, the presence of mosaic perfusion, air trapping, and ancillary CT findings can be diagnostic of OB. It should be emphasized, however, that mosaic perfusion is a nonspecific finding seen in a number of conditions, that mild air trapping is commonly seen in normal subjects, and that there is overlap between the high-resolution CT manifestations of OB and the findings seen in other causes of airway obstruction such as asthma and emphysema *(19)*.

A)

B)

C)

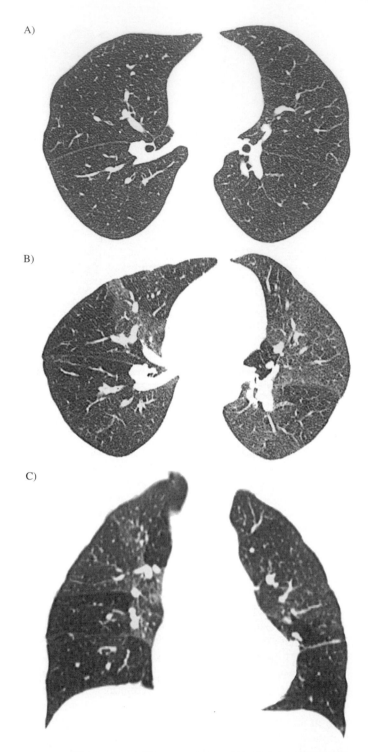

Fig. 7. Normal inspiratory CT in obliterative bronchiolitis. (**A**) High-resolution CT scan obtained at end-inspiration on a multidetector CT scanner is within normal limits. (**B**) Expiratory image at the same level as (**A**) demonstrates patchy lobular and segmental areas of air trapping. (**C**) Coronal reformatted image better demonstrates the extent of air trapping. The patient was a 54-year-old woman with postinfectious obliterative bronchiolitis.

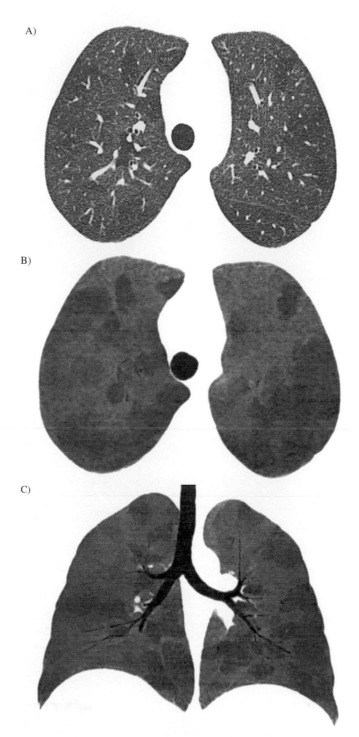

Fig. 8. Minimum intensity projection (MinIP) in the assessment of obliterative bronchiolitis. (**A**) High-resolution CT scan obtained in a multidetector CT scanner at the level of aortic arch shows subtle lobular areas of decreased attenuation and vascularity. (**B** and **C**) Cross-sectional and coronal minimum intensity projection (MinIP) reformation images improve the detection of lobular areas of decreased attenuation. The patient was a 29-year-old woman with chronic graft-versus-host disease and obliterative bronchiolitis 1 year after allogeneic hematopoietic stem-cell transplantation.

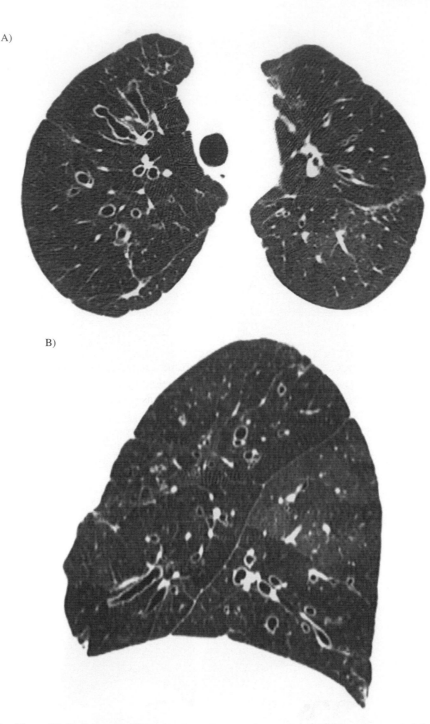

Fig. 9. Ancillary CT findings of obliterative bronchiolitis. Cross-sectional (**A**) and sagittal (**B**) reformatted high-resolution CT images obtained on multidetector CT scanner show diffuse areas of decreased attenuation and vascularity with associated cylindrical and varicose bronchiectasis and bronchial wall thickening. The patient was a 21-year-old woman with severe airflow obstruction and obliterative bronchiolitis 8 years after lung transplantation for cystic fibrosis.

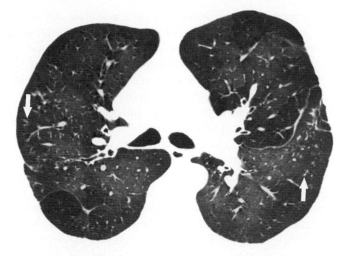

Fig. 10. Obliterative bronchiolitis. High-resolution CT image shows mosaic perfusion pattern and centrilobular nodules and tree-in-bud opacities (arrows) representing thick-walled bronchioles with or without intraluminal debris (same patient as Fig. 5).

Mosaic perfusion can be seen in various airway diseases including OB, asthma, and bronchiectasis; in occlusive pulmonary vascular disease (particularly chronic pulmonary thromboembolism) (Fig. 11); and infiltrative lung disease, such as hypersensitivity pneumonitis (45,52,63–66). The differential diagnosis requires careful analysis of associated findings such as bronchial dilatation and enlargement of the main pulmonary artery and interpretation of the CT images in the proper clinical context. Airway diseases that cause mosaic perfusion can usually be distinguished from vascular causes such as chronic pulmonary thromboembolism by the presence of bronchial dilatation, seen in more than 70% of patients with airway abnormalities, and the lack of enlargement of the main pulmonary artery, a finding seen in the majority of patients with chronic pulmonary thromboembolism associated with mosaic perfusion (45). It should be noted however that bronchial dilatation may also occur

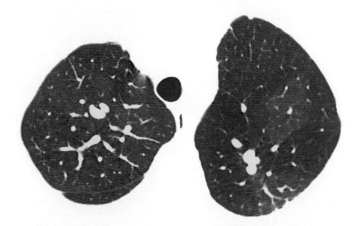

Fig. 11. Mosaic perfusion pattern in chronic pulmonary thromboembolism. High-resolution CT image shows mosaic perfusion in the upper lobes with enlargement of the segmental arteries in areas of increased attenuation. The patient was a 57-year-old woman with chronic thromboembolic pulmonary arterial hypertension.

in patients with chronic pulmonary thromboembolism *(67)*, and there are no reliable distinguishing features between mosaic perfusion resulting from OB and mosaic perfusion because of other airway diseases. Furthermore, air trapping can also be seen in patients with pulmonary embolism. In a study by Arakawa et al. *(68)*, air trapping at expiratory images was identified in 9 of 15 (60%) patients with pulmonary embolism, including four with acute pulmonary embolism, one with chronic pulmonary embolism, and four with acute and chronic pulmonary embolism.

Air trapping is frequently seen in asymptomatic subjects with normal pulmonary function *(48,69–73)* particularly in older subjects and smokers (Fig. 12) *(70,73,74)*. Lobular air trapping involving fewer than three adjacent secondary pulmonary lobules *(48)* can be seen in approximately 50% of asymptomatic subjects and in various clinical settings, including OB, cigarette smoking, asthma, bronchiolitis associated with hypersensitivity pneumonitis (Fig. 13), and sarcoidosis *(64–66,73,75–77)*. Extent of air trapping, not simply its presence, therefore needs to be taken into account in the interpretation of expiratory CT scans *(48,73)*. It has been shown that mosaic perfusion and air trapping can be considered abnormal when they affect an area of more than 25% of the total area of the lung *(48,73)* and are not limited to the superior segment of the lower lobe or the lingula tip *(48)*. The presence of additional CT features in areas of decreased attenuation is also valuable in differentiating between abnormal air trapping in patients with OB and normal subjects. In a review of the high-resolution CT findings of 15 patients with pathologically proven OB after lung transplantation and 18 control subjects, the combination of bronchial dilatation on the inspiratory CT scan and air trapping on the expiratory CT scan was seen only in patients with OB and were the two most sensitive and specific findings on high-resolution CT scans of patients with OB *(46)*.

Copley et al. *(19)* assessed the discriminatory value of high-resolution CT to distinguish between OB, asthma, centrilobular emphysema, panlobular emphysema, and normal controls. A correct first-choice diagnosis was made in 199 of 276 (72%) observations, and a correct first-choice diagnosis was made in 35 of 38 (92%) observations in patients with OB. The major sources of diagnostic inaccuracy were difficulty in differentiating between panlobular and centrilobular emphysema, asthma and normality, and asthma and OB. Distinguishing features between OB and panlobular emphysema because of α_1-antitrypsin deficiency were the presence of parenchymal destruction, vascular distortion,

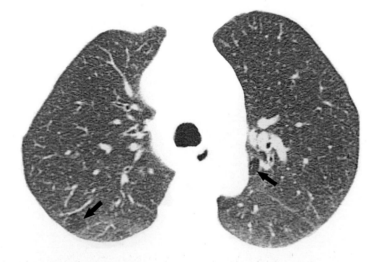

Fig. 12. Normal air trapping on CT. High-resolution CT image at the level of aortic arch obtained at end of maximal expiration shows a few lobular areas of air trapping. The patient was a 56-year-old man with no pulmonary symptoms.

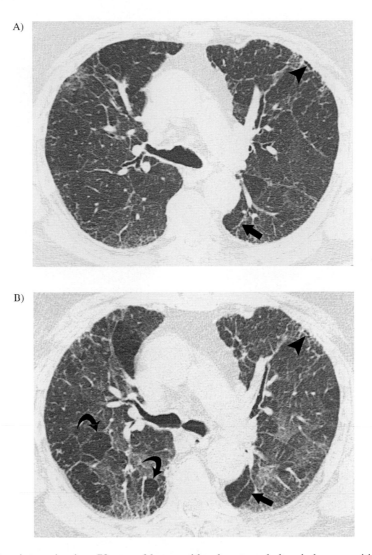

Fig. 13. Lobular air trapping in a 79-year-old man with subacute and chronic hypersensitivity pneumonitis. (**A**) High-resolution CT image shows bilateral patchy ground-glass opacities, fine reticulation, and mild subpleural honeycombing (arrowhead). Also noted are a few lobules with decreased attenuation and vascularity (straight arrow). (**B**) Expiratory high-resolution CT scan at the same level as (A) demonstrates air trapping in lobules that had decreased attenuation on the inspiratory CT (straight arrow) and in other lung regions (curved arrows). The lobular areas of air trapping are presumably related to obliterative bronchiolitis and the ground-glass opacities due to interstitial lymphocytic infiltration.

and linear scars or thickened septa at the lung bases in most patients with panlobular emphysema (Fig. 14). Patients with OB were more likely to have bronchial dilatation and decreased parenchymal attenuation and vascularity than asthmatics patients. The authors concluded that high-resolution CT is helpful to distinguish diseases that cause airflow obstruction, and it is particularly accurate in the identification of OB *(19)*. Jensen et al. *(47)* compared the CT findings in patients with refractory asthma with those of patients with idiopathic OB. A mosaic pattern of lung attenuation was seen in 50% of OB patients compared with only 3% of patients with refractory asthma.

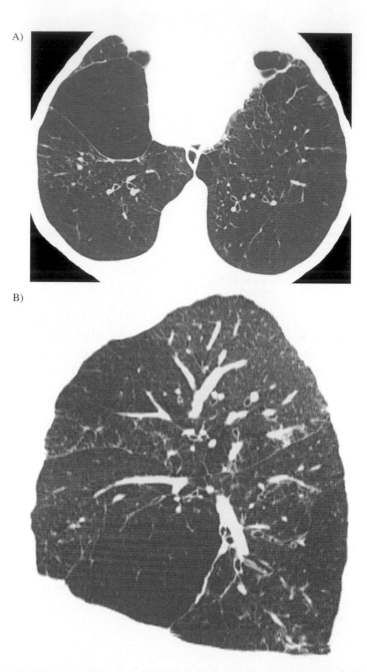

Fig. 14. Severe panlobular emphysema in 53-year-old man with α_1-antitrypsin deficiency. (**A**) High-resolution CT image obtained in a multidetector CT scanner shows extensive areas of decreased attenuation with parenchymal destruction, vascular distortion, and linear scars. (**B**) Sagittal reformatted image shows the predominance of abnormalities in the lower lung regions typical of panlobular emphysema.

7. SPECIFIC CAUSES AND UNDERLYING DISEASES ASSOCIATED WITH OBLITERATIVE BRONCHIOLITIS

A large number of conditions may result in OB (see Table 1). The vast majority of cases, however, occur following childhood viral or mycoplasma infection *(3,40,78)*, hematopoietic stem cell or lung and heart-lung transplantation *(79–82)*, and toxic fume inhalation *(3,5,83)*. Less common causes include connective tissue disorders (especially rheumatoid arthritis) *(84–90)*, drug therapy including D-penicillamine, lamustine and gold *(5,91)*, ingestion of toxines such as Sauropous androgyn *(92–94)*, neuroendocrine cell hyperplasia with multiple carcinoid tumorlets *(95–97)*, inflammatory bowel disease *(98,99)*, eosinophilic fasciitis *(3,5)*, Stevens–Johnson syndrome and paraneoplastic pemphigus *(100,101)*. OB may be seen as a component of interstitial lung disease (hypersensitivity pneumonitis and sarcoidosis) *(64,75,76)* or large airway disease (asthma, bronchiectasis, and cystic fibrosis) *(102–105)*. Rarely OB may be idiopathic *(106)*.

7.1. Postinfectious Obliterative Bronchiolitis

Obliterative bronchiolitis may be a late sequela of lower respiratory tract infections occurring in infancy or childhood, particularly by adenovirus *(40,107,108)*. Other causes include respiratory syncytial virus, parainfluenza virus, influenza virus, measles, and *Mycoplasma pneumoniae (5,109)*. The true prevalence of OB due to infection is unknown; however, it has been estimated that approximately 1% of the patients with acute viral bronchiolitis develop postinfectious OB *(110)*. The diagnosis of postinfectious OB in the childhood is based on history of lower airway infection, usually acute viral bronchiolitis, followed by persistent chronic obstructive pulmonary disease. The time interval between the acute illness and the development of postinfectious OB is generally 6 months (range 1–42 months) *(111)*. In the majority of the cases, the condition does not become apparent until adulthood. Most patients with postinfectious OB are asymptomatic or present with mild-to-moderate clinical findings and have a good prognosis *(40,78,112)*. Occasionally, severe and sometimes fatal disease may occur *(112,113)*. In a prospective study performed to define the clinical course and the prognosis of 31 patients who had symptomatic postinfectious OB during a mean of 3.5 years of follow-up, clinical remission was identified in 23% of the patients, persistence of respiratory symptoms in 68%, and death in approximately 10% *(112)*. Lung transplantation or lung volume reduction surgery should be considered for patients who show persistent and severe obstructive symptoms and progressive impairment in lung function *(114)*. The chest radiograph may be normal or show various findings including unilateral hyperlucency of a lobe or lung; bilateral hyperlucent lungs; complete collapse of the affected lobe; a mixed pattern of hyperlucency and persistent collapse; and peribronchial thickening *(78)*. High-resolution CT usually demonstrates bronchial wall thickening, bronchiectasis, mosaic perfusion, and air trapping (see Figs 7 and 15) *(109,115)*.

Swyer–James (MacLeod) syndrome is an uncommon condition characterized radiographically by a hyperlucent lobe or lung and functionally by normal or reduced TLC and presence of expiratory air trapping. The hyperlucency of the lobe or lung results from decreased pulmonary blood flow secondary to OB. Swyer–James syndrome typically follows lower respiratory tract infection in a developing lung, most commonly adenovirus bronchiolitis or bronchopneumonia. The pulmonary tissue and pulmonary vasculature are hypoplastic. The chest radiograph performed at TLC shows hyperlucency and decreased vascularity of the involved lobe or lung, normal or decreased size of the involved lobe or lung, and decreased size of the ipsilateral hilum (Fig. 16). Expiratory chest radiograph shows air trapping in the involved lobe or lung.

High-resolution CT, similar to the radiograph, shows hyperlucency and decreased vascularity and normal or decreased size of the involved lung or lobe on inspiratory images and air trapping on expiratory images *(116–118)*. In the vast majority of cases, CT demonstrates bronchiectasis and areas of abnormally low attenuation and perfusion and air trapping in the contralateral lung (Fig. 17)

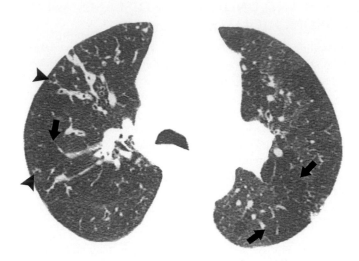

Fig. 15. Obliterative bronchiolitis in 41-year-old man with history of repeated childhood respiratory tract infections. High-resolution CT image shows areas of decreased attenuation and vascularity (straight arrows) interspersed with areas of increased attenuation because of blood flow redistribution (mosaic perfusion pattern), particularly in the left upper lobe. Also noted are bronchial wall thickening and a few centrilobular nodules and tree-in-bud opacities (arrowheads).

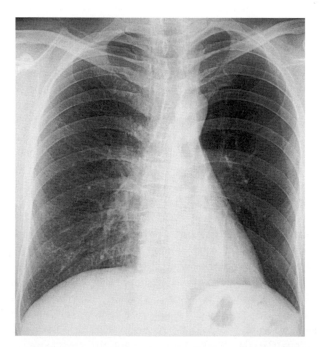

Fig. 16. Swyer–James (MacLeod) syndrome. Posteroanterior chest radiography shows hyperlucency, decreased vascularity, and decreased volume of the left lung with ipsilateral mediastinal shift. The patient was an asymptomatic 40-year-old man with obliterative bronchiolitis following childhood viral infection.

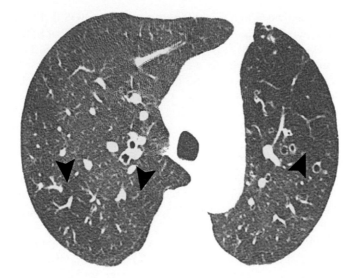

Fig. 17. Swyer–James (Macleod's) syndrome. High-resolution CT image demonstrates extensive areas of decreased attenuation and vascularity in the left upper lobe and to lesser extent in the right upper lobe (arrowheads). Also noted are decreased volume of the left lung and left upper lobe bronchiectasis.

(116,117). Air trapping is seen on CT performed at end-expiration and on dynamic expiratory CT *(119).* The majority of patients with Swyer–James syndrome are asymptomatic adults. Occasionally, patients may present with a history of repeated lower respiratory tract infections or shortness of breath.

7.2. Obliterative Bronchiolitis Associated with Transplantation

Obliterative bronchiolitis is a common and important complication of lung and heart-lung transplantation and remains the single leading cause of morbidity and mortality in these patients. The prevalence of OB following lung transplantation is approximately 20% at 1 year and greater than 50% at 3–5 years *(79,120–123).* OB is the primary cause of death in 30% of the affected individuals after the third postoperative year and more than half of affected individuals after 5 years *(120,121,123,124).* Clinically, OB typically is first recognized 16–20 months after transplantation although it may manifest as early as the second or third month after transplantation *(80,125,126).* OB is believed to be a manifestation of chronic rejection. Although by definition OB is a pathologic diagnosis, histologic confirmation is difficult to obtain. The reported sensitivity of transbronchial biopsy ranges from 15 to 87% and the specificity approximately 75% *(21–23,25,26).* Surgical biopsy is seldom performed on these patients. Bronchoalveolar lavage is usually nonspecific and may show neutrophilic and/or lymphocytic inflammation *(127,128).* However, transbronchial biopsy and bronchoalveolar lavage are important in excluding other possible diagnoses as contributing causes of deteriorating pulmonary function in patients with lung transplantation and heart-lung transplantation, such as acute rejection and infection *(129,130).* Because of the low sensitivity of transbronchial biopsy in demonstrating OB, the International Society for Heart and Lung Transplantation has established the concept of bronchiolitis obliterans syndrome (BOS) and a staging system to quantify the severity of airflow obstruction *(131).* According to the revised classification system, the staging is based on the reduction in the forced expiration volume in 1 s (FEV_1) and mid-expiratory flow rate (FEF_{25-75}), in comparison with baseline post-transplant values, with or without histologic documentation of OB, and the exclusion of other causes for the functional abnormality *(132).* On the basis of the severity of functional impairment, BOS can be subdivided into five different categories: BOS 0 (FEV_1 > 90% of baseline, and FEF_{25-75} > 75% of baseline), BOS 0-p (potential OB; FEV_1 81–90% of baseline, and/or FEF_{25-75} ≤ 75% of baseline), BOS 1 (mild OB; FEV_1 66–80% of baseline), BOS 2 (moderate OB; FEV_1 51–65% of baseline), and BOS 3 (severe OB; FEV_1 ≤ 50% of baseline).

Post-transplant OB has a variable course. Some patients experience a sudden onset with rapid decline of lung function and respiratory failure. Others experience insidious onset with a slow, progressive decline over time or, less commonly, an initial rapid decline in FEV_1 followed by a prolonged period of stability (133,134). Clinical symptoms at onset are usually absent or nonspecific. Some patients present with an asymptomatic fall in FEV_1 and/or biopsy findings of OB. Clinical symptoms include malaise, dry cough, and shortness of breath on exertion. Sputum production at presentation is typically absent; however, repeated episodes of bacterial infection, followed by permanent airway colonization with pathogenic bacteria and fungi (e.g., *Pseudomonas* and *Staphylococcus* spp. and *Aspergillus fumigatus*), may result in productive cough later in the course of the disease (134).

Obliterative bronchiolitis is also the most common noninfectious late pulmonary complication of allogeneic hematopoietic stem-cell transplantation (HSCT) (127,135). OB in these patients typically occurs more than 3 months following transplantation and in the setting of underlying chronic graft-versus-host disease (GVHD) (82,127). OB is estimated to affect approximately 20% of patients who receive allogeneic transplants (81,82) but is rare after autologous transplantation (136). In a recent study, the 5-year survival rate of 47 HSCT recipients with OB was 10%, compared with 40% for those without OB (137). Occasionally, air-leak syndromes including pneumomediastinum, pneumothorax, pneumopericardium, subcutaneous emphysema, and cervical emphysema may complicate severe OB in these patients (17,138–140).

The pathogenesis of OB in lung transplantation and heart-lung transplantation is not well understood. The main risk factors for the development of BOS are acute rejection, particularly when recurrent or severe, lymphocytic bronchitis/bronchiolitis, and cytomegalovirus pneumonitis (132,134,141–144). Gastroesophageal reflux with occult microaspiration that may promote chronic inflammation and bacterial infections in the lower airways may be a potential risk factor for BOS (145,146). The etiology of post-transplant gastroesophageal reflux is probable multifactorial and includes intraoperative vagal injury, drug-induced prolonged gastric emptying, and impaired lower esophageal sphincter function (145–148). Preliminary studies suggest that antireflux surgery, such as fundoplication, may improve lung function in some of these patients (149). Risk factors for OB among allogeneic recipients are probably also multifactorial and include acute and chronic GVHD, older donor and recipient age, myeloablative conditioning, methotrexate use, antecedent respiratory infection, and serum immunoglobulin deficiency (81,82,150).

Early diagnosis of OB in transplanted patients is important because prompt initiation of therapy may help to preserve lung function and improve long-term survival (81,134). The treatment of OB usually consists of corticosteroids and augmented immunosuppression. However, only a minority improve. BOS does not appear to recur in an accelerated manner after retransplantation (151–153). The risk of developing OB is similar to that of first-time lung transplant recipients.

Lung function is currently the gold standard for detecting chronic allograft dysfunction in transplanted patients. High-resolution CT is a valuable tool in the evaluation and follow-up of transplanted patients (Fig. 18). CT is a direct measure of the lung structure and allows the identification of structural abnormalities associated with chronic allograft dysfunction, including bronchiectasis, airway wall thickening, mucus in small and large airways, and air trapping because of small airway abnormalities (see Figs 8 and 9). The presence of air trapping on expiratory high-resolution CT scans is the most sensitive and accurate radiologic indicator of OB following transplantation (46,154–158). High-resolution CT has been used to predict BOS in both adults and children; however, more recent studies have shown that the value of air trapping at expiratory high-resolution CT before the clinical

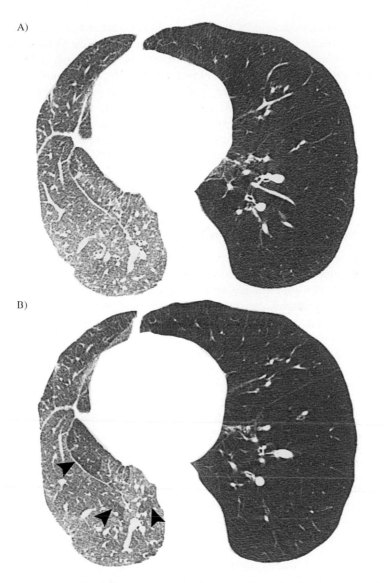

Fig. 18. Obliterative bronchiolitis following unilateral lung transplantation for severe panacinar emphysema. (**A**) Expiratory high-resolution CT image shortly after transplantation shows no definite abnormality in the transplanted lung. The native lung demonstrates diffuse decrease in attenuation and marked hyperinflation due to panacinar emphysema. (**B**) Expiratory image at the same level as (A) 1 year later demonstrates lobular air trapping in the right lower lobe (arrows). The patient was a 60-year-old man with bronchiolitis obliterans syndrome.

appearance and during the early stages of BOS is lower than previously reported *(154,156)*. The reported sensitivities and specificities of air trapping range from 44 to 91% and 80 to 100%, respectively *(46,154–158)*. This variability may be due to differences in the technique used to quantify the extent of air trapping, patient selection with inclusion of heart-lung or bilateral-lung and single-lung transplant recipients and predate the revised criteria for BOS, which are believed to be more sensitive for the detection of early-stage BOS *(132)*. Furthermore, most studies included high-resolution CT scans that were obtained after clinical diagnosis of OB. In a recent study, Konen et al. *(154)* assessed the value of CT findings in predicting BOS before its clinical appearance and during the early stages of BOS. The authors found lower sensitivity for air trapping (44–50%) than previously reported (74–91%) *(155–158)*. The sensitivities of mosaic perfusion, bronchiectasis, and bronchial wall thickening were even lower, not exceeding 25% *(154,158,159)*. The limitations of high-resolution CT are also at least in part because of the inter- and intra-observer variability in the interpretation of the CT images and the different scoring systems used to quantify the extent of air trapping on CT *(154,156,157,160)*. A composite CT score system may have a potential role in the early detection of OB in lung transplant recipients, as demonstrated in a recent study with good intra- and inter-observer agreement *(161)*. Preliminary studies have shown that functional MR imaging using hyperpolarized 3-He detects BOS earlier than spirometry or high-resolution CT *(31,162)*. The main limitations of functional MR imaging are high cost and limited availability. It therefore currently remains an investigational modality.

7.3. Postinhalational Obliterative Bronchiolitis

Obliterative bronchiolitis is a well-described complication of inhalational injury being seen most commonly after inhalation of nitrogen dioxide (Silo filler's disease). The acute phase of Silo filler's disease typically manifests within minutes or hours after exposure and usually resolves within hours *(83)*. The main clinical symptoms consist of cough, dyspnea, fatigue, and cyanosis. Patients may develop pulmonary edema and acute respiratory distress syndrome (ARDS). If the patient survives, a progressive and irreversible obstructive ventilatory defect may be noted 2–5 weeks later *(83)*. At the late stage, the radiologic findings are similar to those of OB because of other causes. Other toxic gases associated with OB include ammonia, chlorine, hydrogen bromide, hydrogen selenide, sulfur dioxide, and fire smoke *(3,5)*. Recently, diacetyl (2,3-butanedione), a ketone with butter-flavor characteristics, was the predominant compound isolated in workers in a microwave popcorn plant *(163,164)*, who developed clinical, histologic, and imaging findings of OB *(163)*. Some of these patients developed severe symptoms and required lung transplantation.

7.4. Obliterative Bronchiolitis Associated with Connective Tissue Disorders

Several connective tissue diseases are associated with an increased risk of bronchiolitis, but OB is seen most commonly in patients with rheumatoid arthritis *(84,85,87,165,166)*. OB in rheumatoid arthritis usually occurs in patients with long-standing disease and is seen most commonly in women in their fifth to sixth decades of life *(84,85)*. OB as the sole and presenting feature of rheumatoid arthritis is rare *(86,167)*.

The course of disease is variable. Penicillamine therapy and, less commonly, gold therapy have been implicated as potential contributive causative agents of OB in some patients with rheumatoid arthritis *(167–169)*.

The radiologic findings of rheumatoid arthritis associated with OB are similar to those of patients with others forms of OB. The most common high-resolution CT findings are mosaic perfusion, air trapping, and bronchiectasis (Fig. 19) *(86,170,171)*.

Occasionally, OB may be seen in association with connective disorders other than rheumatoid arthritis, including Sjögren's syndrome *(172)*, systemic lupus erythematosus *(173)*, and scleroderma *(88–90)*.

7.5. Sauropous androgynus-Related Obliterative Bronchiolitis

Consumption of juice prepared from the uncooked leaves of the vegetable *Sauropous androgynus* (a member of the Euphorbiaceae family), which is alleged to help weight control, has a known association with OB *(92–94,174)*. *S. androgynus* is commonly found in Malaysia, Indonesia, southwest China, and Vietnam. It is not known whether OB results from cytotoxic effect, inflammatory reaction,

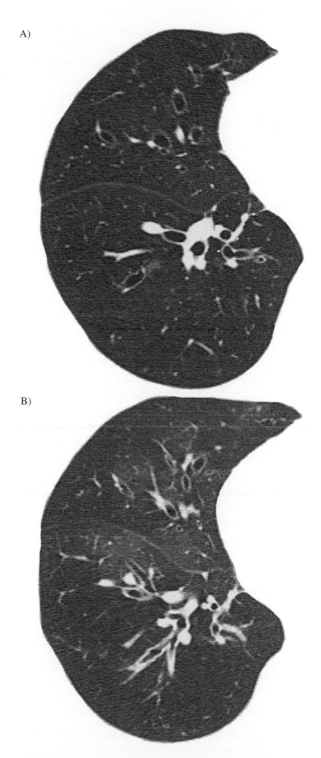

Fig. 19. Obliterative bronchiolitis in a 49-year-old woman with long-standing rheumatoid arthritis. (**A**) High-resolution CT image targeted to the right lung shows extensive areas of decreased attenuation and vascularity and bronchiectasis. (**B**) Expiratory image shows air trapping.

or immunological response. Lai et al. *(94)* reported the clinical and radiologic features of OB associated with consumption of uncooked *S. androgynus* in 23 patients during an outbreak in Taiwan. All patients were young or middle-aged nonsmoking women who developed rapidly progressive shortness of breath and persistent cough 3–4 months after ingestion of blended vegetable juice. The patients had moderate-to-severe airflow obstruction without response to bronchodilator therapy or prednisolone. The chest radiographs were normal, and high-resolution CT demonstrated bilateral bronchiectasis and patchy mosaic perfusion at inspiratory CT in 11 of 23 patients and air trapping at expiratory scans in all patients. Four patients had open lung biopsy findings of OB. OB associated with consumption of *S. androgynus* has a poor prognosis, some patients requiring lung transplantation *(175,176)*.

7.6. Obliterative Bronchiolitis Associated with Diffuse Neuroendocrine Cell Hyperplasia, Carcinoid Tumorlets, and Carcinoid Tumors

Neuroendocrine (Kulchitzky) cells are commonly found in the basal layer of the surface epithelium and in the bronchial glands from the level of the main bronchi to the proximal bronchioles. Diffuse idiopathic pulmonary neuroendocrine cell hyperplasia (DIPNECH) is a rare condition characterized by proliferation of neuroendocrine cells as clusters of cells or as linear arrays along the basement membrane *(95,177)*. DIPNECH is regarded as a precursor to the development of carcinoid tumorlets, which consist of nodular proliferations (diameter <5 mm) of airway neuroendocrine cells that extend beyond the epithelium into the adjacent wall or lung parenchyma. If such a lesion exceeds 5 mm in diameter, it is regarded as a carcinoid tumor *(177–179)*. Aguayo et al. *(95)* reported the clinical and pathologic findings of six lifelong nonsmokers who had diffuse hyperplasia of airway neuroendocrine cells and multiple pulmonary carcinoid tumorlets associated with OB and airway obstruction. The OB in these patients is postulated to be secondary to a combination of intraluminal obstruction by hyperplastic neuroendocrine cells and peribronchiolar fibrosis presumably secondary to peptide secretory products released by the proliferating neuroendocrine cells *(95,180)*. The patients are usually women in their fifth or sixth decade and have history of long-standing progressive respiratory distress (>10 years) and persistent cough with mild-to-moderate airflow obstruction at lung function tests *(96)*. The chest radiograph is usually normal. The most common high-resolution CT findings are mosaic perfusion at inspiratory CT and air trapping at expiratory images. Other high-resolution CT findings include bronchial wall thickening, a few dilated bronchi and occasional well-defined nodules measuring 0.2–1.5 mm in diameter that correspond to the carcinoid tumorlets and carcinoid tumors identified histologically (Fig. 20) *(96,97,178,181)*.

7.7. Cryptogenic Obliterative Bronchiolitis

Cryptogenic (idiopathic) OB is rare and has been described mainly in older women *(106,182)*. Patients with cryptogenic OB usually present with chronic cough, dyspnea, mild-to-severe airway obstruction that may progress to respiratory failure and does not respond to bronchodilators. The radiologic findings of cryptogenic OB are similar to those of patients with other forms of OB (see Fig. 6) *(35,47)*.

7.8. Obliterative Bronchiolitis Associated with Inflammatory Bowel Disease

The most frequent pulmonary complications associated with inflammatory bowel disease are tracheobronchitis, chronic bronchitis, and bronchiectasis *(183–186)*. Occasionally, patients with ulcerative colitis and Crohn's disease may develop OB *(187)*. Colectomy is believed to be a risk factor for the development of pulmonary disease in these patients *(99,183,184,186)*. In a study of 17 patients with inflammatory bowel disease (14 patients with ulcerative colitis and three patients with

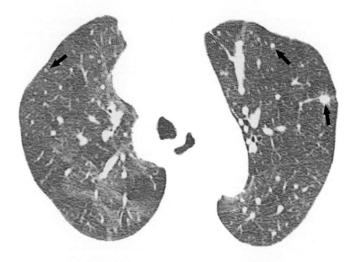

Fig. 20. Diffuse idiopathic pulmonary neuroendocrine cell hyperplasia (DIPNECH). Expiratory high-resolution CT image at the level or aortic arch shows patchy areas of air trapping and bilateral 2–8 mm well-defined soft tissue nodules (arrows). The patient was a 72-year-old woman with biopsy proven obliterative bronchiolitis and DIPNECH and multiple pulmonary carcinoid tumorlets and carcinoid tumors.

Crohn's disease) without active bowel disease at the time of the study, bronchiectasis was seen in 13 patients (76%) including 11 with ulcerative colitis and two with Crohn's disease, nine patients showed evidence of air trapping, and five had tree-in-bud opacities at high-resolution CT *(99)*.

REFERENCES

1. Colby TV. Bronchiolitis. Pathologic considerations. *Am J Clin Pathol* 1998; 109:101–109.
2. Myers JL, Colby TV. Pathologic manifestations of bronchiolitis, constrictive bronchiolitis, cryptogenic organizing pneumonia and diffuse panbronchiolitis. *Clin Chest Med* 1993; 14:611–623.
3. Ryu JH, Myers JL, Swensen SJ. Bronchiolar disorders. *Am J Respir Crit Care Med* 2003; 168:1277–1292.
4. King TE. Overview of bronchiolitis. *Clin Chest Med* 1993; 14:607–610.
5. Travis WD, Colby TV, Koss MN, Rosado-de-Christenson MI., Muller NL, King TE, Jr., eds Bronchiolar disorders. In: *Atlas of Nontumor Pathology. Non-Neoplastic Disorders of the Lower Respiratory Tract.* Washington, DC: American Registry of Pathology and the Armed Forces Institute of Pathology, 2002; 351–380.
6. Muller NL, Miller RR. Diseases of the bronchioles: CT and histopathologic findings. *Radiology* 1995; 196:3–12.
7. Poletti V, Costabel U. Bronchiolar disorders: classification and diagnostic approach. *Semin Respir Crit Care Med* 2003; 24:457–464.
8. Padley SPG, Adler BD, Hansell DM, Müller NL. Bronchiolitis obliterans: high-resolution CT findings and correlation with pulmonary function tests. *Clin Radiol* 1993; 47:236–240.
9. Gosink BB, Friedman PJ, Liebow AA. Bronchiolitis obliterans: roentgenographic-pathologic correlation. *AJR Am J Roentgenol* 1973; 117:816–832.
10. Baar HS, Galindo J. Bronchiolitis fibrosa obliterans. *Thorax* 1966; 21:209–214.
11. Lange W. Ueber eine eigenthumliche Erkrankung der kleinen Bronchien und Bronchiolen (Bronchitis et bronchiolitis obliterans). *Dtsch Arch Klin Med* 1901; 70:342–364.
12. American Thoracic Society/European Respiratory Society International Multidisciplinary Consensus Classification of the Idiopathic Interstitial Pneumonias. *Am J Respir Crit Care Med* 2002; 165:277–304.
13. Schlesinger C, Koss MN. The organizing pneumonias: an update and review. *Curr Opin Pulm Med* 2005; 11:422–430.
14. Schlesinger C, Meyer CA, Veeraraghavan S, Koss MN. Constrictive (obliterative) bronchiolitis: diagnosis, etiology, and a critical review of the literature. *Ann Diagn Pathol* 1998; 2:321–334.
15. Dikensoy O, Bayram N, Bingol A, Filiz A. Bronchiolitis obliterans in a case of juvenile rheumatoid arthritis presented with pneumomediastinum. *Respiration* 2002; 69:100–102.
16. Tanvetyanon T, Toor AA, Stiff PJ. Post-transplant air-leak syndrome. *Br J Haematol* 2004; 126:758.

17. Kumar S, Tefferi A. Spontaneous pneumomediastinum and subcutaneous emphysema complicating bronchiolitis obliterans after allogeneic bone marrow transplantation—case report and review of literature. *Ann Hematol* 2001; 80:430–435.

18. Hansell DM, Rubens MB, Padley SP, Wells AU. Obliterative bronchiolitis: individual CT signs of small airways disease and functional correlation. *Radiology* 1997; 203:721–726.

19. Copley SJ, Wells AU, Muller NL, et al. Thin-section CT in obstructive pulmonary disease: discriminatory value. *Radiology* 2002; 223:812–819.

20. Yousem SA, Berry GJ, Cagle PT, et al. Revision of the 1990 working formulation for the classification of pulmonary allograft rejection: Lung Rejection Study Group. *J Heart Lung Transplant* 1996; 15:1–15.

21. Pomerance A, Madden B, Burke MM, Yacoub MH. Transbronchial biopsy in heart and lung transplantation: clinico-pathologic correlations. *J Heart Lung Transplant* 1995; 14:761–773.

22. Kramer MR, Stoehr C, Whang JL, et al. The diagnosis of obliterative bronchiolitis after heart-lung and lung transplantation: low yield of transbronchial lung biopsy. *J Heart Lung Transplant* 1993; 12:675–681.

23. Trulock EP. Management of lung transplant rejection. *Chest* 1993; 103:1566–1576.

24. Yousem SA, Paradis IL, Dauber JH, Griffith BP. Efficacy of transbronchial lung biopsy in the diagnosis of bronchiolitis obliterans in heart-lung transplant recipients. *Transplantation* 1989; 47:893–895.

25. Yousem SA, Paradis I, Griffith BP. Can transbronchial biopsy aid in the diagnosis of bronchiolitis obliterans in lung transplant recipients? *Transplantation* 1994; 57:151–153.

26. Chamberlain D, Maurer J, Chaparro C, Idolor L. Evaluation of transbronchial lung biopsy specimens in the diagnosis of bronchiolitis obliterans after lung transplantation. *J Heart Lung Transplant* 1994; 13:963–971.

27. Halvorsen RA, Jr., DuCret RP, Kuni CC, Olivari MT, Tylen U, Hertz MI. Obliterative bronchiolitis following lung transplantation. Diagnostic utility of aerosol ventilation lung scanning and high resolution CT. *Clin Nucl Med* 1991; 16:256–258.

28. Cook RC, Fradet G, Muller NL, Worsely DF, Ostrow D, Levy RD. Noninvasive investigations for the early detection of chronic airways dysfunction following lung transplantation. *Can Respir J* 2003; 10:76–83.

29. Muller NL. Advances in imaging. *Eur Respir J* 2001; 18:867–871.

30. de Lange EE, Mugler JP, 3rd, Brookeman JR, et al. Lung air spaces: MR imaging evaluation with hyperpolarized 3He gas. *Radiology* 1999; 210:851–857.

31. McAdams HP, Palmer SM, Donnelly LF, Charles HC, Tapson VF, MacFall JR. Hyperpolarized 3He-enhanced MR imaging of lung transplant recipients: preliminary results. *AJR Am J Roentgenol* 1999; 173:955–959.

32. Lynch DA. Imaging of small airways disease. *Clin Chest Med* 1993; 14:623–634.

33. Garg K, A. LD, Newell JD, King TE. Proliferative and constrictive bronchiolitis: classification and radiologic features. *AJR Am J Roentgenol* 1994; 162:803–808.

34. McLoud TC, Epler GR, Colby TV, Gaensler EA, Carrington CB. Bronchiolitis obliterans. *Radiology* 1986; 159:1–8.

35. Breatnach E, Kerr I. The radiology of cryptogenic obliterative bronchiolitis. *Clin Radiol* 1982; 33:657–661.

36. Morrish WF, Herman SJ, Weisbrod GL, Chamberlain DW. Bronchiolitis obliterans after lung transplantation: findings at chest radiography and high-resolution CT. *Radiology* 1991; 179:487–490.

37. Dawson KP, Long A, Kennedy J, Mogridge N. The chest radiograph in acute bronchiolitis. *J Paediatr Child Health* 1990; 26:209–211.

38. Davies HD, Wang EE, Manson D, Babyn P, Shuckett B. Reliability of the chest radiograph in the diagnosis of lower respiratory infections in young children. *Pediatr Infect Dis J* 1996; 15:600–604.

39. Hansell DM. Small airways diseases: detection and insights with computed tomography. *Eur Respir J* 2001; 17: 1294–1313.

40. Kim CK, Kim SW, Kim JS, et al. Bronchiolitis obliterans in the 1990s in Korea and the United States. *Chest* 2001; 120:1101–1106.

41. Sweatman MC, Millar AB, Strickland B, Turner-Warwick M. Computed tomography in adult obliterative bronchiolitis. *Clin Radiol* 1990; 41:116–119.

42. Eber CD, Stark P, Bertozzi P. Bronchiolitis obliterans on high-resolution CT: a pattern of mosaic oligemia. *J Comput Assist Tomogr* 1993; 17:853–856.

43. Lau DM, Siegel MJ, Hildebolt CF, Cohen AH. Bronchiolitis obliterans syndrome: thin-section CT diagnosis of obstructive changes in infants and young children after lung transplantation. *Radiology* 1998; 208:783–788.

44. Lynch DA, Brasch RC, Hardy KA, Webb WR. Pediatric pulmonary disease: assessment with high-resolution ultrafast CT. *Radiology* 1990; 176:243–248.

45. Worthy SA, Müller NL, Hartman TE, Swensen SJ, Padley SP, Hansell DM. Mosaic attenuation pattern on thin-section CT scans of the lung: differentiation among infiltrative lung, airway, and vascular diseases as a cause. *Radiology* 1997; 205:465–470.

46. Worthy SA, Park CS, Kim JS, Müller NL. Bronchiolitis obliterans after lung transplantation: high resolution CT findings in 15 patients. *AJR Am J Roentgenol* 1997; 169:673–677.

47. Jensen SP, Lynch DA, Brown KK, Wenzel SE, Newell JD. High-resolution CT features of severe asthma and bronchiolitis obliterans. *Clin Radiol* 2002; 57:1078–1085.

48. Webb WR, Stern EJ, Kanth N, Gamsu G. Dynamic pulmonary CT: findings in normal adult men. *Radiology* 1993; 186:117–124.

49. Stern EJ, Webb WR. Dynamic imaging of lung morphology with ultrafast high-resolution computed tomography. *J Thorac Imag* 1993; 8:273–282.

50. Stern EJ, Frank MS. Small-airway diseases of the lungs: findings at expiratory CT. *AJR Am J Roentgenol* 1994; 163:37–41.

51. Sweatman MC, Millar AB, Strickland B, Turner-Warwick M. Computed tomography in adult obliterative bronchiolitis. *Clin Radiol* 1990; 41:116–119.

52. Arakawa H, Webb WR, McCowin M, Katsou G, Lee KN, Seitz RF. Inhomogeneous lung attenuation at thin-section CT: diagnostic value of expiratory scans. *Radiology* 1998; 206:89–94.

53. Stern EJ, Webb WR, Gamsu G. Dynamic quantitative computed tomography: a predictor of pulmonary function in obstructive lung diseases. *Invest Radiol* 1994; 29:564–569.

54. Gotway MB, Lee ES, Reddy GP, Golden JA, Webb WR. Low-dose, dynamic, expiratory thin-section CT of the lungs using a spiral CT scanner. *J Thorac Imaging* 2000; 15:168–172.

55. Lucidarme O, Grenier PA, Cadi M, Mourey-Gerosa I, Benali K, Cluzel P. Evaluation of air trapping at CT: comparison of continuous-versus suspended-expiration CT techniques. *Radiology* 2000; 216:768–772.

56. Remy-Jardin M, Remy J, Gosselin B, Copin MC, Wurtz A, Duhamel A. Sliding thin slab, minimum intensity projection technique in the diagnosis of emphysema: histopathologic-CT correlation. *Radiology* 1996; 200:665–671.

57. Bhalla M, Naidich DP, McGuinness G, Gruden JF, Leitman BS, McCauley DI. Diffuse lung disease: assessment with helical CT–preliminary observations of the role of maximum and minimum intensity projection images [see comments]. *Radiology* 1996; 200:341–347.

58. Yang GZ, Hansell DM. CT image enhancement with wavelet analysis for the detection of small airways disease. *IEEE Trans Med Imaging* 1997; 16:953–961.

59. Fotheringham T, Chabat F, Hansell DM, et al. A comparison of methods for enhancing the detection of areas of decreased attenuation on CT caused by airways disease. *J Comput Assist Tomogr* 1999; 23:385–389.

60. Wittram C, Batt J, Rappaport DC, Hutcheon MA. Inspiratory and expiratory helical CT of normal adults: comparison of thin section scans and minimum intensity projection images. *J Thorac Imaging* 2002; 17:47–52.

61. Wittram C, Rappaport DC. Bronchiolitis obliterans after lung transplantation: appearance on expiratory minimum intensity projection images. *Can Assoc Radiol J* 2000; 51:103–106.

62. Lentz D, Bergin CJ, Berry GJ, Stoehr C, Theodore J. Diagnosis of bronchiolitis obliterans in heart-lung transplantation patients: importance of bronchial dilatation on CT. *AJR Am J Roentgenol* 1992; 159:463–467.

63. Lynch DA, Newell JD, Tschomper BA, Cink TM, Newman LS, Bethel R. Uncomplicated asthma in adults: comparison of CT appearance of the lungs in asthmatic and healthy subjects. *Radiology* 1993; 188:829–833.

64. Hansell DM, Wells AU, Padley SP, Müller NL. Hypersensitivity pneumonitis: correlation of individual CT patterns with functional abnormalities. *Radiology* 1996; 199:123–128.

65. Remy-Jardin M, Remy J, Wallaert B, Müller NL. Subacute and chronic bird breeder hypersensitivity pneumonitis: sequential evaluation with CT and correlation with lung function tests and bronchoalveolar lavage. *Radiology* 1993; 198:111–118.

66. Small JH, Flower CD, Traill ZC, Gleeson FV. Air-trapping in extrinsic allergic alveolitis on computed tomography. *Clin Radiol* 1996; 51:684–688.

67. Remy-Jardin M, Remy J, Louvegny S, Artaud D, Deschildre F, Duhamel A. Airway changes in chronic pulmonary embolism: CT findings in 33 patients. *Radiology* 1997; 203:355–360.

68. Arakawa H, Kurihara Y, Sasaka K, Nakajima Y, Webb WR. Air trapping on CT of patients with pulmonary embolism. *AJR Am J Roentgenol* 2002; 178:1201–1207.

69. Park CS, Müller NL, Worthy SA, Kim JS, Awadh N, Fitzgerald M. Airway obstruction in asthmatic and healthy individuals: inspiratory and expiratory thin-section CT findings. *Radiology* 1997; 203:361–367.

70. Lee KW, Chung SY, Yang I, Lee Y, Ko EY, Park MJ. Correlation of aging and smoking with air trapping at thin-section CT of the lung in asymptomatic subjects. *Radiology* 2000; 214:831–836.

71. Tanaka N, Matsumoto T, Miura G, et al. Air trapping at CT: high prevalence in asymptomatic subjects with normal pulmonary function. *Radiology* 2003; 227:776–785.

72. Lucidarme O, Coche E, Cluzel P, Mourey-Gerosa I, Howarth N, Grenier P. Expiratory CT scans for chronic airway disease: correlation with pulmonary function test results. *AJR Am J Roentgenol* 1998; 170:301–307.

73. Mastora I, Remy-Jardin M, Sobaszek A, Boulenguez C, Remy J, Edme JL. Thin-section CT finding in 250 volunteers: assessment of the relationship of CT findings with smoking history and pulmonary function test results. *Radiology* 2001; 218:695–702.

74. Verschakelen JA, Scheinbaum K, Bogaert J, Demedts M, Lacquet LL, Baert AL. Expiratory CT in cigarette smokers: correlation between areas of decreased lung attenuation, pulmonary function tests and smoking history. *Eur Radiol* 1998; 8:1391–1399.

75. Davies CW, Tasker AD, Padley SP, Davies RJ, Gleeson FV. Air trapping in sarcoidosis on computed tomography: correlation with lung function. *Clin Radiol* 2000; 55:217–221.
76. Terasaki H, Fujimoto K, Muller NL, et al. Pulmonary sarcoidosis: comparison of findings of inspiratory and expiratory high-resolution CT and pulmonary function tests between smokers and nonsmokers. *AJR Am J Roentgenol* 2005; 185:333–338.
77. Magkanas E, Voloudaki A, Bouros D, et al. Pulmonary sarcoidosis. Correlation of expiratory high-resolution CT findings with inspiratory patterns and pulmonary function tests. *Acta Radiol* 2001; 42:494–501.
78. Chang AB, Masel JP, Masters B. Post-infectious bronchiolitis obliterans: clinical, radiological and pulmonary function sequelae. *Pediatr Radiol* 1998; 28:23–29.
79. Hertz MI, Taylor DO, Trulock EP, et al. The registry of the international society for heart and lung transplantation: nineteenth official report-2002. *J Heart Lung Transplant* 2002; 21:950–970.
80. Keller CA, Cagle PT, Brown RW, Noon G, Frost AE. Bronchiolitis obliterans in recipients of single, double, and heart-lung transplantation. *Chest* 1995; 107:973–980.
81. Afessa B, Litzow MR, Tefferi A. Bronchiolitis obliterans and other late onset non-infectious pulmonary complications in hematopoietic stem cell transplantation. *Bone Marrow Transplant* 2001; 28:425–434.
82. Chien JW, Martin PJ, Gooley TA, et al. Airflow obstruction after myeloablative allogeneic hematopoietic stem cell transplantation. *Am J Respir Crit Care Med* 2003; 168:208–214.
83. King TE, Jr. Miscellaneous causes of bronchiolitis: inhalational, infectious, drug-induced, and idiopathic. *Semin Respir Crit Care Med* 2003; 24:567–576.
84. Wells AU, duBois RM. Bronchiolitis in association with connective tissue diseases. *Clin Chest Med* 1993; 14:655–666.
85. Geddes DM, Corrin B, Brewerton DA, Davies RJ, Turner-Warwick M. Progressive airway obliteration in adults and its association with rheumatoid disease. *Q J Med* 1977; 46:427–444.
86. Remy-Jardin M, Remy J, Cortet B, Mauri F, Delcambre B. Lung changes in rheumatoid arthritis: CT findings. *Radiology* 1994; 193:375–382.
87. White ES, Tazelaar HD, Lynch JP, 3rd. Bronchiolar complications of connective tissue diseases. *Semin Respir Crit Care Med* 2003; 24:543–566.
88. Hakala M, Paakko P, Sutinen S, Huhti E, Koivisto O, Tarkka M. Association of bronchiolitis with connective tissue disorders. *Ann Rheum Dis* 1986; 45:656–662.
89. Boehler A, Vogt P, Speich R, Weder W, Russi EW. Bronchiolitis obliterans in a patient with localized scleroderma treated with D-penicillamine. *Eur Respir J* 1996; 9:1317–1319.
90. Yousem SA. The pulmonary pathologic manifestations of the CREST syndrome. *Hum Pathol* 1990; 21:467–474.
91. Turner-Warwick M. Adverse reactions affecting the lung: possible association with D-penicillamine. *J Rheumatol Suppl* 1981; 7:166–168.
92. Chang H, Wang JS, Tseng HH, Lai RS, Su JM. Histopathological study of Sauropus androgynus-associated constrictive bronchiolitis obliterans: a new cause of constrictive bronchiolitis obliterans [see comments]. *Am J Surg Pathol* 1997; 21:35–42.
93. Ger LP, Chiang AA, Lai RS, Chen SM, Tseng CJ. Association of Sauropus androgynus and bronchiolitis obliterans syndrome: a hospital-based case-control study. *Am J Epidemiol* 1997; 145:842–849.
94. Lai RS, Chiang AA, Wu MT, et al. Outbreak of bronchiolitis obliterans associated with consumption of Sauropus androgynus in Taiwan. *Lancet* 1996; 348:83–85.
95. Aguayo SM, Miller YE, Waldron JA, Jr., et al. Brief report: idiopathic diffuse hyperplasia of pulmonary neuroendocrine cells and airways disease. *N Engl J Med* 1992; 327:1285–1288.
96. Lee JS, Brown KK, Cool C, Lynch DA. Diffuse pulmonary neuroendocrine cell hyperplasia: radiologic and clinical features. *J Comput Assist Tomogr* 2002; 26:180–184.
97. Brown MJ, English J, Müller NL. Bronchiolitis obliterans due to neuroendocrine hyperplasia: high-resolution CT and pathologic correlation. *AJR Am J Roentgenol* 1997; 168:1561–1562.
98. Wilcox P, Miller R, Miller G, et al. Airway involvement in ulcerative colitis. *Chest* 1987; 92:18–22.
99. Mahadeva R, Walsh G, Flower CD, Shneerson JM. Clinical and radiological characteristics of lung disease in inflammatory bowel disease. *Eur Respir J* 2000; 15:41–48.
100. Tsunoda N, Iwanaga T, Saito T, Kitamura S, Saito K. Rapidly progressive bronchiolitis obliterans associated with Stevens-Johnson syndrome. *Chest* 1990; 98:243–245.
101. Mar WA, Glaesser R, Struble K, Stephens-Groff S, Bangert J, Hansen RC. Paraneoplastic pemphigus with bronchiolitis obliterans in a child. *Pediatr Dermatol* 2003; 20:238–242.
102. Grenier P, Mourey-Gerosa I, Benali K, et al. Abnormalities of the airways and lung parenchyma in asthmatics: CT observations in 50 patients and inter- and intraobserver variability. *Eur Radiol* 1996; 6:199–206.
103. Silva CI, Colby TV, Muller NL. Asthma and associated conditions: high-resolution CT and pathologic findings. *AJR Am J Roentgenol* 2004; 183:817–824.
104. Lynch DA, Newell J, Hale V, et al. Correlation of CT findings with clinical evaluations in 261 patients with symptomatic bronchiectasis. *AJR Am J Roentgenol* 1999; 173:53–58.

105. Helbich TH, Heinz-Peer G, Eichler I, et al. Cystic fibrosis: CT assessment of lung involvement in children and adults. *Radiology* 1999; 213:537–544.

106. Kraft M, Mortenson RL, Colby TV, Newman L, Waldron JA, Jr., King TE, Jr. Cryptogenic constrictive bronchiolitis. A clinicopathologic study. *Am Rev Respir Dis* 1993; 148:1093–1101.

107. Marrie TJ, Poulin-Costello M, Beecroft MD, Herman-Gnjidic Z. Etiology of community-acquired pneumonia treated in an ambulatory setting. *Respir Med* 2005; 99:60–65.

108. Rocholl C, Gerber K, Daly J, Pavia AT, Byington CL. Adenoviral infections in children: the impact of rapid diagnosis. *Pediatrics* 2004; 113:e51–56.

109. Kim CK, Chung CY, Kim JS, Kim WS, Park Y, Koh YY. Late abnormal findings on high-resolution computed tomography after Mycoplasma pneumonia. *Pediatrics* 2000; 105:372–378.

110. Milner AD, Murray M. Acute bronchiolitis in infancy: treatment and prognosis. *Thorax* 1989; 44:1–5.

111. Yalcin E, Dogru D, Haliloglu M, Ozcelik U, Kiper N, Gocmen A. Postinfectious bronchiolitis obliterans in children: clinical and radiological profile and prognostic factors. *Respiration* 2003; 70:371–375.

112. Zhang L, Irion K, Kozakewich H, et al. Clinical course of postinfectious bronchiolitis obliterans. *Pediatr Pulmonol* 2000; 29:341–350.

113. Chuang YY, Chiu CH, Wong KS, et al. Severe adenovirus infection in children. *J Microbiol Immunol Infect* 2003; 36:37–40.

114. Bloch KE, Weder W, Boehler A, Zalunardo MP, Russi EW. Successful lung volume reduction surgery in a child with severe airflow obstruction and hyperinflation due to constrictive bronchiolitis. *Chest* 2002; 122:747–750.

115. Zhang L, Irion K, da Silva Porto N, Abreu e Silva F. High-resolution computed tomography in pediatric patients with postinfectious bronchiolitis obliterans. *J Thorac Imaging* 1999; 14:85–89.

116. Marti-Bonmati L, Ruiz PF, Catala F, Mata JM, Calonge E. CT findings in Swyer-James syndrome. *Radiology* 1989; 172:477–480.

117. Moore ADA, Godwin JD, Dietrich PA, Verschakelen JA, Henderson WR. Swyer-James syndrome: CT findings in eight patients. *AJR Am J Roentgenol* 1992; 158:1211–1215.

118. Norton KI, Mendelson DS, Hodes D, Kattan M. Computed tomography findings in the Swyer-James syndrome. *Clin Imaging* 1989; 13:48–50.

119. Stern EJ, Samples TL. Dynamic ultrafast high resolution CT findings in a case of Swyer-James syndrome. *Pediatr Radiol* 1992; 22:350–352.

120. Sundaresan S, Trulock EP, Mohanakumar T, Cooper JD, Patterson GA. Prevalence and outcome of bronchiolitis obliterans syndrome after lung transplantation. Washington University Lung Transplant Group. *Ann Thorac Surg* 1995; 60:1341–1346; discussion 1346–1347.

121. Reichenspurner H, Girgis RE, Robbins RC, et al. Stanford experience with obliterative bronchiolitis after lung and heart-lung transplantation. *Ann Thorac Surg* 1996; 62:1467–1472; discussion 1472–1463.

122. Valentine VG, Robbins RC, Berry GJ, et al. Actuarial survival of heart-lung and bilateral sequential lung transplant recipients with obliterative bronchiolitis. *J Heart Lung Transplant* 1996; 15:371–383.

123. Reichenspurner H, Girgis RE, Robbins RC, et al. Obliterative bronchiolitis after lung and heart-lung transplantation. *Ann Thorac Surg* 1995; 60:1845–1853.

124. Dauber JH. Posttransplant bronchiolitis obliterans syndrome. Where have we been and where are we going? [editorial; comment]. *Chest* 1996; 109:857–859.

125. Worthy SA, Flint JD, Müller NL. Pulmonary complications after bone marrow transplantation: high-resolution CT and pathologic findings. *RadioGraphics* 1997; 17:1359–1371.

126. Paradis I, Yousem S, Griffith B. Airway obstruction and bronchitis obliterans after lung transplantation. *Clin Chest Med* 1993; 14:751–763.

127. Clark JG, Crawford SW, Madtes DK, Sullivan KM. Obstructive lung disease after allogeneic marrow transplantation. Clinical presentation and course. *Ann Intern Med* 1989; 111:368–376.

128. St John RC, Gadek JE, Tutschka PJ, Kapoor N, Dorinsky PM. Analysis of airflow obstruction by bronchoalveolar lavage following bone marrow transplantation. Implications for pathogenesis and treatment. *Chest* 1990; 98:600–607.

129. Guilinger RA, Paradis IL, Dauber JH, et al. The importance of bronchoscopy with transbronchial biopsy and bronchoalveolar lavage in the management of lung transplant recipients. *Am J Respir Crit Care Med* 1995; 152: 2037–2043.

130. Aboyoun CL, Tamm M, Chhajed PN, et al. Diagnostic value of follow-up transbronchial lung biopsy after lung rejection. *Am J Respir Crit Care Med* 2001; 164:460–463.

131. Cooper JD, Billingham M, Egan T, et al. A working formulation for the standardization of nomenclature and for clinical staging of chronic dysfunction in lung allografts. International Society for Heart and Lung Transplantation. *J Heart Lung Transplant* 1993; 12:713–716.

132. Estenne M, Maurer JR, Boehler A, et al. Bronchiolitis obliterans syndrome 2001: an update of the diagnostic criteria. *J Heart Lung Transplant* 2002; 21:297–310.

133. Nathan SD, Ross DJ, Belman MJ, et al. Bronchiolitis obliterans in single-lung transplant recipients. *Chest* 1995; 107:967–972.

134. Boehler A, Estenne M. Post-transplant bronchiolitis obliterans. *Eur Respir J* 2003; 22:1007–1018.

135. Watkins TR, Chien JW, Crawford SW. Graft versus host-associated pulmonary disease and other idiopathic pulmonary complications after hematopoietic stem cell transplant. *Semin Respir Crit Care Med* 2005; 26:482–489.

136. Paz HL, Crilley P, Patchefsky A, Schiffman RL, Brodsky I. Bronchiolitis obliterans after autologous bone marrow transplantation. *Chest* 1992; 101:775–778.

137. Dudek AZ, Mahaseth H, DeFor TE, Weisdorf DJ. Bronchiolitis obliterans in chronic graft-versus-host disease: analysis of risk factors and treatment outcomes. *Biol Blood Marrow Transplant* 2003; 9:657–666.

138. Adjaoud D, Dauger S, Yakouben K, et al. Reversible severe air leak syndrome in a child with bronchiolitis obliterans after allogeneic stem cell transplantation. *Eur J Pediatr* 2006; 165:579–580.

139. Galanis E, Litzow MR, Tefferi A, Scott JP. Spontaneous pneumomediastinum in a patient with bronchiolitis obliterans after bone marrow transplantation. *Bone Marrow Transplant* 1997; 20:695–696.

140. Hill G, Helenglass G, Powles R, Perren T, Selby P. Mediastinal emphysema in marrow transplant recipients. *Bone Marrow Transplant* 1987; 2:315–320.

141. Heng D, Sharples LD, McNeil K, Stewart S, Wreghitt T, Wallwork J. Bronchiolitis obliterans syndrome: incidence, natural history, prognosis, and risk factors. *J Heart Lung Transplant* 1998; 17:1255–1263.

142. Sharples LD, McNeil K, Stewart S, Wallwork J. Risk factors for bronchiolitis obliterans: a systematic review of recent publications. *J Heart Lung Transplant* 2002; 21:271–281.

143. Bando K, Paradis IL, Similo S, et al. Obliterative bronchiolitis after lung and heart-lung transplantation. An analysis of risk factors and management. *J Thorac Cardiovasc Surg* 1995; 110:4–13; discussion 13–14.

144. Kroshus TJ, Kshettry VR, Savik K, John R, Hertz MI, Bolman RM, 3rd. Risk factors for the development of bronchiolitis obliterans syndrome after lung transplantation. *J Thorac Cardiovasc Surg* 1997; 114:195–202.

145. Benden C, Aurora P, Curry J, Whitmore P, Priestley L, Elliott MJ. High prevalence of gastroesophageal reflux in children after lung transplantation. *Pediatr Pulmonol* 2005; 40:68–71.

146. Hadjiliadis D, Duane Davis R, Steele MP, et al. Gastroesophageal reflux disease in lung transplant recipients. *Clin Transplant* 2003; 17:363–368.

147. D'Ovidio F, Singer LG, Hadjiliadis D, et al. Prevalence of gastroesophageal reflux in end-stage lung disease candidates for lung transplant. *Ann Thorac Surg* 2005; 80:1254–1260.

148. Young LR, Hadjiliadis D, Davis RD, Palmer SM. Lung transplantation exacerbates gastroesophageal reflux disease. *Chest* 2003; 124:1689–1693.

149. Davis RD, Jr., Lau CL, Eubanks S, et al. Improved lung allograft function after fundoplication in patients with gastroesophageal reflux disease undergoing lung transplantation. *J Thorac Cardiovasc Surg* 2003; 125:533–542.

150. Santo Tomas LH, Loberiza FR, Jr, Klein JP, et al. Risk factors for bronchiolitis obliterans in allogeneic hematopoietic stem-cell transplantation for leukemia. *Chest* 2005; 128:153–161.

151. Novick RJ, Schafers HJ, Stitt L, et al. Recurrence of obliterative bronchiolitis and determinants of outcome in 139 pulmonary retransplant recipients. *J Thorac Cardiovasc Surg* 1995; 110:1402–1413; discussion 1413–1404.

152. Novick RJ, Schafers HJ, Stitt L, et al. Seventy-two pulmonary retransplantations for obliterative bronchiolitis: predictors of survival. *Ann Thorac Surg* 1995; 60:111–116.

153. Novick RJ, Andreassian B, Schafers HJ, et al. Pulmonary retransplantation for obliterative bronchiolitis. Intermediate-term results of a North American-European series. *J Thorac Cardiovasc Surg* 1994; 107:755–763.

154. Konen E, Gutierrez C, Chaparro C, et al. Bronchiolitis obliterans syndrome in lung transplant recipients: can thin-section CT findings predict disease before its clinical appearance? *Radiology* 2004; 231:467–473.

155. Bankier AA, Van Muylem A, Knoop C, Estenne M, Gevenois PA. Bronchiolitis obliterans syndrome in heart-lung transplant recipients: diagnosis with expiratory CT. *Radiology* 2001; 218:533–539.

156. Lee ES, Gotway MB, Reddy GP, Golden JA, Keith FM, Webb WR. Early bronchiolitis obliterans following lung transplantation: accuracy of expiratory thin-section CT for diagnosis. *Radiology* 2000; 216:472–477.

157. Siegel MJ, Bhalla S, Gutierrez FR, Hildebolt C, Sweet S. Post-lung transplantation bronchiolitis obliterans syndrome: usefulness of expiratory thin-section CT for diagnosis. *Radiology* 2001; 220:455–462.

158. Leung AN, Fisher K, Valentine V, et al. Bronchiolitis obliterans after lung transplantation: detection using expiratory HRCT. *Chest* 1998; 113:365–370.

159. Berstad AE, Aalokken TM, Kolbenstvedt A, Bjortuft O. Performance of long-term CT monitoring in diagnosing bronchiolitis obliterans after lung transplantation. *Eur J Radiol* 2006; 58:124–131.

160. Arakawa H, Webb WR. Air trapping on expiratory high-resolution CT scans in the absence of inspiratory scan abnormalities: correlation with pulmonary function tests and differential diagnosis. *AJR Am J Roentgenol* 1998; 170:1349–1353.

161. de Jong PA, Dodd JD, Coxson HO, et al. Bronchiolitis obliterans following lung transplantation: early detection using computed tomographic scanning. *Thorax* 2006; 61:799–804.

162. Zaporozhan J, Ley S, Gast KK, et al. Functional analysis in single-lung transplant recipients: a comparative study of high-resolution CT, 3He-MRI, and pulmonary function tests. *Chest* 2004; 125:173–181.

163. Akpinar-Elci M, Travis WD, Lynch DA, Kreiss K. Bronchiolitis obliterans syndrome in popcorn production plant workers. *Eur Respir J* 2004; 24:298–302.

164. Kreiss K, Gomaa A, Kullman G, Fedan K, Simoes EJ, Enright PL. Clinical bronchiolitis obliterans in workers at a microwave-popcorn plant. *N Engl J Med* 2002; 347:330–338.

165. Perez T, Remy-Jardin M, Cortet B. Airways involvement in rheumatoid arthritis: clinical, functional, and HRCT findings. *Am J Respir Crit Care Med* 1998; 157:1658–1665.

166. Herzog CA, Miller RR, Hoidal JR. Bronchiolitis and rheumatoid arthritis. *Am Rev Respir Dis* 1979; 119:555–560.

167. Schwarz MI, Lynch DA, Tuder R. Bronchiolitis obliterans: the lone manifestation of rheumatoid arthritis? *Eur Respir J* 1994; 7:817–820.

168. Epler GR, Snider GL, Gaensler EA, Cathcart ES, Fitzgerald MK, Carrington CB. Bronchiolitis and bronchitis in connective tissue disease. *JAMA* 1979; 242:528–532.

169. Zitnik RJ, Cooper JA, Jr. Pulmonary disease due to antirheumatic agents. *Clin Chest Med* 1990; 11:139–150.

170. Fujii M, Adachi S, Shimizu T, Hirota S, Sako M, Kono M. Interstitial lung disease in rheumatoid arthritis: assessment with high-resolution computed tomography. *J Thorac Imag* 1993; 8:54–62.

171. Akira M, Sakatani M, Hara H. Thin-section CT findings in rheumatoid arthritis-associated lung disease: CT patterns and their courses. *J Comput Assist Tomogr* 1999; 23:941–948.

172. Papiris SA, Maniati M, Constantopoulos SH, Roussos C, Moutsopoulos HM, Skopouli FN. Lung involvement in primary Sjogren's syndrome is mainly related to the small airway disease. *Ann Rheum Dis* 1999; 58:61–64.

173. Weber F, Prior C, Kowald E, Schmuth M, Sepp N. Cyclophosphamide therapy is effective for bronchiolitis obliterans occurring as a late manifestation of lupus erythematosus. *Br J Dermatol* 2000; 143:453–455.

174. Yang CF, Wu MT, Chiang AA, et al. Correlation of high-resolution CT and pulmonary function in bronchiolitis obliterans: a study based on 24 patients associated with consumption of Sauropus androgynus. *AJR Am J Roentgenol* 1997; 168:1045–1050.

175. Oonakahara K, Matsuyama W, Higashimoto I, et al. Living-donor lobar lung transplantation in Sauropus androgynus-associated bronchiolitis obliterans in Japan. *Intern Med* 2005; 44:1103–1104.

176. Luh SP, Lee YC, Chang YL, Wu HD, Kuo SH, Chu SH. Lung transplantation for patients with end-stage Sauropus androgynus-induced bronchiolitis obliterans (SABO) syndrome. *Clin Transplant* 1999; 13:496–503.

177. Kerr KM. Pulmonary preinvasive neoplasia. *J Clin Pathol* 2001; 54:257–271.

178. Miller RR, Muller NL. Neuroendocrine cell hyperplasia and obliterative bronchiolitis in patients with peripheral carcinoid tumors. *Am J Surg Pathol* 1995; 19:653–658.

179. Travis WD. Pathology of lung cancer. *Clin Chest Med* 2002; 23:65–81, viii.

180. Cohen AJ, King TE, Jr, Gilman LB, Magill-Solc C, Miller YE. High expression of neutral endopeptidase in idiopathic diffuse hyperplasia of pulmonary neuroendocrine cells. *Am J Respir Crit Care Med* 1998; 158:1593–1599.

181. Johney EC, Pfannschmidt J, Rieker RJ, Schnabel PA, Mechtersheimer G, Dienemann H. Diffuse idiopathic pulmonary neuroendocrine cell hyperplasia and a typical carcinoid tumor. *J Thorac Cardiovasc Surg* 2006; 131:1207 1208.

182. Turton CW, Williams G, Green M. Crytogenic obliterative bronchiolitis in adults. *Thorax* 1981; 36:805–810.

183. Camus P, Colby TV. The lung in inflammatory bowel disease. *Eur Respir J* 2000; 15:5–10.

184. Camus P, Piard F, Ashcroft T, Gal AA, Colby TV. The lung in inflammatory bowel disease. *Medicine (Baltimore)* 1993; 72:151 183.

185. Casey MB, Tazelaar HD, Myers JL, et al. Noninfectious lung pathology in patients with Crohn's disease. *Am J Surg Pathol* 2003; 27:213–219.

186. Spira A, Grossman R, Balter M. Large airway disease associated with inflammatory bowel disease. *Chest* 1998; 113:1723–1726.

187. Ward H, Fisher KL, Waghray R, Wright JL, Card SE, Cockcroft DW. Constrictive bronchiolitis and ulcerative colitis. *Can Respir J* 1999; 6:197–200.

14

Smoking-Related Small Airways and Interstitial Lung Disease

David M. Hansell and Athol U. Wells

Summary

The consequences of airways and interstitial inflammation caused by cigarette smoking are many and varied. In addition to well-recognized smoking-related disorders, including chronic bronchitis and emphysema, there is increasing appreciation of the complex relationship between small airways and interstitial damage, typified by respiratory bronchiolitis interstitial lung disease. Individual diseases ascribable to cigarette smoking and their relationship to each other are described.

Key Words: Cigarette smoking; interstitial lung disease; high-resolution computed tomography; pulmonary Langerhans cell hisitiocytosis; desquamative interstitial pneumonia; respiratory bronchiolitis; respiratory bronchiolitis-associated interstitial lung disease; usual interstitial pneumonia.

1. INTRODUCTION

The list of diffuse lung diseases linked to cigarette smoking continues to increase and is no longer confined to the key components of chronic obstructive pulmonary disease, namely chronic bronchitis and emphysema. Early investigations in the 1970s, based on histologic studies, established the concept of subclinical small airways inflammation in cigarette smokers. In the absence of any obvious radiographic correlate of such subtle changes, there was a hiatus in the understanding of the pathogenetic and clinical aspects of cigarette smoking-induced lung disease. High-resolution computed tomography (HRCT) has lifted the veil on many facets of smoking-related disease, notably the distribution and interplay between interstitial and emphysematous diseases, airways changes, and longitudinal changes in the lungs of cigarette smokers.

The close anatomic proximity between the distal airways and the gas-exchanging parts of the lung means that considering cigarette smoking-induced lung disease as exclusively affecting the small airways or interstitium is conceptually unhelpful; although inelegant, the term applied to the prototypical cigarette smokers' disease, respiratory bronchiolitis-associated interstitial lung disease (RB-ILD), does at least encompass both the airways and the interstitium. The continuity between the small and the larger airways is given, but the manifestations of disease of the microscopic and macroscopic (cartilage and mucus gland containing) airways differ, and a section on larger airways abnormalities in cigarette smokers is included later in the chapter for completeness. The interest in the HRCT appearances of cigarette smoking lung disease has coincided with refinement and reclassification of the idiopathic interstitial lung diseases. The synergistic approach of imaging and pathology to the investigation and understanding of smoking-related diseases has led to several new insights, in particular, the coexistence and transformation of several disorders, and these emerging concepts are explored.

From: *Contemporary Medical Imaging: CT of the Airways*
Edited by: P. M. Boiselle and D. A. Lynch © Humana Press, Totowa, NJ

2. RESPIRATORY BRONCHIOLITIS/RESPIRATORY BRONCHIOLITIS-ASSOCIATED INTERSTITIAL LUNG DISEASE

Respiratory bronchiolitis is a very frequent incidental finding in cigarette smokers. The characteristic histologic picture, first described more than 30 years ago in an autopsy study that included 19 young asymptomatic smokers *(1)*, is usually clinically silent. However, in 1987 Myers et al. described a clinically significant diffuse lung disease associated with respiratory bronchiolitis in heavy smokers, characterized by lung crackles, a restrictive ventilatory defect and radiographic findings suggestive of interstitial lung disease *(2)*. Following the publication of further case series *(3,4)*, the term "RBILD" *(4)* was coined to distinguish between this disorder, incidental respiratory bronchiolitis, and the more diffuse smoking-related parenchymal disorder, desquamative interstitial pneumonia (DIP). With recognition of their histologic similarity, RBILD can be viewed as an exaggerated form of respiratory bronchiolitis, resulting in dyspnea, cough, and pulmonary function impairment.

Respiratory bronchiolitis and RBILD are almost invariably associated with smoking. In a landmark study by Fraig et al. *(5)* in which 156 surgical lung biopsy specimens were evaluated, typical respiratory bronchiolitis was present in all 83 current smokers and in 25 of 49 former smokers, sometimes more than 5 years after smoking cessation: respiratory bronchiolitis was not identified in any lifelong non-smoker. The profusion of pigmented macrophages and the likelihood of peribronchial fibrosis both rose with an increasing pack-year smoking history. Earlier reports of a minority of smokers without respiratory bronchiolitis are likely to reflect the grouping together of current and former smokers *(6)* and may also have resulted from differences in histologic definition, as in the study of Remy-Jardin et al. *(7)*, in which the presence of pigmented macrophages in resected lungs was not viewed as indicative of respiratory bronchiolitis. It is increasingly accepted that respiratory bronchiolitis represents a specific physiologic response to smoking, and, to date, there are no convincing reports of this lesion occurring in non-smokers.

The index autopsy series of Niewoehner et al. *(1)*, in which respiratory bronchiolitis was reported in a small group of "non-smokers," as well as in smokers, was limited by the fact that smoking histories were obtained from relatives. In dust-related environmental lung disease and "variant respiratory bronchiolitis" (reported in a handful of non-smokers) *(5)*, the typical peribronchial macrophages do not have the characteristic brown pigmentation of smokers' macrophages. Respiratory bronchiolitis is variably present in former smokers. Bronchoalveolar lavage (BAL) data indicate that, in most cases, BAL macrophage abnormalities regress within 3 years of smoking cessation *(8)*. Histological evidence of respiratory bronchiolitis often disappears within one year of smoking cessation but can occasionally persist for decades *(5)*. RBILD can be considered an almost exclusively a cigarette smoking-related disease; it has been reported in only one non-smoker, who was heavily exposed to solder fumes *(9)*.

2.1. Pathology

Respiratory bronchiolitis and RBILD cannot be distinguished histologically *(2,5)*. In both disorders, alveolar macrophages with brown and finely granular pigmentation (representing constituents of cigarette smoke) accumulate within respiratory bronchioles and neighboring alveoli (Fig. 1). A chronic inflammatory cell infiltrate is commonly present in bronchiolar and surrounding alveolar walls, with septal thickening because of collagen deposition a more variable feature *(5,10)*. The surrounding pulmonary parenchyma is normal, apart from smoking-related emphysematous changes *(11)*. In some series, the diagnosis of RBILD has been primarily made on histologic criteria *(4,9,12)*. However, biopsy appearances are not always a reliable guide to disease severity elsewhere in the lungs ("sampling error"), especially when lung biopsy is directed to localized HRCT abnormalities in otherwise limited respiratory bronchiolitis. More importantly, airway-centred parenchymal fibrosis is often present in asymptomatic current or former smokers. Thus, the diagnosis of RBILD, as opposed

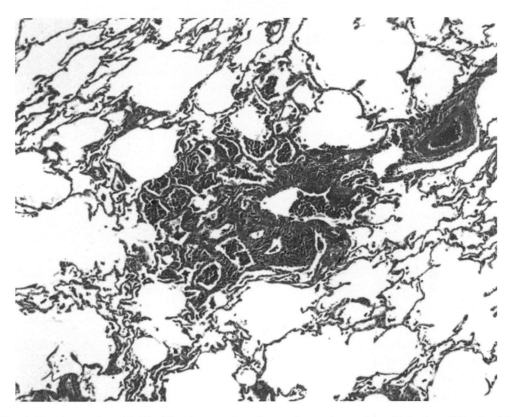

Fig. 1. Respiratory bronchiolitis. The airspaces in and around a respiratory bronchiole show filling by faintly pigmented macrophages with relative sparing of the surrounding lung tissue (courtesy Dr TV Colby).

to respiratory bronchiolitis, is usually based on global disease severity, as judged by symptoms, pulmonary function impairment, and the extent of HRCT abnormalities—and not on lung biopsy in isolation.

2.2. Clinical Aspects

Respiratory bronchiolitis is generally clinically silent. By contrast, patients with RBILD usually present with insidious exertional dyspnea, persistent cough (generally non-productive) between the third and the sixth decade; less frequent symptoms include chest pain and weight loss (2,4,9,11). Bilateral end-inspiratory crackles are common, but clubbing is unusual (9). In asymptomatic patients, functional impairment and chest radiographic or HRCT abnormalities are required to make the diagnosis. Although RBILD is a much more benign disorder than UIP or fibrotic non-specific interstitial pneumonia (NSIP) (13), with no reported deaths, little is known about serial pulmonary function trends. On the basis of small series, RBILD can be expected to improve or remain stable in most cases following smoking cessation, with or without treatment (2), with occasional exceptions (9).

In respiratory bronchiolitis, pulmonary function tests are often normal, and in other cases, mild airflow obstruction is difficult to interpret because of coexisting centrilobular emphysema. Restrictive and obstructive abnormalities have been documented in RBILD (2,4,9). In most cases, a mixed, predominantly restrictive ventilatory defect is associated with mild-to-moderate reduction in measures of gas transfer. The severity of pulmonary function impairment is often a key discriminant between respiratory bronchiolitis and RBILD, but in a few patients with RBILD, diagnosed on the basis of symptoms and HRCT findings, pulmonary function tests may be normal (10).

BAL findings are often useful in the diagnosis of RBILD, as they allow other interstitial lung diseases to be excluded. As in respiratory bronchiolitis, brown pigmentation of macrophages is consistently present. RBILD can usually be distinguished from other idiopathic interstitial pneumonias by increases in macrophage numbers and the absence of a BAL neutrophilia or eosinophilia (14). BAL findings are especially useful in the distinction between RBILD and hypersensitivity pneumonitis, in which a BAL lymphocytosis is the rule (15). A characteristic BAL picture in conjunction with the history and HRCT appearances is usually sufficient for diagnosis, without the need to proceed to surgical lung biopsy.

Apart from smoking cessation, which is often associated with disease regression (16,17), the optimal management of RBILD is uncertain. Corticosteroid therapy, with or without immuno-suppressive treatment, is often employed if disease remains clinically significant despite smoking cessation (2,4,9,11,16), but no proof of efficacy exists and prolonged treatment is seldom warranted in non-responsive disease.

2.3. Imaging

In current and former smokers with respiratory bronchiolitis, the chest radiograph is normal or shows non-specific changes. Radiographic abnormalities may be more obvious in RBILD, with a widespread reticulonodular pattern in some case (2,4) with accompanying bronchial wall thickening and patchy ground-glass attenuation commonly present (16). However, chest radiographic findings are highly non-specific and do not, in themselves, allow RBILD to be diagnosed with any confidence.

The spectrum of HRCT features in respiratory bronchiolitis is identical to that in RBILD (although a diagnosis of RBILD is often partially based on the fact that HRCT abnormalities are more extensive). HRCT abnormalities reported by Remy-Jardin in 98 current smokers [with, by definition, underlying respiratory bronchiolitis (5)] included parenchymal micronodules (27%) (Fig. 2), patchy ground-glass opacities (21%) (Fig. 3), lobular areas of decreased attenuation (34%) (Fig. 4A and B), and emphysema (21%) (Fig. 5), with all these features much more prevalent than in non-smokers (18). Parenchymal micronodules up to 2–3 mm in diameter were ill defined and more profuse in the upper zones. Apart from emphysema, none of these HRCT patterns was associated with pulmonary function impairment. Remy-Jardin was subsequently able to show that ground-glass attenuation on HRCT in current and former smokers (undergoing resections of solitary pulmonary nodules) corresponded to respiratory bronchiolitis (i.e., alveolar space accumulations of pigmented macrophages and mucus, variably associated with mild interstitial inflammation and/or fibrosis) (7). Some ill-defined micronodules were thought to indicate bronchiolectasis with peribronchiolar fibrosis. Thus, HRCT abnormalities in respiratory bronchiolitis correspond with inflammation in terminal bronchioles, with a variable contribution from inflammation and/or fibrosis in the surrounding lung parenchyma (19). On the basis of serial HRCT observations, albeit in a small number of patients, it appears possible that the centrilobular nodules of respiratory bronchiolitis may evolve to emphysema (20).

The HRCT features of respiratory bronchiolitis are more extensive in RBILD. Centrilobular micronodules, ground-glass opacities, atelectasis, reticular elements, linear (including septal thickening) abnormalities, and emphysema were all described in small studies (12,21,22). In the largest HRCT series (containing 21 patients), wall thickening of bronchi proximal to segmental airways was present in 90% (16) (Fig. 6). Other frequent features included peripheral bronchial wall thickening (86%), centrilobular nodules (71%), patchy ground-glass opacification (57%), emphysema

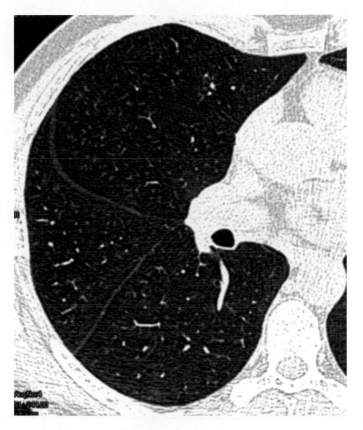

Fig. 2. Micronodular pattern on HRCT ascribed to cigarette smoking in an adult heavy smoker (not biopsy proven). Some of the nodules are indistinct and of ground-glass density others, adjacent to the minor fissure anteriorly, resemble a tree-in-bud pattern.

(57%), and patchy areas of decreased attenuation (most frequently in the lower lobes). Centrilobular nodules and ground-glass opacity were both often diffuse, in contrast to the limited abnormalities of respiratory bronchiolitis in healthy smokers *(18)*. As in healthy smokers, the profusion of centrilobular nodules increases with increasing macrophage accumulation in respiratory bronchioles and increasingly severe chronic inflammation within respiratory bronchiolar walls: ground-glass attenuation is likely to represent intense macrophage accumulation in the alveoli and alveolar ducts *(16)*.

Patchy areas of decreased attenuation on inspiratory HRCT, present in a minority of RBILD cases *(16)*, were under reported in earlier series *(12,18)*. Patchy decreased attenuation on expiratory CT is more readily recognized and is frequently present in RBILD and also in healthy smokers and former smokers *(23,24)*. Segmental air trapping is seen in 25–30% of current and former smokers but very seldom in non-smokers. By contrast, limited lobular air trapping is often present in both smokers and non-smokers and is, thus, highly non-specific. In current smokers, air trapping is often admixed with profuse micronodules. Patchy decreased attenuation on expiratory HRCT is a non-specific feature of small airways disease, also seen in other conditions including hypersensitivity pneumonitis *(25)*.

The extent of disease on HRCT can help to distinguish between respiratory bronchiolitis and RBILD, whereas the nature of HRCT abnormalities *per se* does not. The HRCT diagnosis of

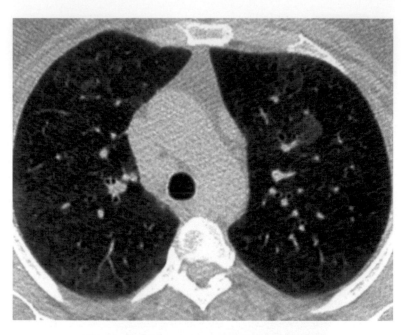

Fig. 3. Cigarette smoker with biopsy proven RBILD. There are patchy ground glass opacities in the upper lobes, corresponding to macrophage infiltration. A nodular pattern is absent. The walls of the subsegmental bronchi are mildly thickened.

A)

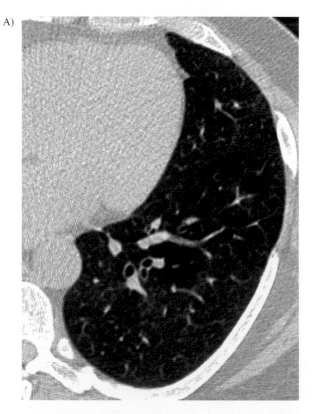

Fig. 4. *(Continued)*

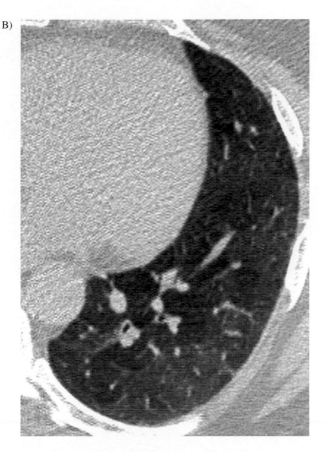

Fig. 4. (**A**) Minor inhomogeneity of the density of the lung parenchyma in the lower zones of a cigarette smoker on inspiratory HRCT. (**B**) On expiratory HRCT, the mosaic pattern reflecting air trapping at a small airways level is accentuated. This individual had no evidence of airflow limitation on pulmonary function testing.

RBILD is essentially a judgment that smoking-related inflammation amounts to a clinically significant diffuse lung disease. In this regard, it should be stressed that limited, but compatible, HRCT abnormalities should not be viewed as indicative of RBILD but as more suggestive of respiratory bronchiolitis *(18,23,24)*. However, there are no agreed HRCT extent criteria on which to base this distinction, and in many patients, the extent of disease on HRCT is diagnostically inconclusive. Thus, a diagnosis of RBILD, as opposed to respiratory bronchiolitis, requires that HRCT findings are integrated with clinical features and the severity of pulmonary function impairment.

HRCT tends to be helpful for excluding alternative diffuse lung disorders. In RBILD, symptoms, clinical signs, and the pattern and level of functional impairment are highly non-specific for identifying alternative conditions, but typical HRCT findings effectively exclude most other diffuse lung diseases. RBILD and DIP occasionally exhibit overlapping features but, as discussed later, DIP is usually characterized by more extensive ground-glass opacity and infrequent or absent nodules *(10,26)*. The HRCT appearances of RBILD most frequently resemble those of subacute hypersensitivity pneumonitis, especially when widespread poorly defined centrilobular nodules and areas of decreased attenuation coexist *(16,25)*, but this distinction can generally be made from the smoking history and BAL findings, without recourse to diagnostic surgical biopsy.

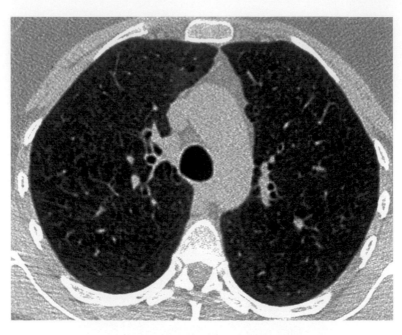

Fig. 5. HRCT through the lung apices of an individual with RBILD showing, in addition to poorly defined micronodules, relatively mild centrilobular emphysema and minor bronchial wall thickening.

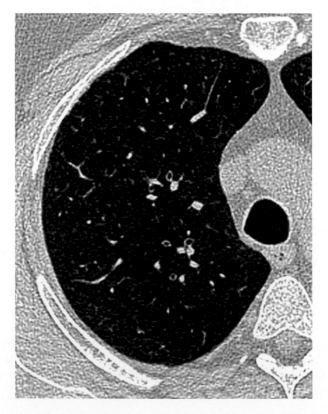

Fig. 6. Thickening of the walls of the subsegmental bronchi of an individual with biopsy proven RBILD (on this section, there are no HRCT features of RBILD such as micronodules or ground glass opacities).

3. DESQUAMATIVE INTERSTITIAL PNEUMONIA

DIP, first described by Liebow in 1965, was widely recognized as a separate clinical entity following the report of Carrington et al., in which the clinical features of DIP and usual interstitial pneumonia were compared *(27)*. Thirty-six of 40 DIP patients (90%) were smokers, with smoking equally prevalent in subsequent smaller DIP series, accounting for the widespread belief that DIP is essentially a smoking-related diffuse lung disorder.

However, DIP is known to occur occasionally in non-smokers, most commonly in the context of pneumoconiosis, drug reactions, or inborn errors of metabolism *(28–31)*. DIP can also develop without an obvious trigger, as observed in a recent series in which eight of 20 DIP patients were lifelong non-smokers *(32)*.

3.1. Pathology

The defining histologic feature of DIP is a diffuse intra-alveolar accumulation of macrophages, associated with type II pneumocyte hyperplasia and, in some cases, diffuse thickening of the alveolar septa *(33)*. Macrophages often contain brown pigment, as in RBILD and respiratory bronchiolitis *(2)*. The essential difference between DIP and RBILD/respiratory bronchiolitis is the diffuse (as opposed to bronchiolocentric) nature of macrophage infiltration (Fig. 7). However, there are considerable histologic similarities between these disorders, and it is argued by some that DIP and RBILD should be amalgamated as a single smoking-related disease *(12)*.

3.2. Clinical Aspects

Patients with DIP usually present in the fourth to sixth decade with non-productive cough, insidious breathlessness, and, occasionally, fatigue or weight loss *(27)*. Bilateral basal or widespread inspiratory crackles are usually present, but clubbing is infrequent. In DIP, the outcome is better than in other

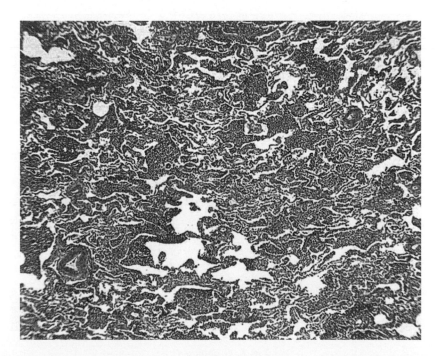

Fig. 7. Desquamative interstitial pneumonia. Scanning power microscopy shows uniform filling of airspaces by macrophages (courtesy Dr TV Colby).

disorders with a similar clinical presentation, including usual interstitial pneumonia *(13,27)* and fibrotic NSIP *(13)*. Most DIP patients have a complete or partial response to corticosteroid therapy, but the treated outcome is occasionally poor, even when there is little or no histologic evidence of concurrent lung fibrosis *(27)*.

Pulmonary function tests usually show a restrictive ventilatory defect in association with a reduction in gas transfer. In occasional cases, the coexistence of emphysema and DIP can result in paradoxically normal lung volumes, even when measures of gas transfer are severely impaired. The BAL profile is often highly cellular, with variable increases in lymphocytes, neutrophils, and eosinophils, but there are no diagnostic features *(14)*. As discussed below, HRCT features are also non-specific, and thus, the diagnosis of DIP requires a surgical biopsy.

Smoking cessation and corticosteroid therapy are the key interventions. In mild disease, a period of observation after smoking cessation can be justified. However, in most cases, a trial of corticosteroid therapy is required, with longer-term treatment approaches guided by the initial response. Immunosuppressive agents are occasionally added, both as steroid-sparing agents and in the hope of additional efficacy in steroid-resistant disease. However, there are no controlled data on which to base management.

3.3. Imaging

The chest radiographic appearances of DIP are highly non-specific and have no useful role in diagnosis, other than confirming the presence of a diffuse lung disease. Because of the low prevalence of DIP, there is only one HRCT series, gleaned from several centers, containing 22 patients *(26)*. Ground-glass opacification, which was invariably present, was usually bilateral and often somewhat symmetrical, peripheral, and predominantly lower zone in distribution (Fig. 8A and B). However, ground-glass opacification was random in distribution in a minority of cases. In over half of cases, limited predominantly basal irregular linear opacities were present, often associated with anatomic

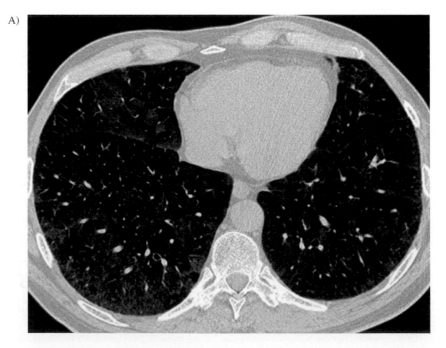

A)

Fig. 8. *(Continued)*

B)

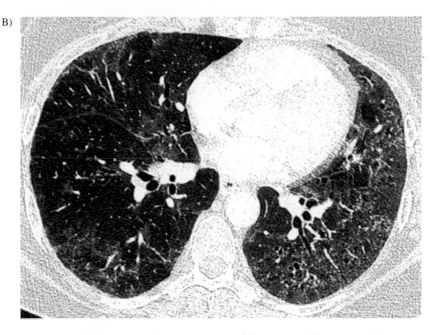

Fig. 8. Two examples of biopsy proven cases of DIP. (**A**) Non-specific pattern of patchy ground glass opacities; in this case, the disease was predominantly lower zone and is more pronounced in the subpleural lung. The dilatation of some of the airways may reflect traction by minor interstitial fibrosis. (**B**) In another case of DIP, there was no obvious predominant distribution. In some areas of ground-glass opacity, there are small cystic air spaces (see also Fig. 9).

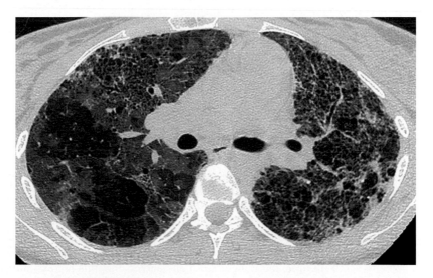

Fig. 9. Microcyst formation in areas of ground glass in a patient with DIP on lung biopsy. These small cysts are thought to represent either bronchiolectasis or background centrilobular emphysema. The distribution of ground-glass opacities in this case was random.

distortion, traction bronchiectasis, and small peripheral cystic spaces (possibly representing dilated bronchioles and alveolar ducts) (Fig. 9). More widespread honeycomb change, commonly present in usual interstitial pneumonia, is not a feature of DIP, and thus, HRCT is often useful in excluding the diagnosis of UIP. However, as the HRCT features of DIP overlap with many other disorders with prominent ground-glass attenuation, including hypersensitivity pneumonitis and RBILD *(12)*, the diagnosis of DIP should not be made using HRCT without histologic confirmation.

4. LANGERHANS CELL HISTIOCYTOSIS

Pulmonary Langerhans cell histocytosis (PLCH) is a disease of cigarette smokers, particularly younger individuals with an impressive smoking history. It is characterized by abnormal collections of Langerhans cells in a peribronchiolar location: These foci undergo cavitation and scarring, and the characteristic morphology of these nodules is well demonstrated on HRCT. The airway centered distribution of the PLCH lesion, and the "interstitial" fibro-emphysematous destruction of the later stages of PLCH has led to controversy over whether PLCH should be regarded as a predominantly small airways, as opposed to interstitial, disease. However, the concept that PLCH affects both the interstitium and small airways is now generally accepted *(34)*. Although the full-blown and pure form of PLCH is considered relatively rare, the incidence of forme fruste manifestations of PLCH, particularly in individuals with other forms of smoking-related diffuse lung disease, is unknown but likely quite common. At both histopathologic examination and on HRCT, coexisting patterns of smoking-related lung damage are frequent, and this theme is more fully explored in the section on the spectrum of smoking-related lung disease.

4.1. Pathology

In healthy individuals, the Langerhans cell is found ubiquitously in epithelial surfaces, notably the skin, but its function remains elusive. The identification of proliferations of similar cells in various systemic disorders has led to various classifications over the years. The term histiocytosis X was introduced in 1953 to encompass three clinical conditions: Hand–Schüller–Christian disease, Letterer–Siwe disease, and eosinophilic granuloma disorders *(35)*, and although the lungs may be involved in these disseminated diseases, lone involvement of the lungs (PLCH) is the most common pulmonary presentation, and this will be the only manifestation of the Langerhans cell disorders discussed here.

The Langerhans cell is only rarely identified at pathologic examination in normal lungs, but the numbers of Langerhans cells increase in response to cigarette smoke. It is thought that alterations in airway epithelium secondary to cigarette smoke attract Langerhans cells and promote their proliferation. The macroscopic appearances of PLCH change over time: in the early stages, there are numerous bronchocentric nodules that later cavitate (Fig. 10) and become cystic as the disease progresses. The cellularity of the PLCH lesions diminishes as the disease "burns out." The final appearances are of stellate scars (Fig. 11) and extensive fibrobullous destruction *(36)*.

The fundamental lesion consists of a nodular aggregation of Langerhans cells many of which show mitoses, with admixed eosinophils and, to a lesser degree, neutrophils and lymphocytes. The infiltration by eosinophils may be striking, to the extent that the pathologic differential diagnosis of eosinophilic pneumonia may be considered. Electron microscopy of the Langerhans cell reveals unique small elongated laminated structures in the cytoplasm (the Birbeck granules). Cavitation of PLCH lesions is characteristic, and the cavity in the nodule may be shown to be in continuity with a dilated airway lumen *(37)*. With time, the Langerhans cells and eosinophils regress and are replaced by pigment-laden macrophages (the pigment is partly derived from cigarette smoke), lymphocytes, plasma cells, and fibroblasts. Both old scarring and active lesions often coexist in the same lung biopsy specimen. When there are no cellular lesions, the histopathologic diagnosis can sometimes be inferred

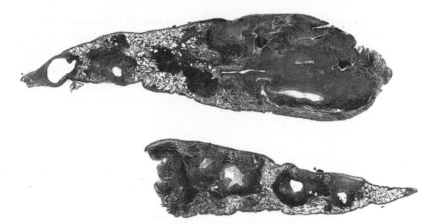

Fig. 10. Pulmonary Langerhans cell histiocytosis—low power. In this active case, there are numerous cellular nodules, some of which are solid and some of which show early cavitation (courtesy Dr TV Colby).

from the architectural features of bronchocentric fibrosis (stellate scars), and the gross appearances of mid- and upper zone fibrobullous involvement. Immunocytochemical staining for Langerhans cells using antibodies to CD1a or S100 protein can be helpful, particularly when Langerhans cells are sparse. Nevertheless, positive results have to be interpreted with care because Langerhans cells and similar interdigitating dendritic cells are increased in other reactive and neoplastic disorders *(38)*.

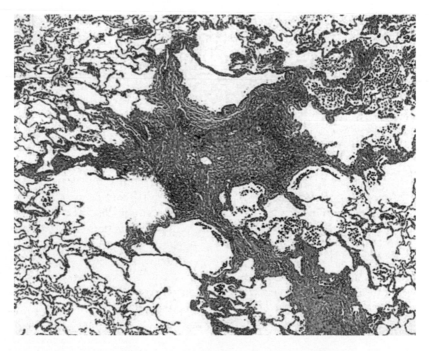

Fig. 11. Healed pulmonary Langerhans cell histiocytosis. There is a stellate scar with surrounding pericicatricial emphysema in the lung tissue. At this advanced stage, Langerhans' cells are absent (courtesy Dr TV Colby).

Given the bronchiolocentric distribution of the LCH lesions *(39)*, scarring of the small airways likely contributes to the hyperinflation, cavitation, and cystic change. A further consequence of this microscopic peribronchovascular distribution of LCH lesions is pulmonary hypertension that has been reported in some patients with LCH *(40)*. It is therefore possible that a few patients thought to have smoking-related "emphysema" and disproportionately severe pulmonary hypertension, actually have this rare LCH-related vasculopathy.

4.2. Clinical Aspects

PLCH usually affects young adults (male : female 4:1) although the age range is a wide. The great majority of affected individuals are cigarette smokers (>95%) *(39)*. Non-specific chest symptoms of dyspnea and cough are common, sometimes accompanied by pneumothorax or systemic symptoms such as weight loss and fever. Some individuals are asymptomatic despite obvious radiographic evidence of PLCH.

4.3. Imaging

The typical radiographic appearances of PLCH at presentation are reticulonodular shadowing in the mid and upper zones of normal size or increased volume lungs *(41)*. The nodules vary in size from micronodular to approximately 1 cm in diameter, and cavitation of some of the larger nodules may be visible on chest radiography (more readily appreciated on HRCT). Overinflation of the lungs becomes evident as the disease progresses *(41)*. The cavitating nodules become thin-walled airspaces that finally coalesce, resulting in emphysematous or fibrobullous lung destruction. Rarely, LCH may present as a solitary pulmonary nodule or mass-like lesion, without background diffuse lung involvement *(42)*. A mediastinal mass or lymph node involvement with or without PLCH has also been reported but is extremely uncommon *(43)*.

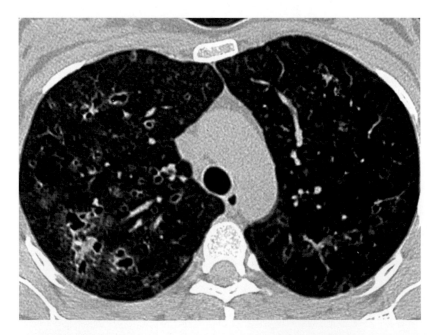

Fig. 12. Numerous cavitating nodules (most profuse in the upper lobes) on HRCT in a patient with Langerhans cell histiocytosis. Some of the nodules have an odd shape, and occasionally, they may superficially resemble bronchiectatic airways.

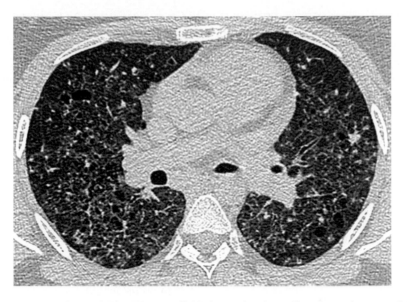

Fig. 13. Micronodular form of Langerhans cell histiocytosis. As well as some larger nodules, there are reticular elements and a few thin-walled cystic airspaces. Some of the very small nodules have cavitated.

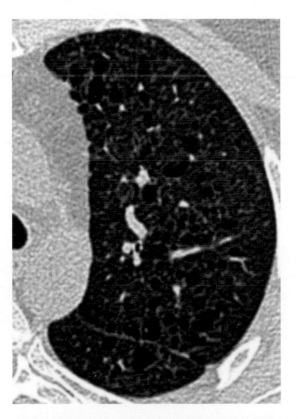

Fig. 14. Thin-walled cystic air spaces in a patient with Langerhans cell histiocytosis. The appearances resemble centrilobular emphysema, but some of the cysts retain the unusual shapes of the precursor cavitating nodular lesions.

The typical mid and upper zone distribution of PLCH is clearly shown on computed tomography with the classic CT appearance being nodules, ranging in size from a few millimeters to 2 cm, some of which show cavitation; the cavitating nodules often have bizarre shapes, especially the larger ones (Fig. 12). The cavitating nodules can resemble bronchiectatic airways (because of their strange elongated shapes), and it cannot be disproved with certainty that some of these lesions do indeed reflect dilated distorted airways (as noted above, at a pathologic level, some of the cavities are in continuity with dilated airways). Nevertheless, frank bronchiectasis is not a feature of PLCH even in its advanced stages. The predominantly upper lobe distribution of PLCH—with sparing of the extreme lung bases and anterior tips of the right middle lobe and lingula—is a useful diagnostic pointer, and this distribution is preserved even in end-stage disease *(44)*. A less widely recognized pattern of PLCH is the micronodular form of the disease (Fig. 13). Even within the smallest nodules cavitation can occasionally be detected on HRCT that, in conjunction with the typical distribution of the disease, are suggestive of the diagnosis in a cigarette smoker.

Other HRCT patterns that are encountered in patients with LCH are occasionally ground-glass opacities that may reflect a DIP-like reaction to PLCH. The coexistence of centrilobular and paraseptal emphysema, at a time when the LCH is largely nodular or showing early cavitation of the nodules, reflects the fact that almost all patients are cigarette smokers. Later in the evolution of the disease, the distinction between pre-existing smoking-related emphysema and the consequences of end-stage LCH is difficult.

On serial CT, the nodules of PLCH tend to progress through the following stages *(45)*: cavitation of nodules, resulting in thin-walled cystic lesions (Fig. 14) and finally emphysema-like and fibrobullous destruction (Fig. 15) *(46)*. It might therefore be thought that CT could provide a gauge of "disease activity," but a histopathologic study has suggested that even within apparently end-stage cystic lung

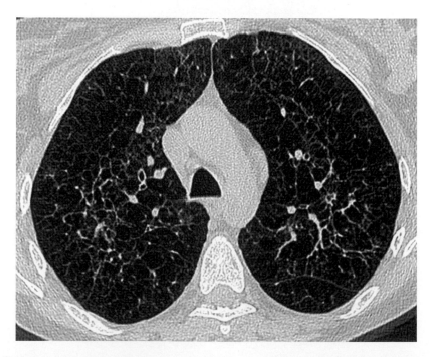

Fig. 15. End-stage Langerhans cell histiocytosis. CT shows widespread fibrobullous destruction of the lung parenchyma. Even at this advanced stage, there tends to be relative sparing of the extreme lung bases in the costophrenic recesses and the medial tips of the right middle lobe and lingula (not shown).

destruction, there may be florid and "active" cellular lesions at a microscopic level *(47)*. Nevertheless, HRCT may be used to monitor the progression, stability, or sometimes the surprisingly complete regression, of PLCH *(46)*. HRCT may also be useful for detecting relapse, which occurs rarely in transplanted lungs *(48)*.

5. MIXED SMOKING-RELATED DISORDERS

Although the various airway and interstitial disorders associated with smoking are dealt with separately in this discussion, there is increasing speculation, based largely on anecdotal evidence, that smoking-related diffuse interstitial lung diseases may be inter-related in their occurrence and pathogenesis *(49)*. As discussed earlier, there is considerable HRCT and histologic overlap between respiratory bronchiolitis and RBILD and between RBILD and DIP. In apparently healthy smokers with respiratory bronchiolitis, areas of DIP-like reaction are histologically indistinguishable from DIP *(5)*. In a recent series, respiratory bronchiolitis and DIP-like change were always present in biopsies from patients with Langerhans cell histiocytosis, resulting in ground-glass attenuation on HRCT in some cases *(50)*. It is known that in occasional current and former smokers, features of Langerhans cell histiocytosis, respiratory bronchiolitis, DIP, emphysema, and pulmonary fibrosis coexist histologically *(10)* (Fig. 16), but the prevalence of this phenomenon is uncertain. Limited coexistent fibrotic HRCT abnormalities are present in DIP in over 50% of cases *(12,26)*, although less frequent in RBILD *(4,16,21)*. In patients with DIP, the HRCT appearances at follow-up evolve into those of fibrotic NSIP in some cases *(32)*. The possible significance of fibrotic NSIP in smokers, including the linkage with RBILD and DIP, under scrutiny in a series of American Thoracic Society/ European Respiratory Society workshops, is as yet uncertain. However, the generic term "smoking-related diffuse lung disease", indicating a mixture of smoking-induced disease processes (Fig. 17), is increasingly in vogue.

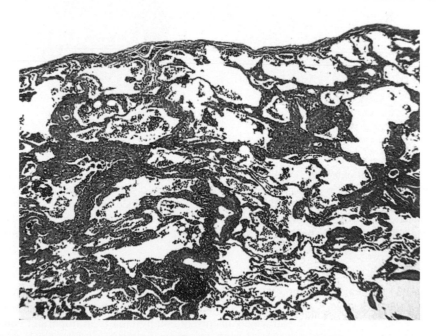

Fig. 16. Smoking-related interstitial lung disease. Patchy stellate centrilobular scarring suggesting PLCH. There is also an increase in airspace macrophages as seen in RB and DIP with some patchy relatively acellular fibrosis involving lung tissue showing background emphysematous change (courtesy Dr TV Colby).

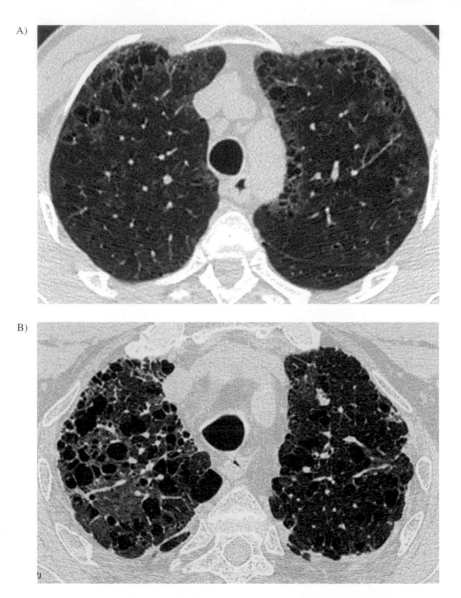

Fig. 17. Two examples of mixed "smoking-related diffuse lung disease" on HRCT. (**A**) Combination of areas of ground-glass opacity, reticular and honeycomb elements. On histologic examination of a lung biopsy, there were features of RBILD, interstitial fibrosis, and emphysema. (**B**) Complex mixture of HRCT patterns, including ground glass, honeycombing, cystic air spaces, and emphysema. The patient was a longstanding heavy smoker. There was no histologic corroboration of these HRCT appearances that were thought to represent "smoking-related diffuse lung disease".

Emphysema, in particular, commonly coexists with other smoking-induced disorders, including DIP, RBILD, and Langerhans cell histiocytosis, and this provides the most suggestive indirect evidence of a common pathogenetic pathway. Concurrent emphysema is an important confounder of the interpretation of pulmonary function tests, giving rise to a predominantly obstructive defect in some patients with DIP or RBILD. In other cases with smoking-related interstitial lung disease, the coexistence of emphysema and fibrotic abnormalities results in paradoxical normality of lung volumes and a disproportionate reduction in gas transfer, exactly as seen when emphysema is associated with idiopathic pulmonary fibrosis (51). Background emphysema is likely to account for the frequent observation of a disproportionate reduction in DLCO noted in two RBILD series (2,9). Pathogenetic links between emphysema and other smoking-related processes are likely to become a major focus of future research. As indicated above, it appears possible that respiratory bronchiolitis/RBILD may evolve to emphysema (20).

There is increasing evidence of an etiological role for smoking in acute eosinophilic pneumonia, with a number of case reports, especially from Japan, of the development of acute eosinophilic pneumonia shortly after starting smoking, usually in teenagers or young adults (52,53). In several cases, strong supportive evidence was obtained by cigarette smoking challenge tests (54). However, linkages between this disorder and the other forms of smoking-related lung disease have yet to be established.

6. LARGE AIRWAYS ABNORMALITIES IN CIGARETTE SMOKERS

All parts of the lower respiratory tract can be affected by cigarette smoking, ranging from the secondary effects of chronic obstructive pulmonary disease on the larger airways, for example, the saber sheath deformity of the trachea (55), to the subtle changes of respiratory bronchiolitis. Chronic bronchitis is the most obvious and frequent consequence of cigarette smoking on the medium-sized airways (for the purposes of this discussion, medium-sized refers to those bronchi directly visible on HRCT). Over the years, the definition of chronic bronchitis has remained a clinical one and is based mainly on the volume and frequency of bronchial secretions expectorated; as a consequence, it is not surprising that a definitive diagnosis of chronic bronchitis is often elusive (56). Difficulties in diagnostic precision are compounded by the fact that, in some parts of the world, environmental pollutants may be equally, or more, important than cigarette smoking as a cause of chronic bronchitis (57). Cigarette smoking and other irritants cause chronic inflammation of the airways, with the cardinal pathologic abnormality being hypertrophy of the mucus glands (which are responsible for abnormally copious sputum production) (Fig. 18). Other changes include squamous metaplasia of the epithelium and a chronic inflammatory cell infiltrate of the bronchial walls. Taken together, these changes result in thickening of bronchial walls, and this is reflected in radiographic and HRCT appearances of individuals with chronic bronchitis. Bronchiectasis does not appear to be secondary to this type of chronic bronchial wall inflammation and, outside the ambit of age-related change (58) and a_1-antitrysin deficiency (59), frank bronchiectasis does not seem to be a direct result of cigarette smoking.

Bronchial wall thickening, even when quite marked, is not readily evident on chest radiography, and the majority of patients with a clinical diagnosis of chronic bronchitis have a normal chest radiograph (60). One of the most subjective and difficult to define radiographic descriptions, "increased lung markings," may in part reflect widespread wall thickening of the airways, but this has not been fully investigated by radiographic pathologic correlative studies (61). Studies using HRCT have predictably shown a higher frequency of bronchial wall thickening (of variable severity) in cigarette smokers (Fig. 19) compared with non-smokers (7,18).

As discussed above, air-trapping can be readily detected in cigarette smokers using expiratory HRCT and can be demonstrated even in those individuals with normal pulmonary function test results (23) (Fig. 4A and B). At least some of this air trapping may be ascribed to bronchial inflammation. For example, it has been shown that the degree of cellular infiltration of peripheral bronchi of cigarette smokers correlates with the degree of air trapping as judged by attenuation differences on inspiratory and expiratory HRCT (62).

It must be emphasized that bronchial wall thickening cannot be regarded as a pathognomonic sign of smoking-related chronic bronchitis because it is non-specific and is encountered in other inflammatory conditions such as asthma (63) and infective or suppurative airways diseases, in

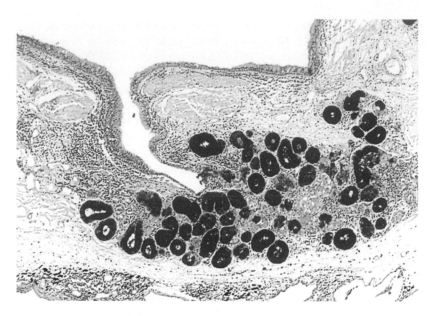

Fig. 18. Chronic bronchitis. An Alcian Blue PAS stain highlights the hypertrophy of the submucosal glands (staining dark reddish) and the increase in goblet cells in the mucosa above (staining pale blue) (courtesy Dr TV Colby).

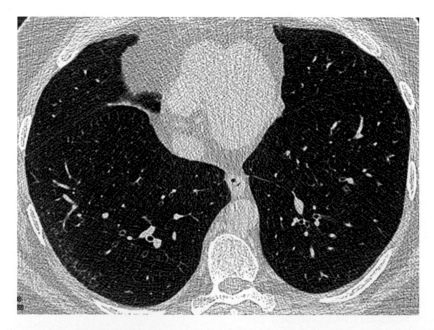

Fig. 19. Non-specific bronchial wall thickening on HRCT in a cigarette smoker. The significance of the peripheral fine reticular pattern in the right lower lobe was uncertain—it likely reflects limited interstitial fibrosis in the spectrum of "smoking-related diffuse lung disease."

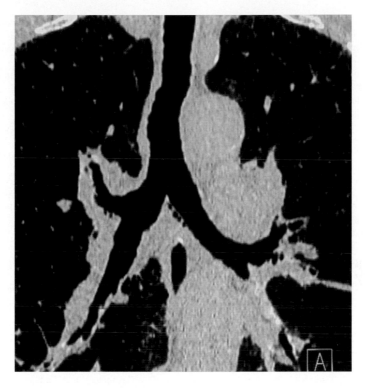

Fig. 20. Coronal reformat of volumetric CT through the major airways of a patient with chronic obstructive pulmonary disease showing bronchial pits along the inferior surface of the left mainstem and right upper lobe bronchi (courtesy Dr N Sverzellati).

particular bronchiectasis *(64)*. A recent study that evaluated wall thickness of airways in patients with chronic obstructive pulmonary disease showed that those patients with symptomatic chronic bronchitis had significantly thicker bronchial walls than those not fulfilling the clinical criteria for chronic bronchitis *(65)*. Automated software has shown that cigarette smokers with functional evidence of COPD have thicker airways than smokers without COPD or non-smokers *(66)*. Quantitative CT studies have shown that bronchial wall thickening, over and above CT evident emphysema, contributes to functional airflow limitation in cigarette smokers *(67,68)*.

Interestingly, one of the signs of chronic bronchitis regarded as a frequent finding in the era of bronchography, namely dilated mucus glands, seen as "bronchial pits" on bronchograms has been revisited by Zompatori et al. *(69)* who have pointed out that these small pits can be identified on CT along the inner surfaces of the large bronchi; furthermore, these are shown to advantage on reformatted volumetric thin-section CT (coronal reconstructions through the major airways) (Fig. 20). Whether this rediscovered sign can be regarded as specific for chronic bronchitis (bearing in mind that Gamsu et al. *(70)* showed that such pits were relatively common in healthy adults on bronchography) remains an open question.

REFERENCES

1. Niewoehner DE, Kleinerman J, Rice DB. Pathologic changes in the peripheral airways of young cigarette smokers. *N. Engl. J. Med.* 1974;291:775–777.
2. Myers JL, Veal CF, Shin MS, Katzenstein ALA. Respiratory bronchiolitis causing interstitial lung disease: a clinico-pathologic study of six cases. *Am. Rev. Respir. Dis.* 1987;135:880–884.

3. Guerry-Force ML, Müller NL, Wright JL, et al. A comparison of bronchiolitis obliterans with organizing pneumonia, usual interstitial pneumonia and small airways disease. *Am. Rev. Respir. Dis.* 1987;135:705–712.

4. Yousem SA, Colby TV, Gaensler EA. Respiratory bronchiolitis-associated interstitial lung disease and its relationship to desquamative interstitial pneumonia. *Mayo Clin. Proc.* 1989;64:1373–1380.

5. Fraig M, Shreesha U, Savici D, Katzenstein AL. Respiratory bronchiolitis: a clinicopathologic study in current smokers, ex-smokers, and never-smokers. *Am J Surg.Pathol* 2002;26:647–653.

6. Cottin V, Streichenberger N, Gamondes JP, et al. Respiratory bronchiolitis in smokers with spontaneous pneumothorax. *Eur. Respir. J.* 1998;12:702–704.

7. Remy-Jardin M, Remy J, Gosselin B, Becette V, Edme JL. Lung parenchymal changes secondary to cigarette smoking: pathologic-CT correlations. *Radiology* 1993;186:643–651.

8. Agius RM, Rutman A, Knight RK, Cole PJ. Human pulmonary alveolar macrophages with smokers' inclusions: their relation to the cessation of cigarette smoking. *Br. J. Exp. Pathol.* 1986;67:407–413.

9. Moon J, Du Bois RM, Colby TV, Hansell DM, Nicholson AG. Clinical significance of respiratory bronchiolitis on open lung biopsy and its relationship to smoking related interstitial lung disease. *Thorax* 1999;54:1009–1014.

10. Elkin SL, Nicholson AG, Du Bois RM. Desquamative interstitial pneumonia and respiratory bronchiolitis-associated interstitial lung disease. *Semin. Respir. Crit Care Med.* 2001;22:387–398.

11. King TE. Respiratory bronchiolitis-associated interstitial lung disease. *Clin. Chest. Med.* 1993;14:693–698.

12. Heyneman LE, Ward S, Lynch DA, Remy-Jardin M, Johkoh T, Müller NL. Respiratory bronchiolitis, respiratory bronchiolitis-associated interstitial lung disease, and desquamative interstitial pneumonia: different entities or part of the spectrum of the same disease process? *AJR* 1999;173:1617–1622.

13. Nicholson AG, Colby TV, Du Bois RM, Hansell DM, Wells AU. The prognostic significance of the histologic pattern of interstitial pneumonia in patients presenting with the clinical entity of cryptogenic fibrosing alveolitis. *Am. J. Respir. Crit. Care Med.* 2000;162:2213–2217.

14. Veeraraghavan S, Latsi PI, Wells AU, et al. BAL findings in idiopathic nonspecific interstitial pneumonia and usual interstitial pneumonia. *Eur. Respir. J.* 2003;22:239–244.

15. Drent M, van Nierop MA, Gerritsen FA, Wouters EF, Mulder PG. A computer program using BALF-analysis results as a diagnostic tool in interstitial lung diseases. *Am. J. Respir. Crit Care Med.* 1996;153:736–741.

16. Park JS, Brown KK, Tuder RM, Hale VA, King TE Jr, Lynch DA. Respiratory bronchiolitis-associated interstitial lung disease: radiologic features with clinical and pathologic correlation. *J. Comput. Assist. Tomogr.* 2002;26:13–20.

17. Prigent A, Lamblin C, Copin MC, Wallaert B. [Respiratory bronchiolitis with diffuse interstitial lung disease]. *Rev. Mal Respir.* 2001;18:201–204.

18. Remy-Jardin M, Remy J, Boulenguez C, Sobaszek A, Edme JL, Furon D. Morphologic effects of cigarette smoking on airways and pulmonary parenchyma in healthy adult volunteers: CT evaluation and correlation with pulmonary function tests. *Radiology* 1993;186:107–115.

19. Müller NL, Miller RR. Diseases of the bronchioles: CT and histopathologic findings. *Radiology* 1995;196:3–12.

20. Remy-Jardin M, Edme JL, Boulenguez C, Remy J, Mastora I, Sobaszek A. Longitudinal follow-up study of smoker's lung with thin-section CT in correlation with pulmonary function tests. *Radiology* 2002;222:261–270.

21. Holt RM, Schmidt RA, Godwin JD, Raghu G. High resolution CT in respiratory bronchiolitis-associated interstitial lung disease. *J. Comput. Assist. Tomogr.* 1993;17:46–50.

22. Essadki O, Chartrand-Lefebvre C, Briere J, Grenier P. Respiratory bronchiolitis: radiographic and CT findings in a pathologically proven case. *Eur. Radiol.* 1998;8:1674–1676.

23. Verschakelen JA, Scheinbaum K, Bogaert J, Demedts M, Lacquet LL, Baert AL. Expiratory CT in cigarette smokers: correlation between areas of decreased lung attenuation, pulmonary function tests and smoking history. *Eur. Radiol.* 1998;8:1391–1399.

24. Mastora I, Remy-Jardin M, Sobaszek A, Boulenguez C, Remy J, Edme JL. Thin-section CT finding in 250 volunteers: assessment of the relationship of CT findings with smoking history and pulmonary function test results. *Radiology* 2001;218:695–702.

25. Hansell DM, Wells AU, Padley SPG, Müller NL. Hypersensitivity pneumonitis: correlation of individual CT patterns with functional abnormalities. *Radiology* 1996;199:123–128.

26. Hartman TE, Primack SL, Swensen SJ, Hansell D, McGuinness G, Müller NL. Desquamative interstitial pneumonia: thin-section CT findings in 22 patients. *Radiology* 1993;187:787–790.

27. Carrington CB, Gaensler EA, Coutu RE, Fitzgerald MX, Gupta RG. Natural history and treated course of usual and desquamative interstitial pneumonia. *N. Engl. J. Med.* 1978;298:801–809.

28. Corrin B, Price AB. Electron microscopic studies in desquamative interstitial pneumonia associated with asbestos. *Thorax* 1972;27:324–331.

29. Abraham JL, Hertzberg MA. Inorganic particulates associated with desquamative interstitial pneumonia. *Chest* 1981;80:67–70.

30. Bone RC, Wolfe J, Sobonya RE, et al. Desquamative interstitial pneumonia following long-term nitrofurantoin therapy. *Am. J. Med.* 1976;60:697–701.

31. Amir G, Ron N. Pulmonary pathology in Gaucher's disease. *Hum. Pathol.* 1999;30:666–670.

32. Craig PJ, Wells AU, Doffman S, et al. Desquamative interstitial pneumonia, respiratory bronchiolitis and their relationship to smoking. *Histopathology* 2004;45:275–282.

33. Liebow AA, Steer A, Billingsley JG. Desquamative interstitial pneumonitis. *Am. J. Med.* 1965;39:369–404.

34. Myers JL, Aubry MC. Pulmonary langerhans cell histiocytosis: what was the question? *Am. J. Respir. Crit. Care Med.* 2002;166:1419–1421.

35. Lichtenstein L. Histiocytosis X. Integration of eosinophilic granuloma of bone, 'Letterer-Slwe disease' and 'Schuller-Christian disease' as related manifestations of a single nosologic entity. *Arch. Pathol.* 1953;56:84–102.

36. Colby TV, Lombard C. Histiocytosis X in the lung. *Hum. Pathol.* 1983;14:847–856.

37. Kambouchner M, Basset F, Marchal J, Uhl JF, Hance AJ, Soler P. Three-dimensional characterization of pathologic lesions in pulmonary langerhans cell histiocytosis. *Am. J. Respir. Crit Care Med.* 2002;166:1483–1490.

38. Habib SB, Congleton J, Carr D, et al. Recurrence of recipient Langerhans' cell histiocytosis following bilateral lung transplantation. *Thorax* 1998;53:323–325.

39. Travis WD, Borok Z, Roum JH, et al. Pulmonary Langerhans cell granulomatosis (histiocytosis X). A clinicopathologic study of 48 cases. *Am. J. Surg. Pathol.* 1993;17:971–986.

40. Fartoukh M, Humbert M, Capron F, et al. Severe pulmonary hypertension in histiocytosis X. *Am. J. Respir. Crit. Care Med.* 2000;161:216–223.

41. Lacronique J, Roth C, Battesti JP, Basset F, Chretien J. Chest radiological features of pulmonary histiocytosis X: a report based on 50 adult cases. *Thorax* 1982;37:104–109.

42. Khoor A, Myers JL, Tazelaar HD, Swensen SJ. Pulmonary Langerhans cell histiocytosis presenting as a solitary nodule. *Mayo Clin. Proc.* 2001;76:209–211.

43. Donnelly LF, Frush DP. Langerhans' cell histiocytosis showing low-attenuation mediastinal mass and cystic lung disease. *AJR Am. J. Roentgenol.* 2000,174.877–878.

44. Primack SL, Hartman TE, Hansell DM, Muller NL. End-stage lung disease: CT findings in 61 patients. *Radiology* 1993;189:681–686.

45. Brauner MW, Grenier P, Mouelhi MM, Mompoint D, Lenoir S. Pulmonary histiocytosis X: evaluation with high-resolution CT. *Radiology* 1989;172:255–258.

46. Brauner MW, Grenier P, Tijani K, Battesti JP, Valeyre D. Pulmonary Langerhans cell histiocytosis: evolution of lesions on CT scans. *Radiology* 1997;204:497–502.

47. Soler P, Bergeron A, Kambouchner M, et al. Is high-resolution computed tomography a reliable tool to predict the histopathological activity of pulmonary Langerhans cell histiocytosis? *Am. J. Respir. Crit. Care Med.* 2000;162:264–270.

48. Gabbay E, Dark JH, Ashcroft T, et al. Recurrence of Langerhans' cell granulomatosis following lung transplantation. *Thorax* 1998;53:326–327.

49. Selman M. The spectrum of smoking-related interstitial lung disorders: the never-ending story of smoke and disease. *Chest* 2003;124:1185–1187.

50. Vassallo R, Jensen EA, Colby TV, et al. The overlap between respiratory bronchiolitis and desquamative interstitial pneumonia in pulmonary Langerhans cell histiocytosis: high-resolution CT, histologic, and functional correlations. *Chest* 2003;124:1199–1205.

51. Wells AU, King AD, Rubens MB, Cramer D, Du Bois RM, Hansell DM. Lone cryptogenic fibrosing alveolitis: a functional-morphologic correlation based on extent of disease on thin-section computed tomography. *Am. J. Respir. Crit. Care Med.* 1997;155:1367–1375.

52. Shintani H, Fujimura M, Yasui M, et al. Acute eosinophilic pneumonia caused by cigarette smoking. *Intern. Med.* 2000;39:66–68.

53. Nakajima M, Manabe T, Niki Y, Matsushima T. Cigarette smoke-induced acute eosinophilic pneumonia. *Radiology* 1998;207:829–831.

54. Watanabe K, Fujimura M, Kasahara K, et al. Acute eosinophilic pneumonia following cigarette smoking: a case report including cigarette-smoking challenge test. *Intern. Med.* 2002;41:1016–1020.

55. Greene R. "Saber-sheath" trachea: relation to chronic obstructive pulmonary disease. *AJR Am. J. Roentgenol.* 1978;130:441–445.

56. Bobadilla A, Guerra S, Sherrill D, Barbee R. How accurate is the self-reported diagnosis of chronic bronchitis? *Chest* 2002;122:1234–1239.

57. Sunyer J, Jarvis D, Gotschi T, et al. Chronic bronchitis and urban air pollution in an international study. *Occup. Environ. Med.* 2006;63:836–843.

58. Matsuoka S, Uchiyama K, Shima H, Ueno N, Oish S, Nojiri Y. Bronchoarterial ratio and bronchial wall thickness on high-resolution CT in asymptomatic subjects: correlation with age and smoking. *AJR Am. J. Roentgenol.* 2003;180: 513–518.

59. Guest PJ, Hansell DM. High resolution computed tomography in emphysema associated with alpha-1-antitrypsin deficiency. *Clin. Radiol.* 1992;45:260–266.

60. Gamsu G, Nadel JA. The roentgenologic manifestations of emphysema and chronic bronchitis. *Med. Clin. North Am.* 1973;57:719–733.
61. Guckel C, Hansell DM. Imaging the 'dirty lung'–has high resolution computed tomography cleared the smoke? *Clin. Radiol.* 1998;53:717–722.
62. Berger P, Laurent F, Begueret H, et al. Structure and function of small airways in mokers: relationship between air trapping at CT and airway inflammation. *Radiology* 2003;228:85–94.
63. Grenier P, Mourey-Gerosa I, Benali K, et al. Abnormalities of the airways and lung parenchyma in asthmatics: CT observations in 50 patients and inter- and intra-observer variability. *Eur. Radiol.* 1996;6:199–206.
64. Diederich S, Jurriaans E, Flower CDR. Interobserver variation in the diagnosis of bronchiectasis on high-resolution computed tomography. *Eur. Radiol.* 1996;6:801–806.
65. Orlandi I, Moroni C, Camiciottoli G, et al. Chronic obstructive pulmonary disease: thin-section CT measurement of airway wall thickness and lung attenuation. *Radiology* 2005;234:604–610.
66. Berger P, Perot V, Desbarats P, Tunon-de-Lara JM, Marthan R, Laurent F. Airway wall thickness in cigarette smokers: quantitative thin-section CT assessment. *Radiology* 2005;235:1055–1064.
67. Nakano Y, Muro S, Sakai H, et al. Computed tomographic measurements of airway dimensions and emphysema in smokers. Correlation with lung function. *Am. J. Respir. Crit. Care Med.* 2000;162:1102–1108.
68. Aziz ZA, Wells AU, Desai SR, et al. Functional impairment in emphysema: contribution of airway abnormalities and distribution of parenchymal disease. *AJR Am. J. Roentgenol.* 2005;185:1509–1515.
69. Zompatori M, Sverzellati N, Gentile T, Spaggiari L, Laporta T, Fecci L. Imaging of the patient with chronic bronchitis: an overview of old and new signs. *Radiol. Med. (Torino)* 2006;111:634–639.
70. Gamsu G, Forbes AR, Ovenfors CO. Bronchographic features of chronic bronchitis in normal men. *AJR Am. J. Roentgenol.* 1981;136:317–322.

IV Pediatric Airways Disorders

15

Large Airways

Edward Y. Lee and Marilyn J. Siegel

Summary

With the recent rapid technological advances, computed tomography (CT), particularly multislice CT, has assumed a greater role in the evaluation of various pediatric airway disorders. With its ability to generate isotropic, high-resolution images as well as high-quality multiplanar and 3D images with faster scan times, CT is especially helpful in evaluating the large airways in children. This chapter addresses patient preparation and CT imaging techniques for evaluating large airway disorders in children. The main focus of this chapter is to illustrate CT appearances of common large airway disorders, which occur in a diverse spectrum of conditions including congenital anomalies, neoplasm, infection and acquired cause such as tracheobronchial stricture

Key Words: Large airway disorders; computed tomography (CT); multislice CT; pediatric patients; multiplanar and three-dimensional (3-D) images.

1. INTRODUCTION

With the development and widespread availability of multislice scanners, computed tomography (CT) has assumed a greater role in the evaluation of pediatric large airway disorders. Multislice CT allows isotropic, high-resolution images, faster scan times, and high-quality multiplanar and three-dimensional (3-D) images of the airway. Faster scan times enable the central airway to be imaged in a few seconds, reducing sedation rates and motion artifact. The high-quality CT reconstructions have enhanced the display of airway stenosis, the assessment of the craniocaudal extent of disease, and the evaluation of complex airway disorders. In addition, they have improved communication between radiologists and clinicians.

In this chapter, we address multislice techniques for performing airway CT, emphasizing the role of multiplanar and 3-D images. The CT appearances of the common large airway disorders in a pediatric population also are highlighted.

2. PATIENT PREPARATION/TECHNIQUE

2.1. Sedation

Pediatric patients pose several challenges for airway imaging, including patient motion, small body size, lack of perivisceral fat, and greater sensitivity to radiation. These problems can be minimized by appropriate use of sedation and intravenous contrast medium (1,2).

Early experience suggests that the sedation rate for young children undergoing multidetector CT is equal to or less than 5% (3,4). These studies have included small patient populations, so further

From: *Contemporary Medical Imaging: CT of the Airways*
Edited by: P. M. Boiselle and D. A. Lynch © Humana Press, Totowa, NJ

assessment will be needed to determine the precise sedation rate in children. Undoubtedly, sedation still will be required for some uncooperative infants and young children. As a general rule, children older than 5 years of age will cooperate after verbal reassurance and explanation of the procedure.

Sedation for imaging examinations is nearly always conscious sedation *(5)*. Conscious sedation is defined as a minimally depressed level of consciousness that retains the patient's abilities to maintain a patent airway, independently and continuously, and respond appropriately to physical stimulation and/or verbal command. The most commonly used sedative drugs are oral chloral hydrate and intravenous pentobarbital sodium. Regardless of the choice of drug, the use of parenteral sedation requires the facility and ability to resuscitate and maintain adequate cardiorespiratory support during and after the examination *(6,7)*.

2.2. Intravenous Contrast Material

Intravenous contrast material is not needed for evaluation of airway stenosis or tracheobronchomalacia, but it is indicated in the evaluation of extrinsic causes of airway disease, such as the vascular anomalies, and in the evaluation of neoplasms, particularly hemangiomas. If intravenous contrast material is to be administered, it is helpful to have an intravenous line in place when the child arrives in the radiology department. This reduces patient agitation that is typically associated with a venipuncture.

The contrast dose is 2 mL/kg (not to exceed 4 mL/kg or 125 mL). A nonionic contrast medium should be used to minimize discomfort at the injection site, side effects such as nausea and vomiting, and patient motion during contrast administration.

Contrast can be administered by mechanical or hand injection. Mechanical administration can be performed if a 22-gauge or larger cannula can be placed into an antecubital vein. Contrast is infused at 1.5–2.5 mL/s for a 22-gauge catheter and 2.0–4.0 mL/s for a 20-gauge catheter. The site of injection is closely monitored during the initial injection of contrast to minimize the risk of contrast extravasation. The contrast medium should be administered by a hand injection using a bolus technique if intravenous access is through a central access line or a smaller caliber antecubital catheter. The complication rates for manual and power injections are similar (<0.4%), provided that the catheter is positioned properly and functions well *(8)*.

3. IMAGING TECHNIQUE

3.1. Technical Considerations of Multislice CT

Although technical parameters somewhat vary based on the type of CT scanner used, there are basic principles that apply for evaluation of large airways in pediatric patients regardless of the type of equipment. Strategies that minimize radiation dose are essential for CT examinations in children. The parameters that influence the radiation exposure include tube current or milliamperage (mAs), kilovoltage peak (kVp), table speed, and detector collimation. The mAs for pediatric CT examinations must be at the lowest possible level while also maintaining image quality *(9–12)*. Guidelines for tube current based on patient weight are shown in Table 1. Kilovoltage also affects scan quality and radiation dose. A kVp of 80 should be considered for patients weighing less than 50 kg. In larger patients, a kVp of 100–120 is needed to compensate for the higher noise *(13)*. The gantry rotation time should be 1-s or less. Fortunately, most state-of-the-art scanners are now equipped with gantry rotation times of 0.5 s or less.

One of the most important advantages of multislice CT is the capability to routinely use thin collimation, which allows retrospective reconstructions to be made without the need for rescanning. Detector collimation along with table speed will vary depending on the type of scanner. For a four-row detector scanner, a 1.0–1.25-mm collimation with a pitch of 1.5–2.0 is adequate for routine scanning.

Table 1
Tube Current by Patient Weight

Weight (kg)	Tube current (mA)
<10	40
10–25	60
26–50	80
51–70	100–120

For a 16-row detector, a 0.75-mm collimation with a pitch of 1.0–1.5 suffices, whereas for a 64-row detector, a 0.5–0.6-mm collimation and a pitch of 1.0–1.5 suffices.

CT scans of the large airway in pediatric patients are acquired from the vocal cords to below the carina. In cooperative pediatric patients, usually children over 5–6 years of age, CT scans are obtained in a single breath-hold at end-inspiration. In sedated pediatric patients, CT scans are obtained at resting lung volume. For evaluation of tracheobronchial malacia, dynamic CT imaging during inspiration and expiration is useful in evaluating changes in airway caliber.

4. POST-PROCESSING TECHNIQUES

The narrow collimation sections (see Section 3.1) are overlapped and used to create multiplanar and 3-D images *(14–16)*. The original volumetric data are reconstructed with a 3-mm slice thickness at 2-mm reconstruction intervals or with a 2-mm thickness at 1-mm reconstruction interval to enhance the quality of the reconstructed images.

4.1. Multiplanar Reformation Methods

Multiplanar images are 1-voxel-thick CT sections that use all pixels in the data set regardless of attenuation. Multiplanar reformations (MPR) can be created along any plane: orthogonal, coronal, sagittal, and in a curved fashion along the airway axis (Fig. 1). Curved reformatting of a stack of CT images is particularly useful in evaluating curved tubular structures, such as the large airway (Fig. 2). A curved coronal MPR is obtained by drawing a reference line through the center of the airway on a sagittal image reconstructed from the original data set, whereas a curved sagittal MPR is obtained by drawing a line through the center of airway on a coronal image reconstructed from the original volumetric data. The advantage of MPR is that it requires virtually no reconstruction time and can be easily obtained at the CT console. Its disadvantage is that it is only a 2-D image.

4.2. Maximum and Minimum Intensity Projection Images

Maximum intensity projection (MIP) images and minimum intensity projection (MinIP) images are created by an image reconstruction algorithm using a CT subvolume data set along parallel rays based on either the highest or the lowest individual CT voxel values. MIP emphasizes the visualization of the bronchial wall in comparison with the bronchial lumen by using the highest available attenuation values. MinIp accentuates the visualization of the bronchial lumen in comparison with the bronchial wall by using the lowest available attenuation values and has also proven to be useful for evaluating the lung parenchyma (Fig. 3). Similarly to MPR, the advantage of MIP and MinIP is that they do not require extensive reconstruction time or skill. However, as they are still a 2-D representation of 3-D volumetric CT data set, they lack depth information of 3-D imaging.

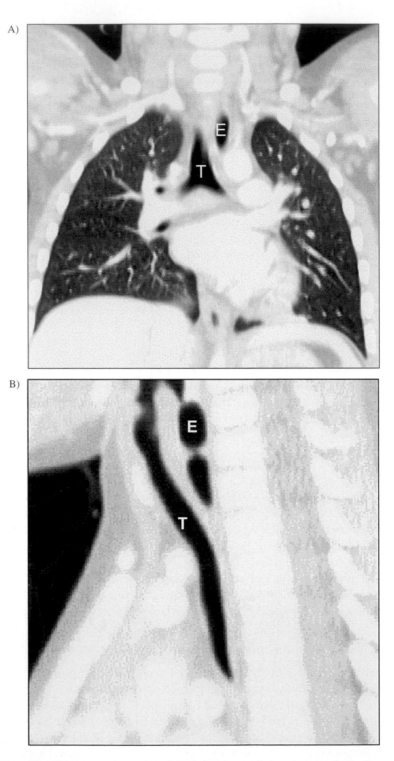

Fig. 1. (**A**) Coronal multiplanar reformation (MPR) CT lung window image of the airway demonstrating that the trachea (T) is not visualized in its entirety because the trachea is usually not completely parallel to the coronal axis. On this coronal lung window MPR CT image, a portion of esophagus (E) is also visualized. (**B**) Sagittal MPR CT lung window image of airway showing trachea (T) and a portion of esophagus (E).

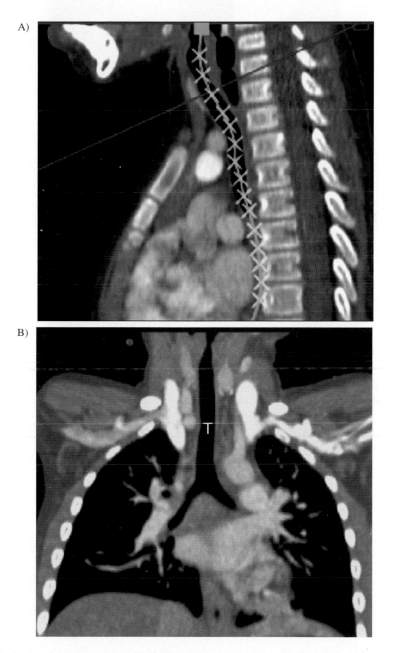

Fig. 2. (**A**) Sagittal multiplanar reformation (MPR) CT image demonstrating a reference line through the center of the airway for reconstruction of a curved coronal MPR image. (**B**) Curved coronal MPR image showing the entire trachea (T), which is unlike the coronal MPR CT image (Fig. 1A), where only a portion of trachea is visualized.

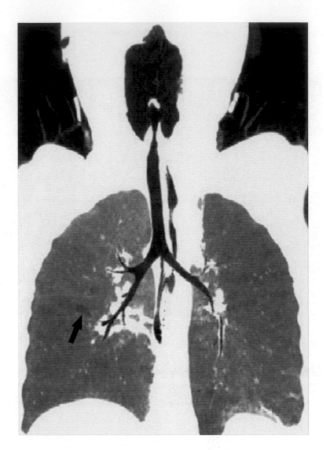

Fig. 3. Minimum intensity projection (MinIP) image demonstrating the entire central airway and lung parenchyma. Air-trapping (arrow) within the lung parenchyma is well visualized on MinIP image.

4.3. Three-Dimensional Volume Rendering

Volume-rendering is currently the most widely used 3-D reconstruction for assessing the airway. Volume rendering uses the entire attenuation composition and spatial relationships in the data set. The data can be manipulated, so that the width, opacity, brightness, and color of the image can be altered. Such post-processing permits the data to be displayed from an external or internal perspective (Figs 4 and 5).

External volume rendering, also referred to as CT tracheobronchography, allows for an opaque or transparent depiction of the airways that helps to define the external surface of the airway. Internal volume rendering, also known as virtual bronchoscopy, enables navigation of the internal lumen of the airway and depiction of the air–lumen interface, simulating the appearance of conventional bronchoscopy *(17)*.

Before the introduction of volume-rendered technology, the shaded-surface display had been widely used to create 3-D images of the airway. With the shaded-surface technique, only structures within a selected threshold range are displayed; and unfortunately, a large amount of data are lost. By comparison, volume rendering utilizes all voxel information acquired in the data set, so that it has become the reconstruction of choice for creating 3-D images. The principle limitation of volume rendering it that it is potentially time-consuming and requires a separate workstation. However, pre-set

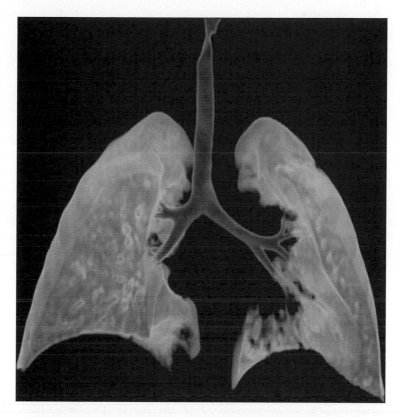

Fig. 4. Three-dimensional external volume rendered image demonstrating the entire large airway.

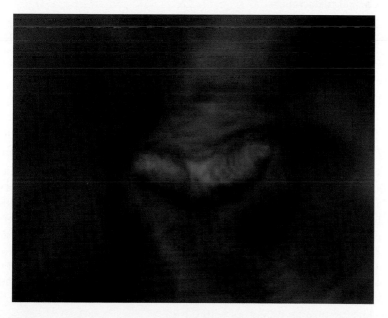

Fig. 5. Three-dimensional internal volume rendered image showing virtual bronchoscopic view of the central airway at the carina level.

airway reconstruction algorithms available with current commercially available software programs allow a series of reconstructions to be performed in only a few minutes.

5. IMAGE INTERPRETATION

Interpretation of CT scans of the large airway in pediatric patients requires careful evaluation of axial, multiplanar, and 3-D images *(18)*. Axial images are important for assessing extraluminal disorder such as adjacent mediastinal structures and lung parenchyma. However, they are limited in detecting subtle airway stenoses and can underestimate the longitudinal extent of disease. Moreover, they have limited ability to display complex airway anatomy. Axial images are also helpful for identifying the presence and extent of airway wall thickening, as well as for identifying artifacts that may simulate true pathology on 3-D images.

Multiplanar and external volume-rendered images can improve the assessment of subtle airway stenoses, the craniocaudal extent of airway narrowing, and the anatomy of complex relationships *(18,19)*. They also are useful for localizing stents and detecting stent complications, including malpositioning, migration, and fracture *(20)*, and for displaying the craniocaudal extent of airway collapse in patients with tracheal or bronchial malacia.

Virtual bronchoscopic images, although not necessary for diagnosis, offer the benefit of viewing the airway distal, a high-grade stenosis or large obstructing neoplasm, areas that otherwise can be difficult to visualize by conventional bronchoscopy *(19,21)*. Other applications for virtual bronchoscopy include localizing foreign bodies and determining sites for performing transbronchial needle aspirations and biopsies.

6. CLINCIAL APPLICATIONS FOR CT

The most common indications prompting CT of the airway are: (i) evaluation of congenital tracheobronchial anomalies, (ii) assessment of tracheal narrowing, and (iii) detection or confirmation of tracheal or bronchial malacia.

7. CONGENITAL MALFORMATIONS OF THE TRACHEA AND BRONCHI

Congenital anomalies of the large airways may result from a primary embryologic error in the formation of these structures or may be secondary to errors in the development of the surrounding vasculature *(22)*. Symptoms usually appear within the first few weeks or months of life.

7.1. Congenital Tracheobronchial Anomalies

7.1.1. Tracheal and Supernumerary Bronchi

Anomalies of tracheobronchial branching include ectopic and supernumerary bronchi arising form the trachea or main bronchi, bronchial isomerism, and bronchial hypoplasia or agenesis. Anomalous bronchi arising from the trachea are more often ectopic than supernumerary. The most common site for bronchial ectopia is the right upper lobe bronchus. Ectopic origin of the right upper lobe bronchus, also termed tracheal bronchus (Fig. 6), has an incidence of 0.1–2% *(22–24)*. A tracheal bronchus is usually discovered incidentally on imaging studies or bronchoscopy performed for other clinical indications, but patients can present with recurrent right upper lobe infection. On CT, the anomalous right upper bronchus arises above the carina on the right lateral wall of the trachea, rather than from the right main bronchus. Consolidation and atelectasis affecting the portion of lung supplied by the anomalous bronchus can also be visualized with CT.

The cardiac bronchus is a supernumerary bronchus *(25,26)*. It arises from the medial wall of the bronchus intermedius, and it may be blind ending or it may ventilate a hypoplastic lobule. Most cardiac bronchi are asymptomatic and discovered during evaluation of other clinical symptoms or signs.

7.1.2. Bronchial Agenesis, Aplasia, and Hypoplasia

Bronchial agenesis results in complete agenesis of the bronchus, lung, and vascular supply (Fig. 7). In bronchial aplasia, there is a rudimentary bronchus and absence of the distal lung. In bronchial hypoplasia, the bronchus is rudimentary and the lung develops, but it is hypoplastic. The pulmonary

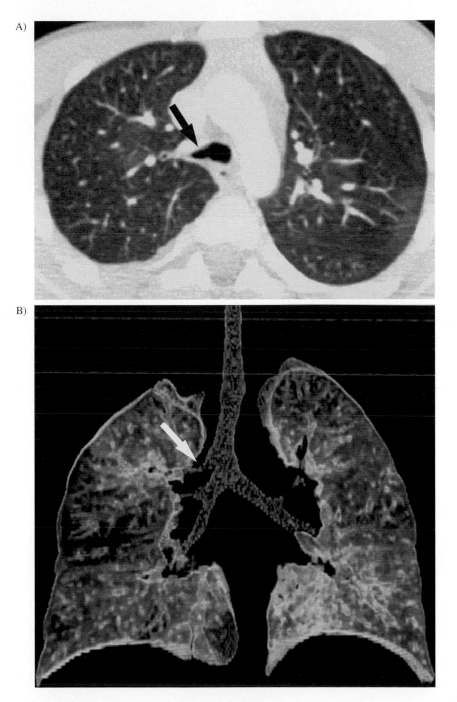

Fig. 6. *(Continued)*

C)

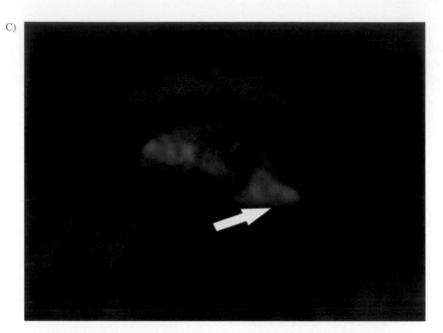

Fig. 6. (**A**) Axial CT image demonstrating anomalous right upper lobe bronchus (arrow), tracheal bronchus, arising from the right lateral wall of the trachea. (**B**) 3-D external volume rendered image showing tracheal bronchus (arrow). Also noted is the volume loss in the right upper lung because of chronic right upper lobe infections. (**C**) 3-D internal volume rendered image demonstrating tracheal bronchus (arrow) arising from the right side of trachea before the carina.

arteries may be absent or hypoplastic in both aplasia and hypoplasia. Other anomalies of the skeletal, cardiovascular, gastrointestinal, and urinary system are common. CT can easily show the extent of bronchial and parenchymal development *(27,28)*.

A)

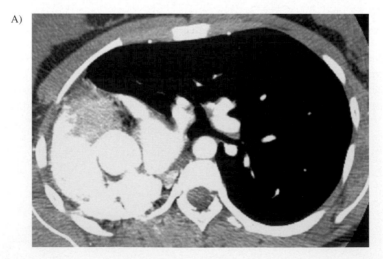

Fig. 7. *(Continued)*

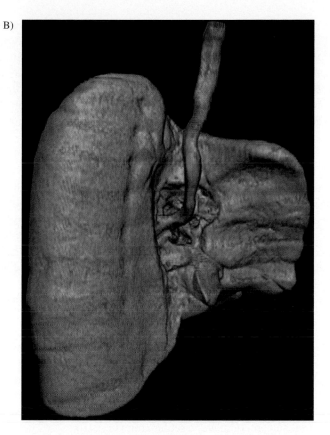

Fig. 7. (A) Axial CT image showing right-sided bronchial agenesis. The entire mediastinum is shifted to the right side of hemithorax. Also noted is the absence of right bronchus, lung, and vascular supply. **(B)** 3-D volume rendered image of the large airway from the posterior view demonstrating absent right bronchus and right lung. Also noted is the hypertrophied and hyperinflated left lung.

7.1.3. Cartilaginous Stenosis

Congenital tracheobronchial stenosis is a rare disorder because of complete tracheal rings associated with absent or deficient tracheal membranes *(29)*. The onset varies with the severity of stenosis. In general, symptoms usually develop in the first year of life and include stridor, wheezing, cyanosis, and recurrent pneumonia. Although plain radiographs and fluoroscopy can often show tracheal narrowing, CT is more sensitive for showing the length and extent of narrowing, and it also can identify associated tracheal or cardiovascular anomalies (Fig. 8). Treatment of short stenoses is resection and end-to-end anastomosis. Longer stenoses may require a patch or tracheal autograft repair *(30,31)*. Survival rate is approximately 77% in the series reported *(30)*. In addition, for those patients who are only minimally symptomatic at the time of diagnosis, it has been reported that they may benefit from observation to monitor airway growth and symptoms rather than proceeding directly to surgery *(32)*. CT could potentially be used in place of the more invasive procedure of bronchoscopy for monitoring such patients.

7.2. Congenital Vascular Anomalies

Congenital anomalies of the aorta and its branch vessels are found in 0.5–3% of the population *(22,33)*. Most vascular malformations result from errors in the formation of the fourth and sixth branchial arch vessels. Fourth arch defects lead to vascular rings encircling the trachea (e.g., right aortic arch with aberrant left subclavian artery and double aortic arch), whereas sixth arch defects lead to anomalous development of the left pulmonary artery (pulmonary sling).

Mediastinal vascular anomalies can compress the large airways resulting in respiratory symptoms, including stridor, chronic cough, recurrent pneumonia, and dysphagia. Patients, however, can be asymptomatic, and the anomaly may be an incidental finding on studies performed for other clinical indications. Chest radiographs can suggest the diagnosis of a vascular ring, but contrast-enhanced CT scan provides the definite diagnosis and can show the precise anatomy for surgical planning *(18,34–37)*.

7.2.1. Right Aortic Arch with Anomalous Left Subclavian Artery

There are two main types of right arches: right arch with aberrant left subclavian artery and right arch with mirror-image branching. In the right arch with aberrant left subclavian artery, the great arteries originate in the following order: left carotid, right carotid, right subclavian, and aberrant left subclavian. The aberrant left subclavian artery arises as the last branch from the aortic arch and traverses the mediastinum behind the esophagus to reach the left arm. Patients are symptomatic when there is a left ligamentum arteriosum, resulting in a vascular ring. In addition, the diverticulum of Kommerel (the remnant of the embryonic dorsal left arch) can further compress the posterior aspect of the trachea (Fig. 9). Approximately 10% of these patients have associated congenital heart disease.

In the right arch with mirror-image branching, the great arteries originate in the following order: left innominate, right carotid, and right subclavian. The descending aorta usually is right-sided. The majority of infants and children with this anomaly have associated cyanotic heart disease. Although there is a rare variant of the right arch with mirror-image branching associated with a diverticulum of Kommerel and left ligamentum resulting in vascular ring, stridor and dysphagia are usually absent in patients with right arch with mirror-image branching because there is no structure posterior to the trachea or esophagus to result in complete vascular ring (Fig. 10).

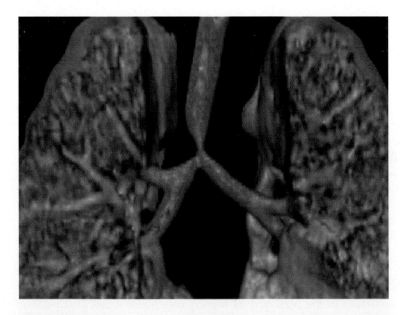

Fig. 8. Three-dimensional external volume rendered image demonstrating congenital tracheobronchial stenosis involving the distal trachea and proximal bilateral main stem bronchi.

7.2.2. Double Aortic Arch

Double aortic arch is characterized by the presence of two aortic arches arising from a single ascending aorta. The two limbs of the arch encircle the trachea and esophagus, resulting in compression of both structures (Fig. 11). Each arch gives rise to a subclavian and carotid artery; with the aorta usually descending on the left. Usually, both limbs are patent, and the right limb is larger and more cephalad than the left. Occasionally, a portion of the left limb is atretic with a fibrous band completing the ring. Three-dimensional reconstructions are particularly helpful for demonstrating an atretic segment. In symptomatic patients, the smaller arch is divided. Following surgery, symptoms may persist for some time because of associated tracheomalacia. *(38)* Dynamic airway CT can be used to document the tracheomalacia.

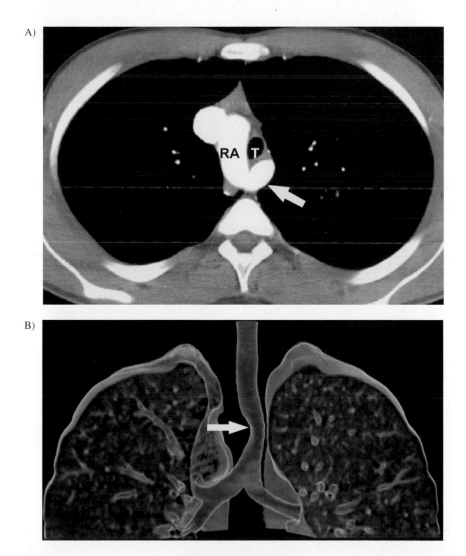

Fig. 9. *(Continued)*

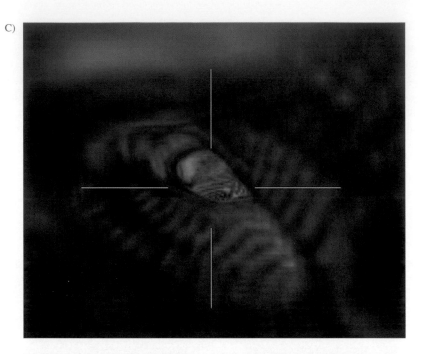

Fig. 9. (A) Axial CT image showing right aortic arch (RA) with aberrant left subclavian artery (arrow). The aberrant left subclavian artery courses behind the trachea (T) to the left side of the chest. **(B)** 3-D external volume rendered image showing compression of the trachea (arrow) because of the right aortic arch with aberrant left subclavian artery. **(C)** 3-D internal volume rendered image demonstrating tracheal compression because of the right aortic arch with aberrant left subclavian artery.

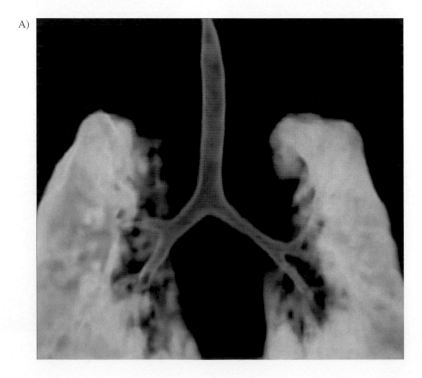

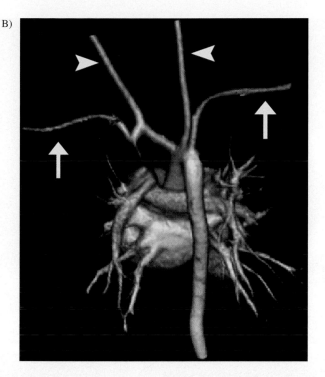

Fig. 10. (**A**) Three-dimensional external volume rendered image showing patent trachea in a patient with right aortic arch with mirror imaging branching. (**B**) Posterior view of a 3-D volume rendered image of the mediastinal vessel in a patient with right aortic arch with mirror imaging branching demonstrating the absence of posterior vascular structure to result in airway compression. Short arrows = bilateral common carotid arteries. Long arrows = bilateral subclavian arteries. Reprinted with permission from Siegel MJ. Great Vessels. In: Siegel MJ, ed. Pediatric Body CT, Second Edition. Philadelphia: Lippincott Williams & Wilkins, 2007:126.

7.2.3. Innominate Artery Syndrome

The innominate artery arises from the left aortic arch and crosses anterior and to the right of the trachea. As it crosses the mediastinum, it can compress the trachea, resulting in stridor, cough, and dyspnea *(39)*. This syndrome predominantly affects infants who have decreased anterior mediastinal space because of the presence of a relatively large thymus. On CT images, anterior compression of the trachea by the innominate artery is seen at or just below the level of the thoracic inlet (Fig. 12). Symptoms usually decrease with patient growth. However, surgical treatment, such as innominate arteriopexy, which creates more anterior mediastinal space, can be beneficial in severely symptomatic patients. Following surgery, some patients may remain symptomatic because of the associated tracheomalacia.

7.2.4. Pulmonary Sling

In pulmonary artery sling, the left pulmonary artery arises from the right and courses between the esophagus and trachea to reach the left hilum. There are two types of pulmonary sling. Type 1 pulmonary sling is associated with characteristic compression of the posterior aspect of the trachea, right main bronchus, and anterior aspect of the esophagus, which can be seen on CT (Fig. 13). Type 2 pulmonary sling is low in location and associated with congenital long segment tracheal stenosis, a horizontal course of the main bronchi (i.e., T-shaped carina), bridging bronchus, and

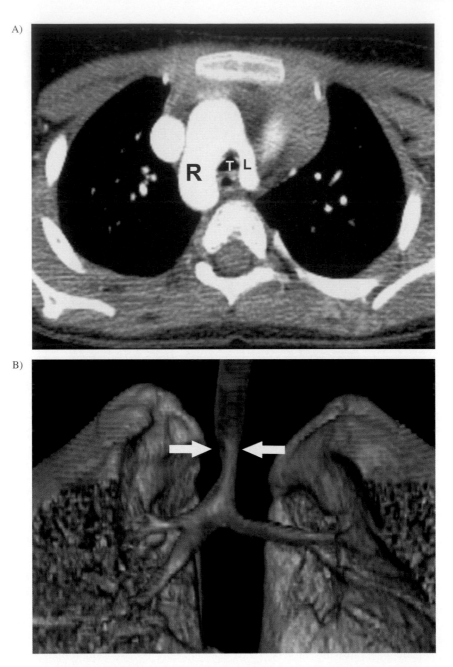

Fig. 11. (A) Axial CT image demonstrating double aortic arch with tracheal compression (T) by the right limb (R) and left (L) limbs of aorta. **(B)** 3-D external volume rendered image of the large airway showing tracheal narrowing (arrows) by the double aortic arch.

multiple other congenital anomalies *(40,41)*. Symptomatic patients are treated with surgical division and reimplantation of the anomalous pulmonary artery *(42)*. Tracheoplasty is also performed in patients with complete cartilaginous rings.

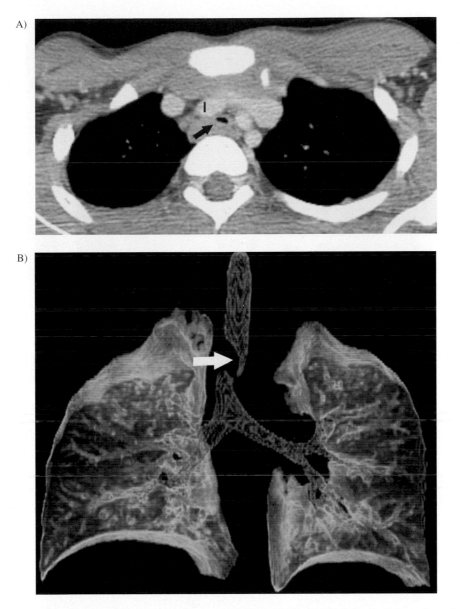

Fig. 12. (**A**) Axial CT image shows innominate artery (I) arising from the left aortic arch and crossing anterior and to the right of the trachea resulting in tracheal compression (arrow). (**B**) 3-D external volume rendered image of large airway demonstrating tracheal compression (arrow) by the innominate artery.

8. ACQUIRED TRACHEAL NARROWING

8.1. Tracheal Stricture

The most common cause of acquired tracheal stricture or stenosis is prior intubation or tracheostomy tube placement. The two most common sites of stenosis or stricture occur at the level of the endotracheal or tracheostomy tube balloon and at the level of the tracheostomy stoma *(43)*.

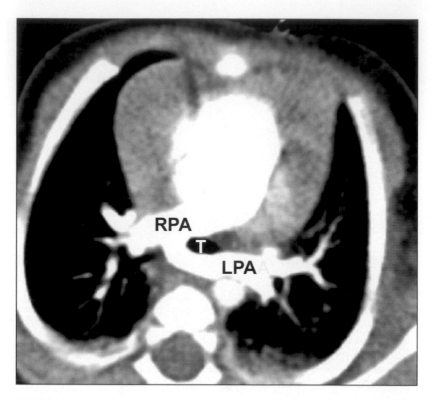

Fig. 13. Axial CT image shows anomalous left pulmonary artery (LPA) arising from the right pulmonary artery (RPA) which courses behind the trachea (T) resulting in the posterior tracheal compression.

The stenosis usually results from pressure necrosis, which causes ischemia and ultimately fibrosis, but it also can result from granulomatous tissue.

8.2. Bronchial Stricture

Acquired bronchial stenosis can be seen after partial lung resection with bronchial anastomosis and after lung transplantation (Fig. 14) *(44–46)*. Similar to tracheal stricture, bronchial stenosis can be due to fibrotic tissue or granulomatous tissue.

8.3. Primary Airway Neoplasms

Neoplasms involving the large airways in pediatric patients are relatively rare. These lesions usually come to the physician's attention because of airway obstruction. Symptoms include stridor, cough, wheezing, and parenchymal infection. Primary airway neoplasms in children are usually benign, unlike those in adults. Benign tumors occur more frequently in the larynx or upper trachea, whereas malignant tumors occur more distally.

Bronchoscopy can identify the intraluminal and mucosal components of airway tumors as well as provide a histologic diagnosis, but often it cannot determine the true extent of the lesion, especially the extent of the tumor outside the tracheal lumen. CT with multiplanar and 3-D reconstructions is useful for showing the mass and its longitudinal and extraluminal extent, but it cannot assess the presence of mucosal or submucosal spread.

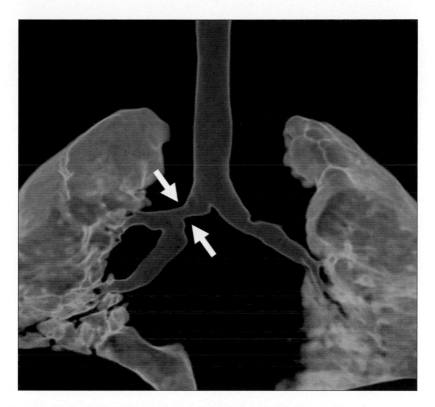

Fig. 14. Three-dimensional external volume rendered image of the large airway demonstrates right main stem bronchial stricture at the anastomosis site in a pediatric lung transplant patient. Also noted is less severe narrowing at the surgical anastomotic site in the left main stem bronchus.

8.3.1. Benign Tumors of the Airway

The CT appearance of a benign neoplasm is nonspecific, but generally benign lesions are relatively small, well circumscribed, smooth, and of soft tissue attenuation *(47)*. Benign lesions do not show extraluminal growth.

The most common benign tumors are papillomas and hemangiomas *(47)*. Papillomas of the respiratory tract in children are usually caused by human papillomavirus, usually types 6 and 11 *(48)*. The average onset of juvenile onset respiratory papillomatosis is approximately 4 years with 75% of cases diagnosed by 5 years of age *(49)*. The larynx, particularly the glottis, is affected in virtually all cases. Distal extension to the trachea and lung can occur, affecting approximately 17 and 5% of patients, respectively *(48)*. Although this is a benign lesion, it is difficult to treat because it tends to recur locally and spread throughout the respiratory tract. Laser bronchoscopy is used most often for tumor debulking. CT demonstrates intrauminal polypoid masses and may show lung lesions (Fig. 15) *(47)*. Lung lesions may appear as nodules, air-filled cysts, or thick-walled cavities (Fig. 16). Although rare, malignant transformation in chronic invasive papillomatosis has also been reported *(50)*.

Hemangiomas arise from mesodermal rests. Although airway hemangiomas are present at birth, symptoms usually develop between 1 and 6 months of age *(47,48)*. Classically, lesions occur in the subglottic region. In rare instances, hemangiomas have been reported to extend into the upper part of the trachea. Laser treatment has been used in symptomatic patients. On CT, hemangiomas appear as rounded soft tissue masses. There is marked contrast enhancement (Fig. 17).

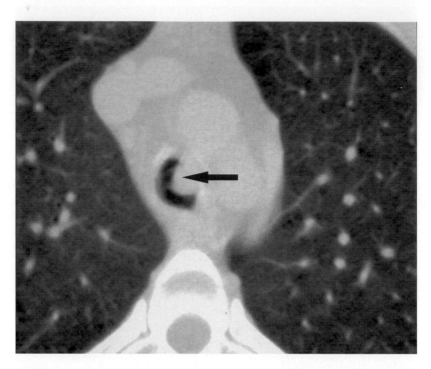

Fig. 15. Axial CT image shows the left-sided polypoid tracheal mass (arrow) which was found to be papilloma confirmed by biopsy in a pediatric patient who presented with progressive stridor and wheezing. Reprinted with permission from Siegal MJ, Coley B. Mediastinum In: Core Curriculum. Lippincott Williams & Wilkins. Philadelphia 2006, page 51.

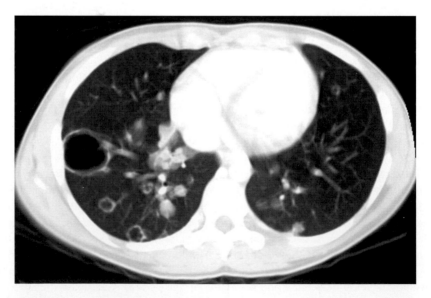

Fig. 16. Axial CT image demonstrates a combination of cavitary and non-cavitary nodules in the bilateral lower lobes in a pediatric patient with known papillomatosis.

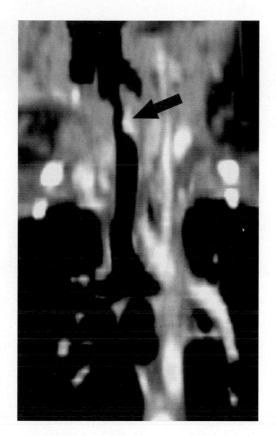

Fig. 17. Coronal multiplanar reformation (MPR) CT image shows subglottic hemangioma (arrow) with a marked contrast enhancement. Location, extension, and degree of airway narrowing are well visualized on coronal MPR CT image. Reprinted with permission from the Journal of Thoracic Imaging Aug; 22(3); 300–309.

Neurofibroma, fibrous histiocytoma, and chondroma are examples of other extremely rare airway tumors in children *(48)*. Local resection or laser therapy is the methods of treatment. On CT, these tumors appear as pedunculated or sessile soft tissue masses. Chondromas may contain calcifications.

8.3.2. Malignant Tumors of the Airways

Although extremely rare in pediatric patients, malignant tumors include malignant fibrous histiocytoma, mucoepidermoid carcinoma, adenoid cystic carcinoma (cylindroma), and rhabdomyosarcoma. Surgical resection is the mode of treatment *(48)*.

Malignant tumors are relatively large masses. They may be smooth or irregular and sessile or pedunculated. Malignant tumors may breech the tracheal wall. CT differentiation between malignant and benign neoplasms is not possible unless the tumor extends beyond the tracheal wall.

8.3.3. Mucus Plugs

Mucus plugs are a diagnostic pitfall, because they can mimic a tracheal or bronchial tumor (Fig. 18). They appear as intraluminal soft-tissue masses mixed with air and will change location or resolve after the patient coughs to clear secretions.

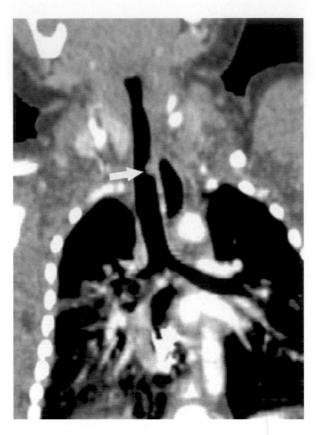

Fig. 18. Coronal multiplanar reformation image demonstrates small low attenuation lesion within the trachea (arrow). The absence of luminal mass on subsequent MRI supported the diagnosis of a mucus plug. Consolidation and atelectatic lung changes in the right lower lobe are also noted.

8.4. Secondary Airway Tumors

The trachea and main bronchi may be secondarily narrowed by mediastinal masses, usually as a result of extrinsic compression or less often by direct invasion. Foregut cysts (i.e., esophageal or bronchogenic duplication cysts) and lymphangiomas are the common non-neoplastic mediastinal masses that can locate close to the central airways with resultant airway compression in pediatric patients. The common tumors of the mediastinum are lymphoma and teratoma (Fig. 19). Metastatic disease in the mediastinum can also result in central airway narrowing (Fig. 20). Hematogenous metastases to the trachea from distant tumors are extremely rare in children.

8.5. Infection

8.5.1. Tuberculosis

Airway involvement by tuberculosis can be caused by direct infection of tubercle bacilli in the tracheobronchial wall or by extension or extrinsic compression from adjacent infected mediastinal lymph nodes (Fig. 21). Histologic findings in early infection show lymphocytic infiltration, ulceration, and caseous necrosis of the airway wall with luminal narrowing *(51,52,53)*. The late sequelae of infection are fibrosis and luminal stenosis. Tuberculous infection typically involves the distal

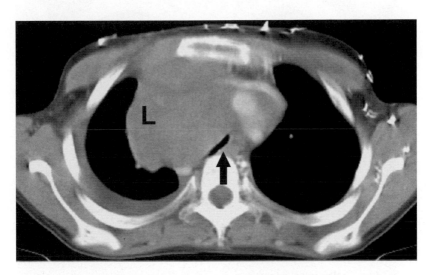

Fig. 19. Axial CT image showing a large anterior mediastinal lymphoma (L) resulting in marked tracheal compression (arrow). Also noted is the prominent anterior chest wall collateral vessel formation from the superior vena cava syndrome.

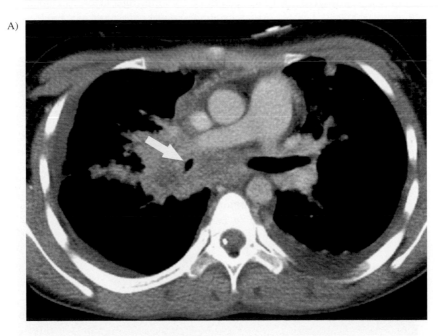

Fig. 20. *(Continued)*

B)

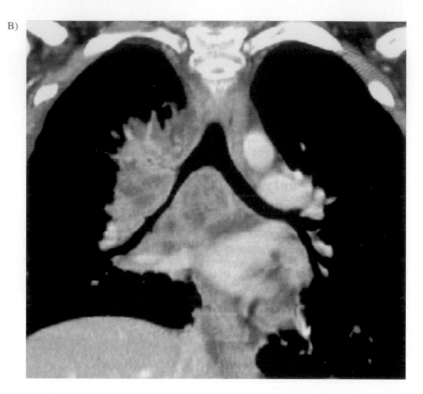

Fig. 20. (A) Axial CT image showing metastatic lung cancer in the mediastinum resulting in right main stem bronchial narrowing (arrow). **(B)** The degree and extension of the right main stem bronchial narrowing is better visualized using a coronal CT image. Also seen are obstructed right upper lobe bronchus and narrowing of bronchus intermedius.

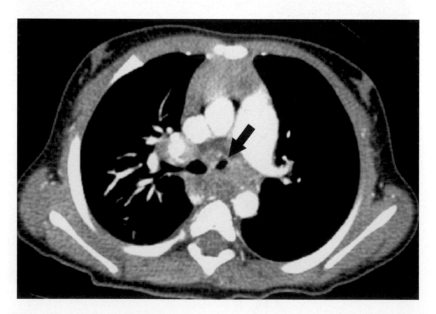

Fig. 21. Axial CT image showing left main stem bronchial narrowing (arrow) from mediastinal lymphadenopathy in a pediatric patient with TB.

trachea and proximal main bronchi. Cough with sputum production are the common presenting symptoms.

In the acute stage of infection, CT shows thickened tracheobronchial walls and airway narrowing (Fig. 22). Wall thickening may be irregular or less commonly smooth and may enhance after administration of intravenous contrast medium. Rim enhancement of adjacent lymph nodes also may be noted. In chronic inactive disease, the CT findings are also tracheobronchial narrowing with wall thickening, but the wall thickening is often smooth. The airway walls and adjacent mediastinal structures no longer enhance. Tuberculosis often involves the left more than the right main bronchus, likely because of its greater length. Areas of calcification can be present in late-stage fibrotic disease. With appropriate treatment, the findings of active disease are often reversible.

8.5.2. Fibrosing Mediastinitis

Fibrosing mediastinitis is a disorder in which exuberant proliferation of dense fibrous tissue encases and compresses mediastinal structures *(54)*. Most cases in children in the USA are caused by *Histoplasma capsulatum*. The fibrotic process is thought to represent a rare hypersensitivity response either to Histoplasma organisms or to an antigen in the lymph nodes rather than a primary infection. There are two types of fibrosing mediastinitis: focal and diffuse. The focal type appears on CT as a localized, calcified mass in the paratracheal or subcarinal areas or in the pulmonary hila. The diffuse form manifests as a diffusely infiltrating soft tissue mass in the paratracheal, hilar, and/or subcarinal regions that encases and narrows the central airways, vessels (superior vena cava and pulmonary arteries and veins), and esophagus (Fig. 23) *(54)*. Calcifications within the soft tissue masses are common. Atelectasis or pneumonitis, attributed to bronchial narrowing or occlusion, tracheoesophageal fistulas, and broncholiths also may occur. Pulmonary venous obstruction can result in parenchymal infarction. In addition to histoplasmosis, other causes of fibrosing mediastinitis include aspergillosis, mucormycosis, blastomycosis, cryptococcosis, Behcet disease, and methysergide maleate use *(54)*.

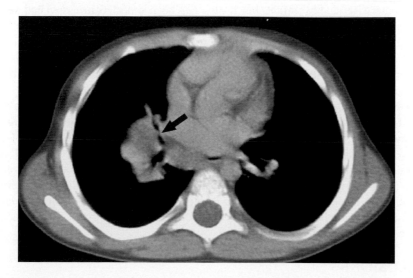

Fig. 22. Right middle lobe bronchial narrowing (arrow) on axial CT image in a pediatric patient with acute stage of TB infection.

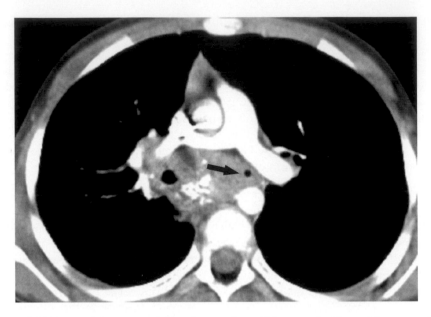

Fig. 23. Axial CT image demonstrates left main stem bronchial narrowing (arrow) because of mediastinal lymphadenopathy. Also noted is the associated calcification.

9. TRACHEOMALACIA AND BRONCHOMALACIA

Tracheomalacia refers to softness of the trachea, usually because of deficient integrity of the supporting cartilages or to atrophy of the longitudinal elastic fibers of the pars membranacea. The resultant effect is weakness of the tracheal walls, which leads to excessive collapse of the airway *(55)*. The term bronchomalacia refers to weakness and exaggerated collapse of one or both main bronchi (Fig. 24).

Tracheomalacia can be congenital or acquired. Congenital or primary tracheomalacia can be isolated in an otherwise healthy infant, but it also has been reported in associated with congenital tracheoesophageal fistula and the mucopolysaccharidoses, such as Hurler and Hunter syndromes *(55)*. Acquired or secondary causes include prior endotracheal intubation, tracheotomy, extrinsic compression from vascular rings, trauma, infection, and surgery. Symptoms and signs usually occur at birth or in the first few weeks of life. The common symptoms include stridor, barking cough, wheezing, cyanosis, and recurrent pulmonary infection.

The hallmark for the diagnosis of tracheobronchomalacia is a greater than 50% reduction in the cross-sectional luminal area of the trachea on expiration. Radiographs, including inspiratory and expiratory views, have been used to diagnose tracheomalacia, but the sensitivity of plain radiography is only 62%, compared with the reference standard of bronchoscopy *(56)*. CT in inspiratory and expiratory phases with sagittal 2-D images along the axis of the trachea have been shown to be helpful in displaying the presence and craniocaudal extent of exaggerated airway collapse associated with tracheomalacia *(57,58,59,60)*. It is important to note that CT scanning during dynamic forced exhalation may be more sensitive for detecting tracheomalacia than CT scans acquired during conventional end-expiration *(58,59)*.

10. CONCLUSIONS

With the rapid advances in CT technology in recent years, CT has assumed a greater role in the evaluation of various pediatric large airway disorders. In particular, multislice CT can produce isotropic, high-resolution images as well as high-quality multiplanar and 3-D images with faster

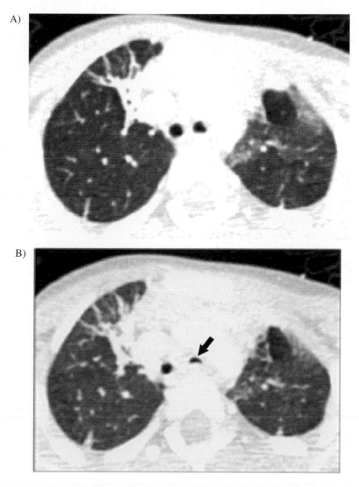

Fig. 24. (**A**) Axial CT image during inspiration demonstrates patent bilateral main stem bronchi. (**B**) Axial CT image during expiration shows more than 50% collapse of the left main stem bronchus (arrow), whereas the right main stem bronchus is still patent. Subsequently performed bronchoscopy confirmed left main stem bronchomalacia. Also noted are postoperative changes from a left upper lobe congenital lobar emphysema surgical resection.

scan times. The advantages of multislice CT are especially helpful in evaluating the large airways in children because they improve the display of airway stenosis, the assessment of the craniocaudal extent of disease, the evaluation of complex airway disorders, as well as the communication between radiologists and clinicians.

REFERENCES

1. Siegel MJ. Techniques. In: Siegel MJ (ed.), *Pediatric Body CT*. Philadelphia: Lippincott Williams & Wilkins, 1999:1–41.
2. Siegel MJ. Pediatric chest applications. In: Fishman EK, Jeffrey B (eds), *Multislice Helical CT*, 3rd ed. Philadelphia: Lippincott Williams & Wilkins, 2003:159–182.
3. Kaste SC, Young CW, Holmes TP, Baker DK. Effect of helical CT on the frequency of sedation in pediatric patients. *AJR* 1997;168:1001–1003.
4. Pappas JN, Donnelly LF, Frush DP. Reduced frequency of sedation of young children using new multi-slice helical CT. *Radiology* 2000;215:897–899.
5. Frush DP, Bisset GS III, Hall SC. Pediatric sedation in radiology: the practice of safe sleep. *AJR* 1996;167(6):1381–1387.

6. Committee on Drugs, American Academy of Pediatrics: guidelines for monitoring and management of pediatric patients during and after sedation for diagnostic and therapeutic procedures. *Pediatrics* 1992;89:1110–1115.
7. American Society of Anesthesiologists Task Force. Practice guidelines for sedation and analgesia by non-anesthesiologist: a report by the American Society of Anesthesiologists Task Force on sedation and analgesia by non-anesthesiologists. *Anesthesiology* 1996;84:459–471.
8. Kaste SC, Young CW. Safe use of power injectors with central and peripheral venous access devices for pediatric CT. *Pediatr Radiol* 1995;26:499–501.
9. Donnelly LF, Emery KH, Brody AS, et al. Minimizing radiation dose for pediatric body applications for single-detector helical CT: strategies at a large children's hospital. *AJR* 2001;176:303–306.
10. Haaga JR. Commentary. Radiation dose management weighing risk versus benefit. *AJR* 2001;177:289–291.
11. Patterson A, Frush DP, Donnelly L. Helical CT of the body: are setting adjusted for pediatric patients. *AJR* 2001;176: 297–301.
12. Slovis TL. The ALARA concept in pediatric CT: myth or reality. *Radiology* 2002;223:5–6.
13. Siegel MJ, Suess C, Schmidt B, Bradley D, Hildebolt C. Radiation dose and image quality in pediatric CT: effect of technical factors and phantom size and shape. *Radiology* 2004;233:515–522.
14. Calhoun PS, Kuszyk B, Heath DG, Carley JC, Fishman EK. Three-dimensional volume rendering of spiral CT data: theory and method. *RadioGraphics* 1999;19:745–764.
15. Cody DD. Image processing in CT. *RadioGraphics* 2002;2:1255–1268.
16. Boiselle PM, Lee KS, Ernst A. Multidetector CT of the central airways. *J Thorac Imaging* 2005;20:186–195.
17. Konen E, Katz M, Rozenman J, Ben-Shlush A, Itzchak Y, Szeinberg A. Virtual bronchoscopy in children: early clinical experience. *AJR* 1998;172:1699–1702.
18. Siegel MJ. Multiplanar and three-dimensional row CT of thoracic vessels and airways in the pediatric population. *Radiology* 2003;229: 641–650.
19. Lam WW, Tam PK, Chan F-L, Chan K-L, Cheung W. Esophageal atresia and tracheal stenosis: use of three-dimensional CT and virtual bronchoscopy in neonates, infants, and children. *AJR* 2000;174:1009–1012.
20. Lee KS, Lunn W, Feller-Kopman D, Ernst A, Hatabu H, Boiselle PM. Multislice CT evaluation of airway stents. *J Thorac Imaging* 2005;20:81–88.
21. Sorantin E, Geiger B, Lindbichler F, Eber E, Schimpi G. CT-based virtual tracheobronchoscopy in children—comparison with axial CT and multiplanar reconstruction: preliminary results. *Pediatr Radiol* 2002;32(1):8–15.
22. Bennett EC, Holinger LD. Congenital malformations of the trachea and bronchi. In: Bluestone CD, Stool SES, Alper CM, et al. (eds), *Pediatric Otolaryngology*, 4th ed. Philadelphia: Saunders, 2002:1473–1483.
23. Ghaye B, Szapiro D, Fanchamps J-M, Dondelinger RF. Congenital bronchial abnormalities revisited. *Radiographics* 2001;21:105–119.
24. Wu JW, White CS, Meyer CA, Haramati LB, Mason AC. Variant bronchial anatomy: CT appearance and classification. *AJR* 1999;172:741–744.
25. Ghaye B, Kos X, Dondelinger RF. Accessory cardiac bronchus: 3D demonstration in nine cases. *Eur Radiol* 1999;9: 45–48.
26. McGuiness G, Naidich D, Garay S, Davis AL, Boyd AD, Mizrachi HH. Accessory cardiac bronchus: CT features and clinical significance. *Radiology* 1993;189:563–566.
27. Daltro P, Fricke BL, Kuroki L, Domingues R, Donnelly LF. CT of congenital lung lesions in pediatric patients. *AJR* 2004;183:1497–1506.
28. Woodring JH, Howard TA, Kanga JF. Congenital pulmonary venolobar syndrome revisited. *RadioGraphics* 1994;14: 349–369.
29. Webb WR. The trachea. In: Webb WR, Higgins CB (eds), *Thoracic Imaging*, 1st ed. Philadelphia: Lippincott Williams & Wilkins, 2005: 511–526.
30. Dunham ME, Holinger LD, Becker CL, et al. Management of severe congenital tracheal stenosis. *Ann Otol Rhinol Laryngol* 1994;103(5 Pt 1):351–356.
31. Anton-Pacheoc JL, Cano I, Garcia A, et al. Patterns of management of congenital tracheal stenosis. *J Pediatr Surg* 2003;38(10):1452–1458.
32. Rutter MJ, Willging JP, Cotton RT. Nonoperative management of complete tracheal rings. *Arch Otolaryngol Head Neck Surg* 2004;130:450–452.
33. McLaughlin RB, Wetmore RF, Tavill MA, et al. Vascular anomalies causing symptomatic tracheobronchial compression. *Laryngoscope* 1999;109(2 Pt 1):312–319.
34. Hopkins KL, Patrick LE, Simoneaux SF, et al. Pediatric great vessel anomalies: initial clinical experience with spiral CT angiography. *Radiology* 1996;200:811–815.
35. Katz M, Konen E, Rozenman J, et al. Spiral CT and 3D image reconstruction of vascular rings and associated tracheobronchial anomalies. *J Comput Assist Tomogr* 1995;19:564–568.
36. Lee EY, Siegel MJ, Hildebolt CF, Gutierrez FR, Bhalla S, Fallah JH. MDCT evaluation of thoracic aortic anomalies in pediatric patients and young adults: comparison of axial, multiplanar and 3D images. *AJR* 2004;182:777–784.

37. Remy-Jardin M, Remy J, Mayo JR, Muller NL. Thoracic aorta. In: *CT Angiography of the Chest*. Philadelphia: Lippincott Williams & Wilkins, 2001:29–50.
38. Chan MSM, Chu WCW, Cheung KL, Arifi AA, Lam WWM. Angiography and dynamic airway evaluation with MDCT in the diagnosis of double aortic arch associated with tracheomalacia. *AJR* 2005;185:1248–1251.
39. Adler SC, Isaacson G, Balsara RK. Innominate artery compression of the trachea: diagnosis and treatment by anterior suspension. A 25-year experience. *Ann Otol Rhino Laryngol* 1995;104(12):924–927.
40. Berdon WE: Rings, slings, and other things: vascular compression of the infant trachea updated from the mid-century to the millennium – the legacy of Robert E. Gross, MD, and Edward B.D. Neuhauser, MD. *Radiology* 2000;216:624–632.
41. Newman B, Meza MP, Tobin RB, Del Nido P. Left pulmonary artery sling diagnosis and delineation of associated tracheobronchial anomalies with MR. *Pediatr Radiol* 1996;26:661–668.
42. Fiore AC, Brown JW, Weber TR, Turrentine MW. Surgical treatment of pulmonary artery sling and tracheal stenosis. *Ann Thorac Surg* 2005;79(1):38–46.
43. Zwischenberger JB, Sankar AB. Surgery of the thoracic trachea. *J Thorac Imaging* 195;10:199–205.
44. Lesperance MM, Zalzal GH. Assessment and management of laryngotracheal stenosis. *Pediatr Clin North Am* 1996;43(6):1413–1427.
45. McAdams HP, Palmer SM, Erasmus JJ, et al. Bronchial anastomotic complications in lung transplant recipients: virtual bronchoscopy for noninvasive assessment. *Radiology* 1998;209:689–695.
46. Medina LS, Siegel MJ, Glazer HS, Anderson DJ, Seminkovitch J, Bejarano PA, Mallory GB. Diagnosis of pulmonary complications associated with lung transplantation in children: value of CT vs histopathologic studies. *AJR* 1994;162. 969–974.
47. McCarthy MJ, Rosado-de-Christenson ML. Tumors of the trachea. *J Thorac Imaging* 1995;10:180–198.
48. Pransky SM, Kang DR. Tumors of the larynx, trachea, and bronchi. In: Bluestone CD, Stool SES, Alper CM, et al. (eds), *Pediatric Otolaryngology*, 4th ed. Philadelphia: Saunders, 2002:1558–1572.
49. Benjamin B, Parsons DS. Recurrent respiratory papillomatosis. *J Laryngol Otol* 1988;102(11):1022–1028.
50. Solomon D, Smith RRL, Kashima HK, Leventhal BG. Malignant transformation in non-irradiated recurrent respiratory papillomatosis. *Laryngoscope* 1985;95:900.
51. Kim Y, Lee KS, Yoon JH, et al. Tuberculosis of the trachea and main bronchi: CT findings in 17 patients. *AJR* 1997;168:1051–1056.
52. Lee JH, Park SS, Lee DH, Shin DH, Yang SC, Yoo BM. Endobronchial tuberculosis. Clinical and bronchoscopic features in 121 cases. *Chest* 1992;102:990–994.
53. Moon WK, Im J-G, Yeon, KM, Han MC. Tuberculosis of the central airways: CT findings of active and fibrotic disease. AJR *1997*;169:649–653.
54. Rossi SE, McAdams HP, Rosado-de-Christenson ML, Franks TJ, Galvin JR. Fibrosing mediastinitis. *Radiographics* 2001;21:737–757.
55. Cardin K, Boiselle PM, Walz D, Ernst A. Tracheomalacia and tracheobronchomalacia in children and adults: an in-depth review of a common disorder. *Chest* 2005;127:984–1005.
56. Walner DL, Ouanounou S, Donnelly LF, et al. Utility of radiographs in the evaluation of pediatric upper airway obstruction. *Ann Otol Rhinol Larhyngol* 1999;108:378–383.
57. Frey EE, Smith WL, Grandgeorge S, et al. Chronic airway obstruction in children: evaluation with cine CT. *AJR* 1987;148:347–352.
58. Baroni RH, Feller-Kopman D, Nishino M, et al. Tracheobronchomalacia: methods for evaluation of central airway collapse. *Radiology* 2005;635–641.
59. Boiselle PM, Feller-Kopman D, Ashiku S, et al. Tracheobronchomalacia. Evolving role of dynamic multislice helical CT. *Radiol Clin North Am* 2003;41:626–636.
60. Gilkeson RC, Ciancibello LM, Hejal RB, Montenegro HD, Lange P. Tracheobronchomalacia dynamic airway evaluation with multidetector CT. *AJR* 2001;176:205–210.

16

Computed Tomography of Pediatric Small Airways Disease

Alan S. Brody

Summary

Imaging small airways disease in children differs from imaging adults. The lungs are morphologically different with smaller peripheral airways and thicker airway walls. Lung development continues after birth with new alveoli developing until 3–6 years of age. Imaging techniques need to be optimized for smaller patients who often cannot follow instructions. High-resolution CT is the imaging modality of choice, and expiratory images are very important in identifying the air trapping that characterized many of the pediatric small airways diseases. Children are more radiation sensitive than adults, and radiation dose is an important consideration when determining CT technique. Pediatric small airways disease includes a broad range of disorders. Asthma and acute bronchiolitis are common pediatric diseases that rarely require imaging other than chest radiographs. Bronchiolitis obliterans (BO) and neuroendocrine cell hyperplasia of infancy (NEHI) are best evaluated with HRCT and have imaging appearances that strongly suggest the specific diagnosis. In follicular bronchiolitis, there are less data available in children than in adults, and the imaging appearance is less well characterized. Many of the diseases seen in children are also seen in adults, but the appearance may differ. BO organizing pneumonia has a nodular appearance more often in children than in adults. NEHI is only seen in the pediatric population. Optimizing the examination for children and familiarity with the disorders that affect children allows the best imaging care in pediatric small airways disease.

Key Words: High-resolution computed tomography; children; diagnostic imaging; airway obstruction; air trapping; bronchiolitis obliterans; follicular bronchiolitis; neuroendocrine cell hyperplasia of infancy.

1. ANATOMY AND DEVELOPMENT

In children as in adults the small airways are defined as airways less than 2 mm in diameter. Anatomically, these are distal bronchi. The transition from bronchi that contain cartilage and mucous glands to bronchioles that do not occurs with an airway diameter of about 1 mm (1). Terminal bronchioles are the most distal purely conducting airways: they branch into respiratory bronchioles from which the alveoli and alveolar ducts extend directly. Smooth muscle is seen in the wall of all airways and provides support for airways without cartilage.

The lung continues its growth and development throughout childhood and into early adulthood. In infants and young children, peripheral airway resistance is a larger component of overall airway resistance than in older children and adults. The airway walls are thicker in young children at each airway generation. The peripheral airways are smaller in young children (2). New alveoli continue to develop until between 3 and 6 years of age. After the age of 6, alveoli increase in size but do not increase in number (3). The size of the bronchioles remains stable from age 6 as well, supporting the use of the same size criteria for small airways in children and adults.

From: *Contemporary Medical Imaging: CT of the Airways*
Edited by: P. M. Boiselle and D. A. Lynch © Humana Press, Totowa, NJ

The classification of disease processes into those primarily affecting the small airways, the large airways, or the lung parenchyma provides a framework for approaching these processes, but it is important to recognize that rarely if ever is only one of these anatomic areas involved. The diseases discussed in this chapter are included because they have a major effect on the small airways. In children, smoking-associated diseases are much less common and will not be discussed in this chapter. Diseases primarily affecting the bronchioles or small airways in children include acute bronchiolitis, constrictive or obliterative bronchiolitis (OB), follicular bronchiolitis (FB), neuroendocrine cell hyperplasia of infancy (NEHI), bronchiolitis obliterans organizing pneumonia (BOOP), and hypersensitivity pneumonitis (HP).

2. IMAGING OVERVIEW

Airways in the range of 1–2 mm are the smallest that can be seen with CT *(4)*, so changes in the small airways are not usually seen directly. Air trapping, best seen on expiratory images, is the most common finding in small airways disease and is the predominant finding in OB. In FB and NEHI, ground-glass opacity predominates, likely because of the peribronchiolar lymphocytic infiltration in FB, whereas in NEHI, the etiology of the ground-glass opacity is less clear. In acute bronchiolitis, there is lower airway inflammation that predominantly affects but is not limited to the bronchioles, so the imaging appearance includes air trapping, atelectasis, and consolidation.

In children, as in adults, areas of air trapping can be seen as a normal finding. In adults, areas of expiratory air trapping have been reported in as many as 64% of normal subjects *(5)*. These are usually small, although one study found segmental or larger areas of air trapping in 14% of normal adults *(6)*. Air trapping in normal children is also common; in our experience, subsegmental air trapping in a subpleural location is the most common appearance (Fig. 1). At our center, a high-resolution CT (HRCT) with more than two or three such areas, or with areas segmental in size or larger would suggest abnormal air trapping rather than normal variation (Fig. 2).

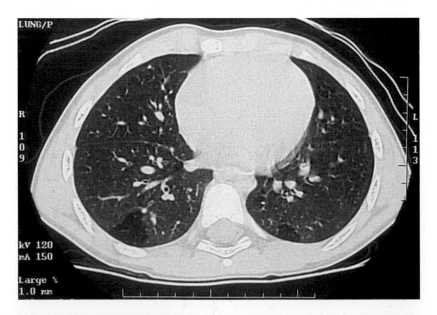

Fig. 1. Expiratory image demonstrates subsegmental air trapping in a posterior subpleural location bilaterally. In children and adults, small areas of air trapping are seen as a normal finding.

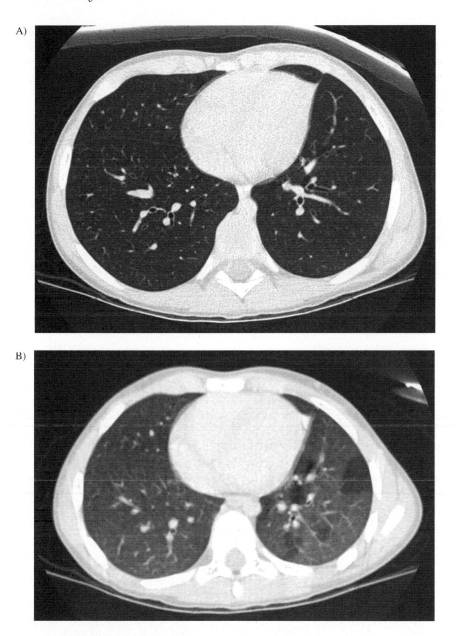

Fig. 2. Inspiratory (**A**) and expiratory (**B**) images in a 7-year-old girl with a history of prior left-sided pneumonia. The inspiratory scan appears almost normal, but on the expiratory image, multiple areas of subsegmental air trapping are seen in the left lower lobe. The number of areas and their unilateral distribution suggests abnormal air trapping, possibly because of obliterative bronchiolitis, rather than normal air trapping. These images show the need for expiratory images as these areas are very difficult to identify on the inspiratory images.

2.1. Technique

CT scanning requires the use of ionizing radiation and therefore carries the possibility of inducing cancer. The actual risk is unclear, but with a possible risk, the ALARA principle (As Low As Reasonably Achievable) should guide the choice of CT parameters. Guidelines for milliamperage (mA) and kilovoltage (kVp) settings have been published *(7–9)*. These guidelines take advantage of the fact that if technique remains constant, image noise decreases with decreasing patient size. Below a certain level, noise has little effect on image quality, so radiation dose can be decreased without degrading the quality of the CT image *(10,11)*. To use the lowest appropriate CT technique, mA settings must be adjusted for patient size. This adjustment can be on the basis of age, height, weight, or body diameter; with body diameter the parameter most directly affecting the relationship between technique and image noise *(12,13)*. Most guidelines adjust mA without adjusting kVp. Radiation dose varies linearly with mA and with the square of kVp, so changes in kVp have a relatively larger effect on radiation dose. Some authors have suggested that improved image contrast with decreasing kVp provides an image quality benefit that does not occur with a similar dose reduction produced by decreasing mA *(14,15)*. Beam hardening artifact has been reported at 80 kVp by some authors *(16)*, suggesting that 100 kVp is a reasonable lower limit except in very small children.

The radiation dose should not be reduced to a point where diagnostic accuracy is compromised. It is important to recognize that mA and kVp settings that produce adequate quality when all other factors are optimal may limit interpretation when other limitations are present. Streak artifact, which increases when kVp and mA are decreased, is also increased by patient motion. Both decreased lung volume and increased image noise limit evaluation of lung detail. For this reason, continuing evaluation of technique and image quality are necessary to insure adequate image quality and the lowest appropriate dose. Table 1 provides a starting point for the development of HRCT protocols for children. Differences in CT scanners, patient preparation, and the radiologist's preference will all require adjustment of these guidelines.

Non-contiguous acquisition using HRCT technique with intervals of 5 mm for younger children and 10 mm for older children provides an excellent sampling technique for diffuse lung disease and should be the primary technique for the evaluation of small airways disease. The areas of air trapping caused by small airways disease are large enough to be reliably detected using the HRCT interval technique. These thin sections are also optimal for identifying bronchiectasis or bronchial wall thickening that are often associated with small airways disease. At 10-mm intervals, there is a dose savings of up to 85% when compared with contiguous technique.

With current CT scanners, scan time is 0.5 s or less, and interscan delay is 1–2 s for HRCT. This acquisition speed has dramatically reduced patient motion and the need for sedation. The greatest challenge in imaging the child's lung with CT, particularly when the evaluation of air trapping is required, is obtaining images at full inflation and at end expiration. Children over the age of 5 or 6

Table 1
High-Resolution Chest CT Technique for Children (Inspiratory Images)

Weight (kg)	Mas	kVp	Slice interva
1–7.5	15–25	100	5
7.5–10	25–30	100	7.5
10–12.5	35	100	7.5
12.5–15	30	120	10
15– 20	35	120	10
20–25	40	120	10
25–35	45	120	10
35–50	50	120	10
50–70	60	120	10

Axial technique. Slice thickness = 1.25 mm. High-frequency reconstruction algorithm. Expiratory images: 2× inspiratory intervals or six equally spaced images apices to lung bases.

years can be taught the necessary breathing maneuvers, and high-quality CT scans can be obtained. This level of cooperation requires a child who is able to listen and follow directions. Coaching sessions before the actual CT scan are very helpful. During the scan, it is necessary for a "coach" to remain in the scanner room to encourage the child, ensure that the breathing instructions are followed, and coordinate the timing of scanning with the child's efforts. Children between 6 and 10 years will require varying degrees of support to cooperate with inspiratory and expiratory CT scanning. By the age of 12 years, the same instructions used for adults will work for most children.

In children who cannot cooperate with breathing instructions, three techniques have been suggested to obtain high-quality inspiratory and expiratory images. The first is decubitus CT scanning *(17)*. After an area of concern is identified on an initial supine CT scan, the patient is turned to a decubitus position, and limited images are repeated through the area. The non-dependent lung should increase in volume, whereas the dependent lung should decrease in volume and increase homogeneously in attenuation. Areas of air trapping are easily confirmed with this technique. An additional benefit is that respiratory motion is often decreased with this technique, particularly in the non-dependent lung. This technique has the important advantage that it can be performed in any patient stable enough to tolerate lying on the CT table (Fig. 3).

The second technique is controlled-ventilation CT (CVCT) *(18)*. This technique was developed for infant pulmonary function tests *(19)* and takes advantage of the Hering–Breuer reflex that causes sedated young children to become apneic following several deep breaths that lower CO_2 and stimulate chest stretch receptors. To perform this technique, a child is placed under sedation and a positive pressure system with a pop-off valve that limits inspiratory pressure to 25 cm of water is connected to a mask that is used to administer a series of deep breaths. Following these breaths, the child becomes

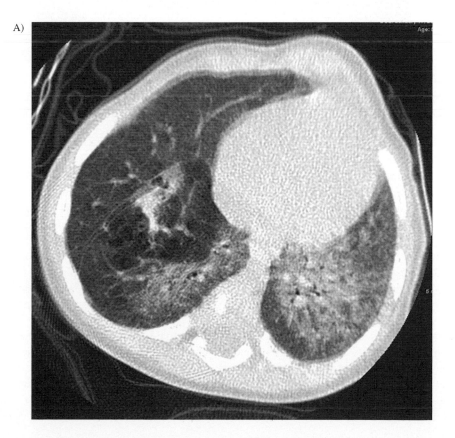

B)

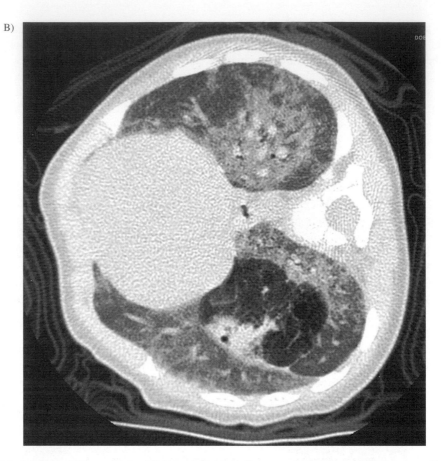

Fig. 3. This 5-month-old boy with familial interstitial lung disease and chronic aspiration was studied without sedation. The initial supine series (**A**) suggested focal air trapping on the right. The right decubitus series (**B**) confirmed the right-sided air trapping and better distinguished central left-sided opacity from dependent atelectasis.

apneic, and if continued positive pressure is administered, inspiratory images can be obtained during the apneic period. If no positive pressure is administered, elastic recoil of the lung allows expiratory images to be obtained. This technique has been safely used in thousands of infant pulmonary function tests. CVCT can be performed using a standard pediatric sedation program. The equipment used for CVCT is readily available in both reusable and disposable forms. A respiratory therapist or other health care professional must be available to perform the technique, and there is a learning curve as the breaths must be administered to assist the patient's own respiration. Owing to the relatively short apneic period, careful coordination with the CT technologist is necessary. Extremely high-quality images can be obtained using this technique on small children with rapid respiratory rates (Fig. 4).

The third method is general anesthesia (GA). The effective use of GA in a radiology department depends on the availability of personnel with anesthesia training. In addition, the necessary equipment and support personnel must be available. If this capability is available, there are a number of advantages of GA. GA provides complete control of breathing. This allows consistent motionless images at the desired lung volume. Skilled airway and ventilation management is immediately available. Recovery times are much shorter with GA than with sedation, allowing less need for

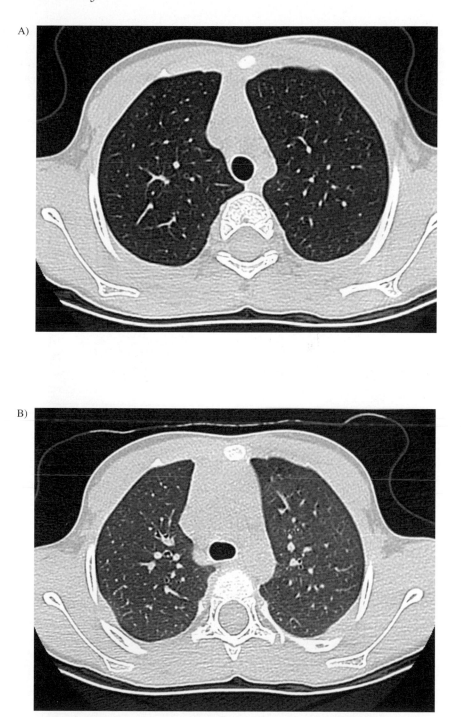

Fig. 4. Inspiratory (**A**) and expiratory (**B**) images, obtained using controlled ventilation technique in a 3-year-old child with a baseline respiratory rate of 70. The images are motion free with excellent parenchymal detail. No abnormality is seen on the inspiratory image. A small area of subsegmental air trapping is seen in the anterior left upper lobe.

recovery care and often a better experience for patients and families. The greatest imaging difficulty with GA is atelectasis. Atelectasis can be minimized by administering frequent deep sigh breaths as soon as induction and intubation are complete. Scanning should begin as soon as possible. We have found that in children atelectasis can suggest nodules or linear opacities as well as airspace opacity. If there is any question, prone images should be obtained (Fig. 5).

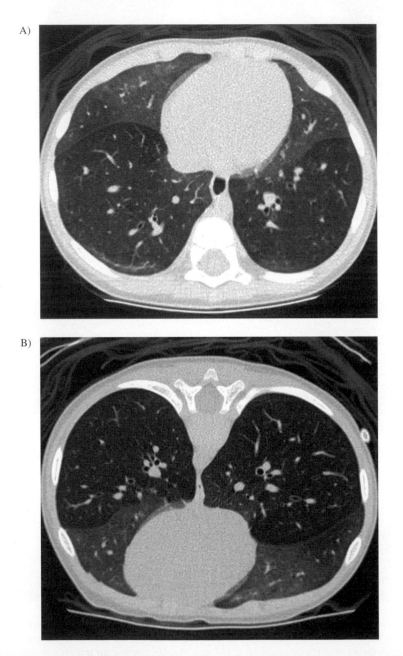

Fig. 5. Linear atelectasis that could be interpreted as fibrosis in a child with neuroendocrine cell hyperplasia of infancy. (**A**) Linear opacity seen in the posterior right lung on the initial supine images. (**B**) Opacity disappeared on prone images obtained after 5 min of deep breathing.

3. INHALATIONAL DISEASE

Inhalation of toxic fumes and particulate matter is associated with small airways disease in children. Air pollution is the most common inhalational insult to the lungs. Air pollution contains ozone and nitrogen dioxide gas as well as particulate matter. Pulmonary function tests have shown decreases in both forced expiratory volume in 1 s, which reflects the large airways, and midexpiratory flow, which reflects the small airways *(20)*. Chest radiography (CXRs) have shown significantly more hyperinflation and increased peribronchial markings when children in areas of high air pollution were compared to controls *(21)*. CT scans performed in 25 children with abnormal CXRs showed peribronchial thickening in 40%, air trapping in 32%, and prominent central airways in 16% *(22)*. Chlorine gas inhalation, most commonly seen because of accidents at swimming pools, is a cause of acute pneumonitis in children with long-term effects documented by restrictive changes on PFTs at 4 months. Both acute and chronic bronchiolar disease has been reported in exposure to sulfur mustard gas *(23)*.

4. ASTHMA

Asthma is a one of the most common pediatric chronic disorders. Asthma is an inherited disorder that requires genetic environment interaction *(24)*. Eosinophils are believed to be the primary inflammatory cells of the asthmatic airway, and 80% of children with asthma have allergies *(25)*. The "hygiene hypothesis" suggests that decreased exposure to childhood infections allows the allergic immunologic system to develop before the infection fighting immunologic system, resulting in an increased sensitivity to allergens *(26)*. Asthma can present at any time, but most patients are diagnosed by age 5 with up to half diagnosed by age 2 *(26)*. Although mortality is low, morbidity is very high. Asthma is the third leading cause of preventable hospitalization in the USA *(24)*. A 1992 study reported 200,000 hospitalizations per year in the USA for asthma *(27)*.

Asthma is characterized by partially or completely reversible airflow obstruction. Most children with asthma wheeze, although cough is common and may be the only symptom. Recurrent episodes of inflammation cause airway remodeling, which is felt to be an important part of the pathophysiology of asthma. Remodeling includes thickening of the basement membrane and airway wall with increased smooth muscle mass in the larger airways *(28)*. Asthma can affect both large and small airways. In some patients, the small airways are the sole or primary site of obstruction *(29)*.

The role of CT in the clinical care of asthma is limited. In severe disease, CT may be requested to exclude other disease processes or less commonly to evaluate complications of asthma. The differential diagnosis for wheezing is broad, and if wheezing is refractory or response to treatment is poor, CT scanning may be requested to evaluate possible etiologies including bronchogenic cysts, tracheal stenosis, vascular rings or slings, and occult aspirated foreign bodies. Because of these possibilities, conventional CT acquisition technique with contrast is recommended rather than high-resolution technique.

CT scanning has been used as a research tool to study the pathophysiology of asthma including the evaluation of airway remodeling *(30)*, bronchial reactivity *(31)*, and air trapping *(32)*. The small airway component of asthma has been quantitatively evaluated using HRCT by calculating the percentage of pixels below −856 HU and −910 HU on a single expiratory image. Both HU thresholds produced similar results. The pixel index correlated with plethysmography, eosinophilic cationic protein, and daytime albuterol use *(32)*.

5. ACUTE BRONCHIOLITIS

Acute bronchiolitis is a common childhood disease that is one of the most common causes of hospital admission in children under 1 year of age. Infants between 2 and 6 months of age are most commonly affected *(33)*. Approximately 2–3% of all infants under 1 year of age are admitted to the hospital with acute bronchiolitis *(34)*. Respiratory syncytial virus (RSV) is the most common cause, with other viruses including adenovirus, parainfluenza, enterovirus, and influenza viruses all less common causes of acute bronchiolitis *(35)*.

The pathologic changes identified in children who have died with bronchiolitis show acute inflammation of bronchioles 75–300 microns in diameter. Epithelial necrosis is followed by an inflammatory infiltrate, largely of lymphocytes. Mucous secretion in larger airways causes mucous plugging.

Children usually present with a several day viral prodrome followed by tachypnea, increased respiratory effort, and wheezing. Mild bronchiolitis is treated at home, whereas more severely ill children are hospitalized. The primary role of hospitalization is to support the infant. Antibiotics and bronchiodilators are ineffective *(34,36)*. The role of antiviral agents and corticosteroids remains unclear. Mortality is low in otherwise healthy children, approximately 1%. In children with other medical conditions, mortality is higher, with a 1982 study reporting a mortality of 37% for children with congenital heart disease *(37)*.

Chest radiographs are frequently obtained in children with bronchiolitis. Common findings include hyperinflation, peribronchial thickening, and areas of infiltrate or atelectasis that are frequently fleeting. Pleural fluid is rare. The chest radiographic findings do not correlate well with the clinical severity, as chest radiographs may be normal in children admitted to the hospital.

CT scanning is rarely performed in acute bronchiolitis but may be appropriate in individual cases for indications such as suspected bacterial superinfection and the differentiation of hyperexpanded lung from large pulmonary cysts. CT findings in such cases have included hyperinflation, air trapping, and areas of consolidation and ground-glass opacity. (Fig. 6)

A)

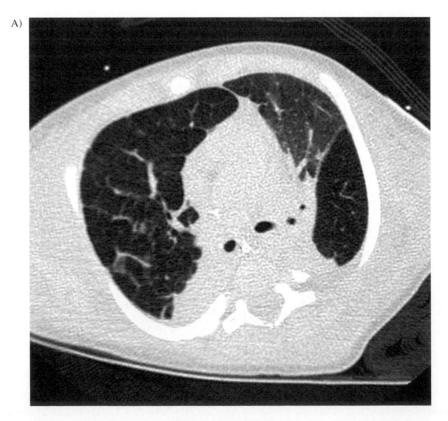

Fig. 6. *(Continued)*

B)

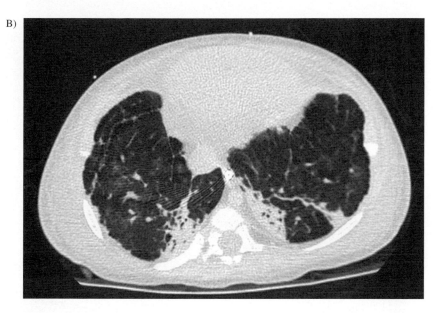

Fig. 6. Two different RSV-positive patients who required intubation and ICU care. (**A**) Inspiratory CT image at the mid-lung level shows mosaic attenuation, linear opacities, and bibasilar consolidation in a 3-month-old girl who presented with acute bronchiolitis. (**B**) CT image at the lung base in a 4-month-old boy with sudden respiratory deterioration shows patchy ground-glass opacity and bibasilar areas of volume loss with air bronchograms.

6. BRONCHIOLITIS OBLITERANS

Bronchiolitis obliterans (BO) can occur secondary to a number of pulmonary insults including infection, drugs, allergic reactions, collagen vascular disease *(38–40)*, exposure to inhaled toxins *(41)*, and organ transplantation. Infection and organ transplantation are the most common etiologies in children.

The term Swyer–James or Swyer–James–McLeod syndrome is frequently used to describe BO in children, particularly where involvement is unilateral. In 1952, Swyer and James reported a case of unilateral pulmonary emphysema in a 6-year-old boy. The right lung was hyperlucent compared with the left, despite shift of the lung to the right. Bronchography showed bronchiectasis and angiography showed decreased blood flow to the right lung. The affected lung was resected and showed emphysematous alveoli, cystic changes, dilated bronchi and bronchioles, and chronic inflammatory changes. Obliteration of peripheral capillaries, but not bronchioles, was described. In 1954, MacLeod presented the clinical and radiographic findings of nine patients 18–41 years old with unilateral hyperlucent lung. He described decreased breath sounds and lung markings in addition to increased lucency of the affected lung. He distinguished these cases from unilateral emphysema by a normal size of the affected lung. He described the bronchial tree as "almost normal" on bronchography *(42)*.

Continued experience and the use of CT scanning have shown that Swyer–James syndrome is one of the various possible appearances of post-infectious BO (Figs 7 and 8). In a study of 13 children with a diagnosis of Swyer–James syndrome in whom CT was performed, nine had bronchiectasis and six who had unilateral disease on CXR were shown to have bilateral disease on CT scanning *(43)*. As would be expected, children with saccular bronchiectasis had more infections than children with cylindrical or no bronchiectasis.

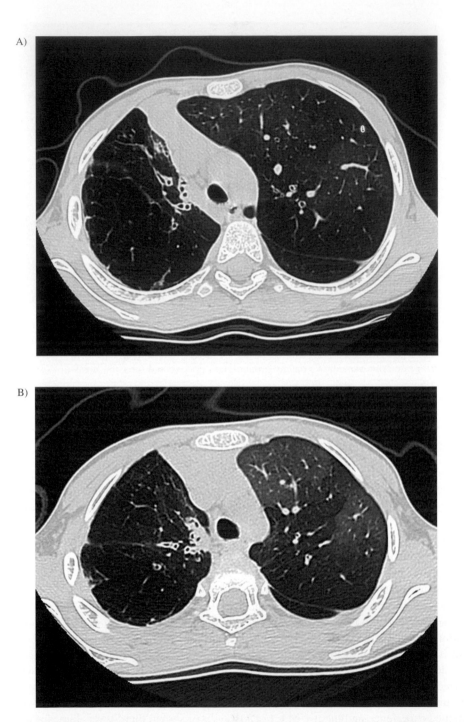

Fig. 7. Post-infectious bronchiolitis obliterans in a 7-year-old boy with chronic respiratory symptoms. (**A**) Inspiratory CT image through the upper lungs shows large bilateral areas of decreased attenuation with attenuated vessels. Bronchiectasis is seen bilaterally. (**B**) Expiratory image shows an increase in attenuation in the area of higher attenuation with no change in the areas of decreased attenuation confirming the expected air trapping in the low attenuation areas.

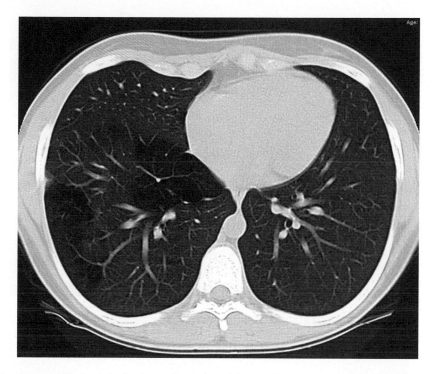

Fig. 8. Inspiratory CT through the lower lungs in a 15-year-old girl shows segmental areas of decreased attenuation with attenuated vessels consistent with post-infectious bronchiolitis obliterans.

Post-infectious BO can occur following multiple infectious agents with adenovirus the most common. In a case control study of 109 cases of BO in children under 3 years of age, bronchiolitis caused by adenovirus and the need for mechanical ventilation were independently and strongly associated with the development of OB *(44)*. In a 5-year follow-up study of 45 hospitalized infants with adenoviral pneumonia, 38 were alive at 5 years. Almost half developed CT evidence of BO. Those children with more severe illness were more likely to develop BO *(45)*. Other agents include RSV, measles, varicella, mycoplasma *(46,47)*, and pertussis *(48)*. In a report of 20 cases, gastroesophageal reflux was diagnosed in 12 *(46)*, suggesting that either a combination of insults or an increased susceptibility to damage from aspiration following the initial infection may contribute to the development of BO.

Multiple causes other than BO can produce a unilateral lucent lung. In children, these include aspirated foreign body, pulmonary sling, bronchogenic cyst or other cause of extrinsic bronchial compression, and Poland syndrome (unilaterally absent pectoralis muscle).

Post-transplant BO (PTBO) is a well-described complication of organ transplantation, particularly allogeneic lung and bone marrow transplantation (Fig. 9). PTBO develops in approximately 50% of patients following lung transplantation and is responsible for more than 40% of deaths occurring more than 1 year after transplant *(49)*. Pathologically, PTBO appears to develop through a series of steps *(50)*. The initial stage of the development of PTBO is believed to be a lymphocyte infiltration of the submucosa, followed by migration through the basement membrane of the airways into the respiratory mucosa. Epithelial necrosis follows, with development of exudates, and proliferation of fibroblasts and other cells forming intraluminal polypoid masses of granulation tissue. This granulation tissue can either re-epithelialize and be incorporated into the airway wall or can develop into dense scar tissue that narrows the airway causing obstructive lung disease and may progress to obliteration of

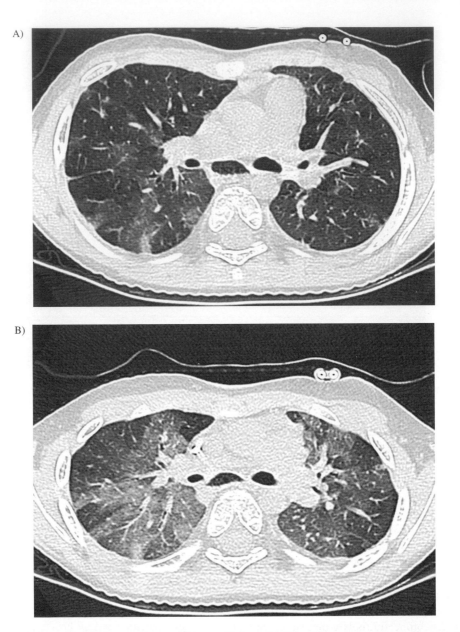

Fig. 9. CT images obtained on a 7-year-old boy with bronchiolitis obliterans on biopsy 3 years after lung transplantation. (**A**) Inspiratory image shows mosaic attenuation more marked in the right lung. Esophageal dilation is secondary to positive pressure administered by mask for controlled ventilation CT. (**B**) Expiratory image shows multiple areas of peripheral air trapping.

the airway lumen. Chronic rejection is believed to be the etiology of lung transplant-related BO *(51)*. Recurrent episodes of acute cellular rejection are risk factors for the development of PTBO *(52)*. The onset of PTBO following acute rejection episodes is more rapid than that following chronic rejection, suggesting that more than one mechanism may lead to PTBO. Gastroesophageal reflux is an additional risk factor *(53)*.

The diagnosis of PTBO is made pathologically, and this can be a difficult diagnosis. Transbronchial biopsy is routinely performed following lung transplant, but because of sampling error, transbronchial biopsy is an insensitive means of diagnosing BO. Owing to the patchy involvement often seen in PTBO, even open-lung biopsy may not be able to make the diagnosis. For these reasons, the diagnosis of BO syndrome (BOS) is usually made on clinical grounds, based on otherwise unexplained development of obstructive changes in pulmonary function (54). A decrease of 20% in FEV1 is strongly suspicious for PTBO. In children, it has been noted that because of continuing growth, changes in FEV1 should be based on normative data rather than the absolute change in volume (55). The onset of PTBO is usually gradual. Transplant recipients often have limited physical activity, so that limited exercise capability is not identified. Authors have reported that symptoms were present for long periods before the clinical diagnosis was made (56). CT scanning may therefore be appropriate in patients with only minor respiratory symptoms if early BOS is suspected.

Studies have differed on their assessment of the ability of CT to predict the development of BOS (57,58). In a recent longitudinal study of 40 patients followed for a median of 36 months, CT scanning did not provide an earlier indication of the development of BOS than PFTs (59). CT scanning does have an important role in evaluating the lungs for other causes of obstructive changes on PFTs.

Only 5% of lung-transplant recipients are less than 18 years old (60), so most of the information available on post-transplantation BO comes from experience with adults. In a CT study of children under 8 years imaged during quiet sleep, children with BOS were compared to children with normal PFTs. Mosaic attenuation was seen in both groups but was more common in those with BOS (83 vs. 40%). Bronchial dilation was seen in 50% of children with BOS and in none of the children with normal PFTs (61). A later study at the same institution found that the use of expiratory CT to evaluate air trapping had little effect on positive predictive value but improved negative predictive value from 84 to 100% (62).

As noted above, the diagnosis of BOS requires a decrease in lung function and then becomes a diagnosis of exclusion, as other conditions can also produce a PFT change must be excluded. CT scanning has the important role of supporting the clinical diagnosis by demonstrating an appearance consistent with BO and of assessing the patient for other abnormalities when the diagnosis of BOS is considered. For example, in a study of open-lung biopsy in pediatric lung-transplant recipients, a different diagnosis was made in 39% of children with a prebiopsy suspicion of PTBO, with pneumonia being the most common new diagnosis (63).

In bone marrow transplantation, improvement in BO has been shown following high-dose corticosteroid therapy (56) and following tumor necrosis factor alpha blockade (64). Thus, early diagnosis of BO by CT may be helpful in this population.

7. FOLLICULAR BRONCHIOLITIS

Follicular bronchiolitis is a disease of unknown etiology characterized by bronchiolar narrowing caused by the development of lymphoid follicles in the peribronchiolar lung. Children can present with symptoms similar to bronchiolitis with wheezing or with crackles. A prolonged course with exacerbations and a history of recurrent pneumonias are common. The onset of disease can range from infancy to adolescence (65). In adults, FB is often associated with collagen vascular disease, immunodeficiencies, and hypersensitivity reactions (66). In the small number of cases reported in children, there has usually been no associated condition (65–69).

The pathologic diagnosis of FB requires the identification of lymphoid follicles with reactive germinal centers distributed along the bronchioles. This disorder likely represents one part of the spectrum of lymphoid infiltrative disorders of the lung that ranges from non-specific lymphoid infiltration to lymphoid interstitial pneumonitis (LIP). In adults, the most common HRCT findings of FB are centrilobular and peribronchial nodules, followed by areas of ground-glass opacity (66).

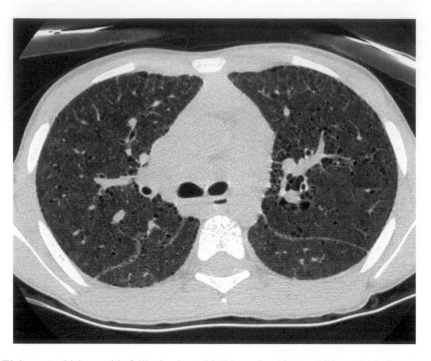

Fig. 10. Eight-year-old boy with follicular bronchiolitis and a history of juvenile inflammatory arthritis. Single CT image at the level of the carina shows diffuse ground-glass attenuation with an ill-defined peripheral nodular appearance on the right. Small thin-walled cysts are seen throughout the lungs.

Very limited reports are available on the imaging appearance of FB in children. One report described findings similar to the adult appearance with nodules and ground-glass opacity *(68)*. A second report described marked hyperinflation throughout the lungs with geographic areas of ground-glass opacity *(69)*. In this second report, no nodules were described. We have seen several cases with extensive ground-glass opacity and parenchymal cysts (Fig. 10). Our experience and the limited studies in the literature suggest that the imaging appearance of FB is more diverse in children than in adults. The appearance seems to extend from the same appearance as seen with NEHI, described below, to the appearance of LIP that is characterized by ground-glass opacity and cysts.

Our understanding of FB may also be limited by difficulty in consistently distinguishing the different lymphoid infiltrative disorders that range from mild lymphocytic infiltration through LIP. In individual cases, a review of the pathologic specimen may be useful in suggesting where in the spectrum of pathologic abnormality a certain patient's lung disease lies.

8. NEUROENDOCRINE CELL HYPERPLASIA OF INFANCY

NEHI is a recently described interstitial lung disease of children that is characterized pathologically by an increased number of neuroendocrine cells in the small airways. These cells are difficult to detect on standard preparations, appearing as small clear cells in the airway epithelium. Bombesin immunostaining is required for accurate assessment. The pathologic features are otherwise non-specific, with either a normal appearance or a mild inflammatory or lymphocytic infiltrate *(70)*.

These patients have a very characteristic clinical presentation with the onset of symptoms in the first year of life and unrevealing auscultation. The children are often markedly tachypneic and hypoxic. The discordance between the clinical status of the patient and the findings on both physical examination and lung biopsy is usually striking *(70)*.

Although a relatively small number of patients with NEHI have been evaluated, there is a strikingly consistent appearance on CT in NEHI *(71)* (Fig. 11). Ground-glass opacity is the most prominent finding, often seen adjacent to the mediastinum with irregular sharply defined margins. The lingula

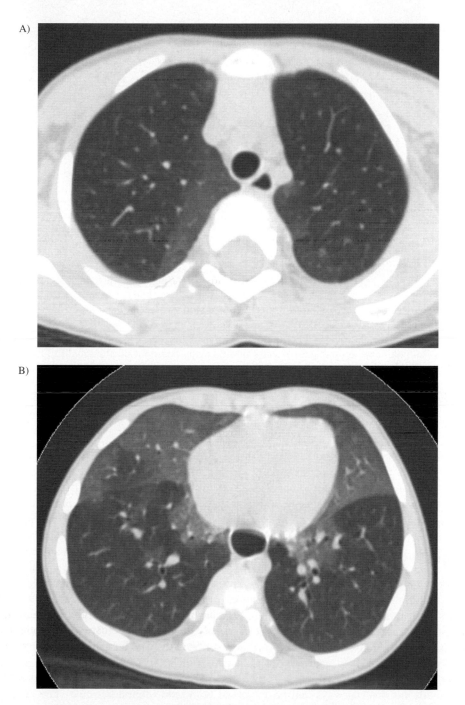

Fig. 11. *(Continued)*

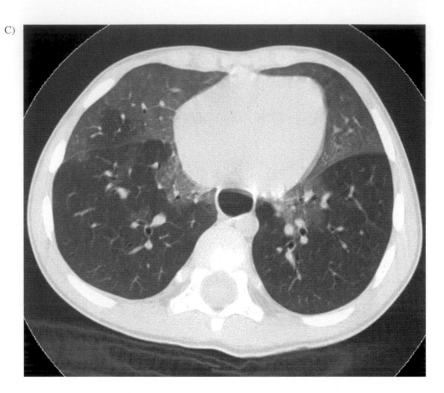

Fig. 11. Three-year-old boy with biopsy proven neuroendocrine cell hyperplasia of infancy (NEHI). This appearance is highly typical of NEHI. (**A**) Inspiratory image through the upper lobes shows a geographic appearance of ground-glass opacity adjacent to the mediastinum. (**B**) Inspiratory image through the lower lobes shows disproportionate ground-glass opacity in the lingula and right middle lobe. Esophageal dilation is secondary to positive pressure administered by mask for controlled ventilation CT. No abnormality other than the ground-glass opacity is seen. (**C**) Expiratory image through the lower lobes shows little relative change in the appearance of the areas of higher and lower attenuation. This reflects diffuse air trapping throughout the lungs.

and right middle lobe are affected more diffusely. The remainder of the lung appears normal on inspiratory images. Expiratory images usually show diffuse air trapping: the expiratory images often appear very similar to the inspiratory images, rather than showing the increase in attenuation difference seen with focal air trapping or the decrease in attenuation difference seen with pulmonary infiltrates. The visualized airways appear normal, and no other parenchymal or pleural abnormalities are seen.

The etiology of the areas of ground-glass attenuation in NEHI is unknown. Pathologically, these areas show only minimal abnormality, and the ground-glass areas are pathologically very similar to the normal appearing areas. In a very small number of subjects in whom prone and supine CT scanning was performed, the distribution of ground-glass opacity did not change with position. Neuroendocrine cells have multiple functions including regulation of pulmonary blood flow *(72)*. It is possible that the ground-glass areas represent plethoric lung because of increased blood flow to these areas.

In the literature and in anecdotal cases, there are cases of NEHI and FB with very similar clinical and pathologic descriptions. In earlier reports that describe cases with an appearance suggesting NEHI as FB, the authors were likely unaware of the diagnosis of NEHI *(69)*. We have seen one case with the imaging appearance of NEHI and a pathologic appearance similar to FB with germinal centers associated with the small airways and no increased bombesin immunostaining. The relationship of these two entities is unclear at this time.

9. BRONCHIOLITIS OBLITERANS ORGANIZING PNEUMONIA OR CRYPTOGENIC ORGANIZING PNEUMONIA

The terms BOOP and cryptogenic organizing pneumonia (COP) are both used to describe a rapidly developing pneumonia-like illness characterized pathologically by polypoid fibromyxoid tissue that fills the distal airspaces from the small conducting airways to the alveoli. The tissue resembles granulation tissue and is associated with chronic inflammation in the alveoli with preserved lung architecture *(73)*. Some authors consider COP a subset of BOOP that has no inciting lung insult and responds promptly and dramatically to steroids *(74)*. The two terms are commonly used interchangeably, however.

BOOP usually responds to steroid treatment, although a prolonged course may be required. Pathologic findings have been described that are associated with response to steroid therapy with the presence of scarring and remodeling of the lung parenchyma associated with a poor response to steroids *(75)*. In one child, a patient with BOOP associated with graft versus host disease following bone marrow transplantation was treated successfully with prednisolone with erythromycin used to allow a lower steroid dose.

BOOP is rare in children. Cases of BOOP have most commonly been reported in children with malignancies treated with chemotherapy or bone marrow transplantation *(76,77)*. Numerous other associations have been reported including ulcerative colitis *(78)*, cystic fibrosis *(79)*, systemic lupus erythematosus *(80)*, and asthma *(81)*. In ulcerative colitis and systemic lupus erythematosus, BOOP has been the presenting symptom of the systemic disease. BOOP has also been reported in asymptomatic children with no underlying disease process *(82)*.

Many varying appearances can be seen with BOOP in children as in adults. The most common appearance is one of ill-defined infiltrates. Consolidation and ground-glass opacities may be present (Fig. 12A). Despite the small airways involvement, airway abnormalities such as centrilobular nodules and tree-in-bud opacities are rare. BOOP presenting as single or multiple well-defined nodules seems to be more common in children than in adults (Fig. 12B). There are no specific features that

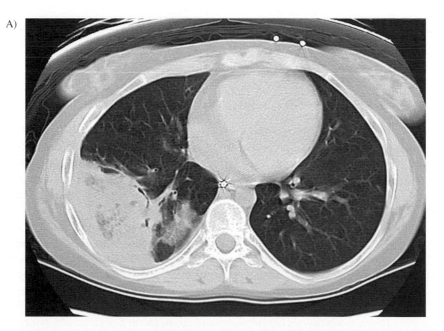

Fig. 12. *(Continued)*

B)

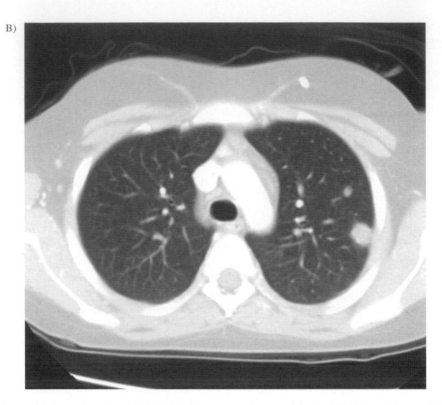

Fig. 12. Two children with bronchiolitis obliterans organizing pneumonia (BOOP) on biopsy. (**A**) Teenage girl with persistent opacity on chest radiographs following bone marrow transplantation. CT scan through the lower lungs shows focal ground glass opacity and consolidation. (**B**) BOOP presenting as pulmonary nodules in a 12-year-old girl with acute lymphocytic leukemia.

suggest BOOP over other causes of parenchymal opacities. In the correct clinical setting, persistent unchanging opacities should suggest the possibility of BOOP.

10. HYPERSENSITIVITY PNEUMONITIS

Although HP typically presents with abnormalities of the lung parenchyma on HRCT, it is included in this chapter because the disease is characterized by a diffuse inflammation of the small airways and surrounding lung parenchyma. Mononuclear cells usually predominate, often associated with poorly formed non-necrotizing granulomas. HP is caused by the repeated exposure to inhaled organic dust. Both immune complex and cell-mediated hypersensitivity are thought to be involved *(83)* but the exact mechanism that results in HP is not well understood.

In most pediatric cases, avian antigens are implicated in the development of HP *(83,84)*. Other agents have been reported to cause HP in children including molds *(85)*, methotrexate *(84)*, and insect repellant *(86)*. As in adults, three forms are described *(87)*. In the acute form, symptoms begin within 4–6 hours of an exposure to a large antigen load with fever, chills, and cough. Imaging studies show diffuse or patchy air space disease. In the subacute form, symptoms follow repeated exposure to the antigen. There is a gradual onset of cough, dyspnea, and malaise. With this presentation, ill-defined nodules and ground-glass opacity are the predominant findings on CT (Fig. 13). If antigen exposure continues, chronic HP can develop. With chronic HP irreversible changes of pulmonary fibrosis

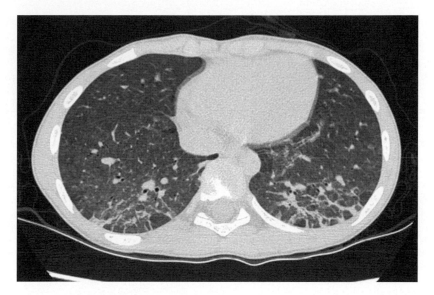

Fig. 13. This 8-year-old boy presented with progressive shortness of breath. His symptoms resolved with steroid treatment and removal of multiple birds from his home. CT image through the lower lobes demonstrates ground-glass opacity and diffuse ill-defined centrilobular nodules throughout the lungs. The reticular opacity at the lung bases resolved on later studies and likely reflects atelectasis rather than fibrosis.

and respiratory insufficiency may develop. Mid-lung changes of pulmonary fibrosis characterize the HRCT appearance in chronic HP.

The development of chronic HP is believed to follow continued exposure to the antigen. To avoid permanent lung damage, it is important to identify acute or subacute HP. HRCT scanning frequently suggests the diagnosis when CXR findings are nonspecific *(88)*. In acute HP, the presentation and history often suggest the diagnosis. In children with persistent and unexplained respiratory symptoms, HRCT should be considered to evaluate for subacute HP.

11. OTHER CAUSES OF BRONCHIOLITIS

In respiratory bronchiolitis-associated interstitial lung disease, symptoms usually begin over the age of 30 years, and this disease is not considered a pediatric disorder. Diffuse panbronchiolitis is a cause of chronic bronchiolitis most common in Japan and very rare outside of Asia. Although most reports are in adults, diffuse panbronchiolitis has been reported in Europe and North America *(89)* and in a child *(90)*. Erythromycin treatment is usually effective, and delayed diagnosis can result in the development of bronchiectasis and respiratory failure *(91)*. In the single pediatric case report, the CT showed centrilobular nodules and bronchial wall thickening with some areas of bronchiectasis and consolidation *(90)*.

REFERENCES

1. Plopper C. Have-Opbroek AWT: Anatomical and histological classification of the bronchioles. In: Epler GR (ed): *Diseases of the Bronchioles*. New York, Raven Press, Ltd.; 1994:15–25.
2. Reid L. Influence of the pattern of structural growth of lung on susceptibility to specific infectious diseases in infants and children. *Pediatr Res* 1977;11(3 Pt 2):210–5.
3. Zeman KL, Bennett WD. Growth of the small airways and alveoli from childhood to the adult lung measured by aerosol-derived airway morphometry. *J Appl Physiol* 2006;100(3):965–71.

4. Long FR, Williams RS, Castile RG. Structural airway abnormalities in infants and young children with cystic fibrosis. *J Pediatr* 2004;144(2):154–61.
5. Chen D, Webb WR, Storto ML, Lee KN. Assessment of air trapping using postexpiratory high-resolution computed tomography. *J Thorac Imaging* 1998;13(2):135–43.
6. Park CS, Muller NL, Worthy SA, Kim JS, Awadh N, Fitzgerald M. Airway obstruction in asthmatic and healthy individuals: inspiratory and expiratory thin-section CT findings. *Radiology* 1997;203(2):361–7.
7. Donnelly LF, Emery KH, Brody AS, et al. Minimizing radiation dose for pediatric body applications of single-detector helical CT: strategies at a large Children's Hospital. *AJR Am J Roentgenol* 2001;176(2):303–6.
8. Donnelly LF, Frush DP. Pediatric multidetector body CT. *Radiol Clin North Am* 2003;41(3):637–55.
9. Kalra MK, Maher MM, Toth TL, et al. Strategies for CT radiation dose optimization. *Radiology* 2004;230(3):619–28.
10. Ravenel JG, Scalzetti EM, Huda W, Garrisi W. Radiation exposure and image quality in chest CT examinations. *AJR Am J Roentgenol* 2001;177(2):279–84.
11. Shah R, Gupta AK, Rehani MM, Pandey AK, Mukhopadhyay S. Effect of reduction in tube current on reader confidence in pediatric computed tomography. *Clin Radiol* 2005;60(2):224–31.
12. Vock P. CT dose reduction in children. *Eur Radiol* 2005;15(11):2330–40.
13. Menke J. Comparison of different body size parameters for individual dose adaptation in body CT of adults. *Radiology* 2005;236(2):565–71.
14. Siegel MJ, Schmidt B, Bradley D, Suess C, Hildebolt C. Radiation dose and image quality in pediatric CT: effect of technical factors and phantom size and shape. *Radiology* 2004;233(2):515–22.
15. Sigal-Cinqualbre AB, Hennequin R, Abada HT, Chen X, Paul JF. Low-kilovoltage multi-detector row chest CT in adults: feasibility and effect on image quality and iodine dose. *Radiology* 2004;231(1):169–74.
16. Cody DD, Moxley DM, Krugh KT, O'Daniel JC, Wagner LK, Eftekhari F. Strategies for formulating appropriate MDCT techniques when imaging the chest, abdomen, and pelvis in pediatric patients. *AJR Am J Roentgenol* 2004;182(4):849–59.
17. Lucaya J, Garcia-Pena P, Herrera L, Enriquez G, Piqueras J. Expiratory chest CT in children. *AJR Am J Roentgenol* 2000;174(1):235–41.
18. Long FR, Castile RG, Brody AS, et al. Lungs in infants and young children: improved thin-section CT with a noninvasive controlled-ventilation technique—initial experience. *Radiology* 1999;212(2):588–93.
19. Jones M, Castile R, Davis S, et al. Forced expiratory flows and volumes in infants. Normative data and lung growth. *Am J Respir Crit Care Med* 2000;161(2 Pt 1):353–9.
20. Horak F Jr, Studnicka M, Gartner C, et al. Particulate matter and lung function growth in children: a 3-yr follow-up study in Austrian schoolchildren. *Eur Respir J* 2002;19(5):838–45.
21. Calderon-Garciduenas L, Mora-Tiscareno A, Chung CJ, et al. Exposure to air pollution is associated with lung hyperinflation in healthy children and adolescents in Southwest Mexico City: a pilot study. *Inhal Toxicol* 2000;12(6):537–61.
22. Calderon-Garciduenas L, Mora-Tiscareno A, Fordham LA, et al. Lung radiology and pulmonary function of children chronically exposed to air pollution. *Environ Health Perspect* 2006;114(9):1432–7.
23. Dompeling E, Jobsis Q, Vandevijver NM, Wesseling G, Hendriks H. Chronic bronchiolitis in a 5-yr-old child after exposure to sulphur mustard gas. *Eur Respir J* 2004;23(2):343–6.
24. Kelly HW. Update on the treatment of childhood asthma. *Curr Pediatr Rev* 2006;2(2):155–64.
25. Akinbami LJ, Schoendorf KC. Trends in childhood asthma: prevalence, health care utilization, and mortality. *Pediatrics* 2002;110(2 Pt 1):315–22.
26. von Mutius E. The environmental predictors of allergic disease. *J Allergy Clin Immunol* 2000;105(1 Pt 1):9–19.
27. Taylor WR, Newacheck PW. Impact of childhood asthma on health. *Pediatrics* 1992;90(5):657–62.
28. Jeffery P. Remodeling in asthma and chronic obstructive lung disease. *Am J Respir Crit Care Med* 2001;164(10):S28-S38.
29. McFadden ER. The chronicity of acute attacks of asthma—mechanical and therapeutic implications. *J Allergy Clin Immunol* 1975;56(1):18–26.
30. de Blic J, Tillie-Leblond I, Emond S, Mahut B, Dang Duy TL, Scheinmann P. High-resolution computed tomography scan and airway remodeling in children with severe asthma. *J Allergy Clin Immunol* 2005;116(4):750–4.
31. Okazawa M, Muller N, McNamara AE, Child S, Verburgt L, Pare PD. Human airway narrowing measured using high resolution computed tomography. *Am J Respir Crit Care Med* 1996;154(5):1557–62.
32. Jain N, Covar RA, Gleason MC, Newell JD Jr, Gelfand EW, Spahn JD. Quantitative computed tomography detects peripheral airway disease in asthmatic children. *Pediatr Pulmonol* 2005;40(3):211–8.
33. Henderson FW, Clyde WA Jr, Collier AM, et al. The etiologic and epidemiologic spectrum of bronchiolitis in pediatric practice. *J Pediatr* 1979;95(2):183–90.
34. Smyth RL, Openshaw PJ. Bronchiolitis. *Lancet* 2006;368(9532):312–22.
35. Welliver RC, Wong DT, Sun M, McCarthy N. Parainfluenza virus bronchiolitis. Epidemiology and pathogenesis. *Am J Dis Child* 1986;140(1):34–40.
36. Wainwright C, Altamirano L, Cheney M, et al. A multicenter, randomized, double-blind, controlled trial of nebulized epinephrine in infants with acute bronchiolitis. *N Engl J Med* 2003;349(1):27–35.

37. MacDonald NE, Hall CB, Suffin SC, Alexson C, Harris PJ, Manning JA. Respiratory syncytial viral infection in infants with congenital heart disease. *N Engl J Med* 1982;307(7):397–400.

38. Geddes DM, Corrin B, Brewerton DA, Davies RJ, Turner-Warwick M. Progressive airway obliteration in adults and its association with rheumatoid disease. *Q J Med* 1977;46(184):427–44.

39. Pegg SJ, Lang BA, Mikhail EL, Hughes DM. Fatal bronchiolitis obliterans in a patient with juvenile rheumatoid arthritis receiving chrysotherapy. *J Rheumatol* 1994;21(3):549–51.

40. Nadorra RL, Landing BH. Pulmonary lesions in childhood onset systemic lupus erythematosus: analysis of 26 cases, and summary of literature. *Pediatr Pathol* 1987;7(1):1–18.

41. Charan NB, Myers CG, Lakshminarayan S, Spencer TM. Pulmonary injuries associated with acute sulfur dioxide inhalation. *Am Rev Respir Dis* 1979;119(4):555–60.

42. Macleod WM. Abnormal transradiancy of one lung. *Thorax* 1954;9(2):147–53.

43. Lucaya J, Gartner S, Garcia-Pena P, Cobos N, Roca I, Linan S. Spectrum of manifestations of Swyer-James-MacLeod syndrome. *J Comput Assist Tomogr* 1998;22(4):592–7.

44. Colom AJ, Teper AM, Vollmer WM, Diette GB. Risk factors for the development of bronchiolitis obliterans in children with bronchiolitis. *Thorax* 2006;61(6):503–6.

45. Castro-Rodriguez JA, Daszenies C, Garcia M, Meyer R, Gonzales R. Adenovirus pneumonia in infants and factors for developing bronchiolitis obliterans: a 5-year follow-up. *Pediatr Pulmonol* 2006;41(10):947–53.

46. Yalcin E, Dogru D, Haliloglu M, Ozcelik U, Kiper N, Gocmen A. Postinfectious bronchiolitis obliterans in children: clinical and radiological profile and prognostic factors. *Respiration* 2003;70(4):371–5.

47. Leong MA, Nachajon R, Ruchelli E, Allen JL. Bronchitis obliterans due to Mycoplasma pneumonia. *Pediatr Pulmonol* 1997;23(5):375–81.

48. Trimis G, Theodoridou M, Mostrou G, Kakavakis K. Swyer-James (MacLeod's) syndrome following pertussis infection in an infant. *Scand J Infect Dis* 2003;35(3):197–9.

49. Boucek MM, Edwards LB, Keck BM, et al. The Registry of the International Society for Heart and Lung Transplantation: Fifth Official Pediatric Report-2001 to 2002. *J Heart Lung Transplant* 2002;21(8):827–40.

50. Yousem SA, Berry GJ, Cagle PT, et al. Revision of the 1990 working formulation for the classification of pulmonary allograft rejection: Lung Rejection Study Group. *J Heart Lung Transplant* 1996;15(1 Pt 1):1–15.

51. Boehler A, Estenne M. Post-transplant bronchiolitis obliterans. *Eur Respir J* 2003;22(6):1007–18.

52. Bando K, Paradis IL, Similo S, et al. Obliterative bronchiolitis after lung and heart-lung transplantation. An analysis of risk factors and management. *J Thorac Cardiovasc Surg* 1995;110(1):4–13; discussion: 4.

53. Hadjiliadis D, Hutcheon MA. Detection of bronchiolitis obliterans syndrome (BOS) in single lung transplant recipients. *J Heart Lung Transplant* 2003;22(7):829–30; author reply: 30–1.

54. Cooper JD, Billingham M, Egan T, et al. A working formulation for the standardization of nomenclature and for clinical staging of chronic dysfunction in lung allografts. International Society for Heart and Lung Transplantation. *J Heart Lung Transplant* 1993;12(5):713–6.

55. Mallory GB, Spray TL. Paediatric lung transplantation. *Eur Respir J* 2004;24(5):839–45.

56. Ratjen F, Rjabko O, Kremens B. High-dose corticosteroid therapy for bronchiolitis obliterans after bone marrow transplantation in children. *Bone Marrow Transplant* 2005;36(2):135–8.

57. Knollmann FD, Ewert R, Wundrich T, Hetzer R, Felix R. Bronchiolitis obliterans syndrome in lung transplant recipients: use of spirometrically gated CT. *Radiology* 2002;225(3):655–62.

58. Konen E, Gutierrez C, Chaparro C, et al. Bronchiolitis obliterans syndrome in lung transplant recipients: can thin-section CT findings predict disease before its clinical appearance? *Radiology* 2004;231(2):467–73.

59. Berstad AE, Aalokken TM, Kolbenstvedt A, Bjortuft O. Performance of long-term CT monitoring in diagnosing bronchiolitis obliterans after lung transplantation. *Eur J Radiol* 2006;58(1):124–31.

60. United Network for Organ Sharing Website www.unos.org (last accessed October 2006).

61. Lau DM, Siegel MJ, Hildebolt CF, Cohen AH. Bronchiolitis obliterans syndrome: thin-section CT diagnosis of obstructive changes in infants and young children after lung transplantation. *Radiology* 1998;208(3):783–8.

62. Siegel MJ, Bhalla S, Gutierrez FR, Hildebolt C, Sweet S. Post-lung transplantation bronchiolitis obliterans syndrome: usefulness of expiratory thin-section CT for diagnosis. *Radiology* 2001;220(2):455–62.

63. Choong CK, Haddad FJ, Huddleston CB, et al. Role of open lung biopsy in lung transplant recipients in a single children's hospital: a 13-year experience. *J Thorac Cardiovasc Surg* 2006;131(1):204–8.

64. Fullmer JJ, Fan LL, Dishop MK, Rodgers C, Krance R. Successful treatment of bronchiolitis obliterans in a bone marrow transplant patient with tumor necrosis factor-alpha blockade. *Pediatrics* 2005;116(3):767–70.

65. Benesch M, Kurz H, Eber E, et al. Clinical and histopathological findings in two Turkish children with follicular bronchiolitis. *Eur J Pediatr* 2001;160(4):223–6.

66. Howling SJ, Hansell DM, Wells AU, Nicholson AG, Flint JD, Muller NL. Follicular bronchiolitis: thin-section CT and histologic findings. *Radiology* 1999;212(3):637–42.

67. Kinane BT, Mansell AL, Zwerdling RG, Lapey A, Shannon DC. Follicular bronchitis in the pediatric population. *Chest* 1993;104(4):1183–6.

68. Reittner P, Fotter R, Lindbichler F, et al. HRCT features in a 5-year-old child with follicular bronchiolitis. *Pediatr Radiol* 1997;27(11):877–9.

69. Oh YW, Effmann EL, Redding GJ, Godwin JD. Follicular hyperplasia of bronchus-associated lymphoid tissue causing severe air trapping. *AJR Am J Roentgenol* 1999;172(3):745–7.

70. Deterding RR, Pye C, Fan LL, Langston C. Persistent tachypnea of infancy is associated with neuroendocrine cell hyperplasia. *Pediatr Pulmonol* 2005;40(2):157–65.

71. Brody AS, Crotty EJ. Neuroendocrine cell hyperplasia of infancy (NEHI). *Pediatr Radiol* 2006;36(12):1328.

72. Van Lommel A. Pulmonary neuroendocrine cells (PNEC) and neuroepithelial bodies (NEB): chemoreceptors and regulators of lung development. *Paediatr Respir Rev* 2001;2(2):171–6.

73. Epler GR. Bronchiolitis obliterans organizing pneumonia. *Arch Intern Med* 2001;161(2):158–64.

74. Cordier JF. Cryptogenic organising pneumonia. *Eur Respir J* 2006;28(2):422–46.

75. Yousem SA, Lohr RH, Colby TV. Idiopathic bronchiolitis obliterans organizing pneumonia/cryptogenic organizing pneumonia with unfavorable outcome: pathologic predictors. *Mod Pathol* 1997;10(9):864–71.

76. Helton KJ, Kuhn JP, Fletcher BD, Jenkins JJ 3rd, Parham DM. Bronchiolitis obliterans-organizing pneumonia (BOOP) in children with malignant disease. *Pediatr Radiol* 1992;22(4):270–4.

77. Hayes-Jordan A, Benaim E, Richardson S, et al. Open lung biopsy in pediatric bone marrow transplant patients. *J Pediatr Surg* 2002;37(3):446–52.

78. Mahajan L, Kay M, Wyllie R, Steffen R, Goldfarb J. Ulcerative colitis presenting with bronchiolitis obliterans organizing pneumonia in a pediatric patient. *Am J Gastroenterol* 1997;92(11):2123–4.

79. Hausler M, Meilicke R, Biesterfeld S, Kentrup H, Friedrichs F, Kusenbach G. Bronchiolitis obliterans organizing pneumonia: a distinct pulmonary complication in cystic fibrosis. *Respiration* 2000;67(3):316–9.

80. Takada H, Saito Y, Nomura A, et al. Bronchiolitis obliterans organizing pneumonia as an initial manifestation in systemic lupus erythematosus. *Pediatr Pulmonol* 2005;40(3):257–60.

81. Barbato A, Panizzolo C, D'Amore ES, La Rosa M, Saetta M. Bronchiolitis obliterans organizing pneumonia (BOOP) in a child with mild-to-moderate asthma: evidence of mast cell and eosinophil recruitment in lung specimens. *Pediatr Pulmonol* 2001;31(5):394–7.

82. Inoue T, Toyoshima K, Kikui M. Idiopathic bronchiolitis obliterans organizing pneumonia (idiopathic BOOP) in childhood. *Pediatr Pulmonol* 1996;22(1):67–72.

83. Patel AM, Ryu JH, Reed CE. Hypersensitivity pneumonitis: current concepts and future questions. *J Allergy Clin Immunol* 2001;108(5):661–70.

84. Fan LL. Hypersensitivity pneumonitis in children. *Curr Opin Pediatr* 2002;14(3):323–6.

85. Bureau MA, Fecteau C, Patriquin H, Rola-Pleszczynski M, Masse S, Begin R. Farmer's lung in early childhood. *Am Rev Respir Dis* 1979;119(4):671–5.

86. Morton R, Brooks M, Eid N. Hypersensitivity pneumonitis in a child associated with direct inhalation exposure of an insect repellant containing DEET. *Pediatr Asthma Allergy Immunol* 2006;19(1):44–50.

87. Venkatesh P, Wild L. Hypersensitivity pneumonitis in children: clinical features, diagnosis, and treatment. *Paediatr Drugs* 2005;7(4):235–44.

88. Hansell DM, Moskovic E. High-resolution computed tomography in extrinsic allergic alveolitis. *Clin Radiol* 1991;43(1):8–12.

89. Randhawa P, Hoagland MH, Yousem SA. Diffuse panbronchiolitis in North America. Report of three cases and review of the literature. *Am J Surg Pathol* 1991;15(1):43–7.

90. Aslan AT, Ozcelik U, Talim B, et al. Childhood diffuse panbronchiolitis: a case report. *Pediatr Pulmonol* 2005;40(4):354–7.

91. Krishnan P, Thachil R, Gillego V. Diffuse panbronchiolitis: a treatable sinobronchial disease in need of recognition in the United States. *Chest* 2002;121(2):659–61.

Index

Printed in the United States of America